100 Questions & Answers About Aging Skin

Robert A. Norman, DO, MPH

Associate Professor of Dermatology
Nova Southeastern University
Fort Lauderdale, FL
Director
Dermatology and Skin Cancer Center
Tampa, FL

JONES AND BARTLETT PUBLISHERS
Sudbury, Massachusetts
BOSTON   TORONTO   LONDON   SINGAPORE

World Headquarters

Jones and Bartlett Publishers
40 Tall Pine Drive
Sudbury, MA 01776
978-443-5000
info@jbpub.com
www.jbpub.com

Jones and Bartlett Publishers
Canada
6339 Ormindale Way
Mississauga, Ontario L5V 1J2
Canada

Jones and Bartlett Publishers
International
Barb House, Barb Mews
London W6 7PA
United Kingdom

Jones and Bartlett's books and products are available through most bookstores and online booksellers. To contact Jones and Bartlett Publishers directly, call 800-832-0034, fax 978-443-8000, or visit our website, www.jbpub.com.

Substantial discounts on bulk quantities of Jones and Bartlett's publications are available to corporations, professional associations, and other qualified organizations. For details and specific discount information, contact the special sales department at Jones and Bartlett via the above contact information or send an email to specialsales@jbpub.com.

The authors, editor, and publisher have made every effort to provide accurate information. However, they are not responsible for errors, omissions, or for any outcomes related to the use of the contents of this book and take no responsibility for the use of the products and procedures described. Treatments and side effects described in this book may not be applicable to all people; likewise, some people may require a dose or experience a side effect that is not described herein. Drugs and medical devices are discussed that may have limited availability controlled by the Food and Drug Administration (FDA) for use only in a research study or clinical trial. Research, clinical practice, and government regulations often change the accepted standard in this field. When consideration is being given to use of any drug in the clinical setting, the healthcare provider or reader is responsible for determining FDA status of the drug, reading the package insert, and reviewing prescribing information for the most up-to-date recommendations on dose, precautions, and contraindications, and determining the appropriate usage for the product. This is especially important in the case of drugs that are new or seldom used.

Production Credits

Senior Acquisitions Editor: Nancy Anastasi Duffy
Editorial Assistant: Sara Cameron
Production Director: Amy Rose
Production Assistant: Tina Chen
Marketing Manager: Ilana Goddess

V.P., Manufacturing and Inventory Control: Therese Connell
Composition: Appingo Publishing Services
Printing and Binding: Malloy, Inc.
Cover Printing: Malloy, Inc.

Cover Credits
Cover Design: Colleen Lamy
Cover Images: © AbleStock , © Ryan McVay/Photodisc/Getty Images

Library of Congress Cataloging-in-Publication Data
Norman, Robert A., 1955-
 100 questions and answers about aging skin / Robert A. Norman.
  p. cm.
 Includes index.
 ISBN-13: 978-0-7637-6245-2
 ISBN-10: 0-7637-6245-8
 1. Skin—Aging—Popular works. 2. Skin—Aging—Miscellanea. 3. Skin—Care and hygiene—Popular works. I. Title. II. Title: One hundred questions and answers about aging skin.
 RL73.A35N67 2009
 616.5—dc22
                          2008052310
6048

Printed in the United States of America
13 12 11 10 09   10 9 8 7 6 5 4 3 2 1

CONTENTS

Many people throughout the world are living well into their old age. A person's physical, as well as psychological, well being is directly affected by his or her general health and the health of his or her skin. Most of us have at least one, if not three or four, skin conditions that can be treated or at least improved with good advice and action.

The skin is a magnificent organ. If you could look quite closely at each square inch of skin, you would find about 19 million cells, 90 oil glands, 600 sweat glands, 65 hairs, and tens of millions of microscopic bacteria, and each square inch is nourished and kept active by 19,000 nerve cells and 19 feet of miniscule blood vessels. All of this amazing collection helps to eliminate one third of the body's waste products and toxins, regulates and maintains water balance and body temperature, uses touch receptors to help us sense pain and avoid harm, and forms a barrier to protect us from outside damage. Clearly, you need to keep this marvelous organ at its best.

More today than ever before, the aesthetic function of our skin has taken the forefront in modern media and our own perceptions. The multibillion-dollar cosmetic industry has brought in wave after wave of new techniques and products and has filled our offices, magazines, and televisions with the promise of a forever youthful glow. This is an uphill battle, however, unless you have the right advice that can cut through the avalanche of information, keep up with the advancements, and capture and use what is important to you and your skin type. Although the constant turnover of skin cells allows for renewal and repair, the skin also keeps its own diary, and the cumulative changes show as we age.

I see many different skin conditions in the older person, whether they're in a nursing home or in my office, and I believe that not enough attention is given to skin problems as we age. A delay in recognition leads to a delay in care of those problems. Also, in many areas, there is little access to specialists.

Albert M. Kligman, MD, PhD (inventor of Retin-A®), wrote, "This traditional neglect of the skin is well-nigh unforgivable and has cruel consequences for the well being of the elderly. These diseases do not kill but they are persistent pestilences which spoil the quality of life. . . . It is the skin more than any other organ which most clearly reveals the cumulative losses which time prints on the visage of the high and low alike."

Dr. Kligman also wrote, "The object of life is to die young, as late as possible," and we now spend billions of dollars to try to reverse the effects of "TMB"—too many birthdays. Because there is an increasing number of options available to maintain your youth, it is important to know what medications, procedures, and daily activities will help.

The goal of this book is to provide a greater understanding of what happens in aging skin and to emphasize that you have enormous opportunities to improve your general and skin health by following what I have included. For more help with your own skin care and comprehensive prevention and treatment, it is important to consult with your local dermatologist and to check the online sites that have been included here.

Robert A. Norman, DO, MPH

DEDICATION

Thank you to my family, friends, and patients for all their wisdom, time, and stories that made this book come to life. Special thanks to Nancy Duffy, Jessica Acox, Sara Cameron, Tina Chen, and all those at Jones and Bartlett Publishers, and to Linda Ruescher and Lawrence Parish for their excellent input and support.

Dedicated to David Daitch, DO, my friend and fellow physician who left this world way too soon and will be greatly missed.

Carpe diem,

Rob Norman

PART ONE

The Basics

What are the layers of the skin, and what are their functions?

Why are geriatric dermatology and aging skin receiving particular attention?

What happens as we age?

More . . .

Epidermis

The outmost layer of the skin. It is visible to the naked eye and is comprised of stratified squamous epithelium.

Dermis

The layer of skin found between the epidermis and the subcutaneous tissue.

Subcutaneous layer

The tissue that separates the dermis from the underlying connective tissue.

Keratinocytes

The cell type that comprises a majority of the epidermis.

According to current U.S. Census statistics, the population that is over 65 years old is increasing, and this trend is expected to continue well into the 21st century.

1. What are the layers of the skin, and what are their functions?

The skin is composed of the **epidermis**, **dermis**, and **subcutaneous layers** (**Plate 1**). The top part of the epidermis is the stratum corneum. The stratum corneum and its surrounding lipid bilayer are composed primarily of ceramides, fatty acids, and cholesterol. When these constituents are present in the proper proportion, they form the "skin barrier," which functions like a brick wall (**keratinocytes**) covered by mortar (the lipid bilayer). This barrier protects the skin and keeps it watertight. Special cells in the epidermis called **melanocytes** produce brown pigment that helps to protect you from ultraviolet light.

The dermis, or middle layer, provides a tough, yet flexible, foundation for the epidermis. Sweat glands and blood vessels help to regulate body temperature, and nerve endings send the sensations of pain, itching, touch, and temperature to the brain. **Sebum** helps to moisturize the skin. Hair has a primarily decorative function in humans. Under the dermis, the fat provides insulation and helps to store calories.

2. Why are geriatric dermatology and aging skin receiving particular attention?

According to current U.S. Census statistics, the population that is over 65 years old is increasing, and this trend is expected to continue well into the 21st century. Additionally, the population of those aged 80 years or older is rapidly increasing. As baby-boomers begin to enter senior citizenship and the older get older, an increased emphasis in geriatric medicine is inevitable. Because the human population is living longer, chronic diseases, including skin diseases, will become more prevalent.

As people age, they may increasingly develop skin-related disorders. Two types of skin aging exist: (1) intrinsic aging, which includes those changes that are due to normal maturity and thus occur in all individuals, and (2) extrinsic aging, which is produced by extrinsic factors such as ultraviolet light exposure, smoking, and environmental pollutants. Decreased mobility, drug-induced disorders, and increased incidences of many chronic diseases are among the reasons that older persons are at heightened risk for skin diseases.

3. What happens as we age?

Many histological changes occur with aging and **photoaging** (see **Tables 1** and **2**). Variation in cell size, shape, and staining results in epidermal dyscrasia of photoaged skin. Melanocytes decline, and **Langerhans' cells** (intradermal macrophages) decrease in density.

The dermis becomes relatively acellular, avascular, and less dense, and the loss of functional elastic tissue results in wrinkles. The nerves, microcirculation, and sweat glands undergo a gradual decline, predisposing them to decreased thermoregulation and sensitivity to burning. Nails undergo a slow decline in growth, with thinning of the nail plate, longitudinal ridging, and splitting. The subcutaneous fat layer atrophies on the cheeks and distal extremities but hypertrophies on the waist of men and thighs of women.

Melanocytes

Cells in the basal layer of epidermis that are involved in the production of dark colored pigment known as melanin.

Sebum

The oily substance produced by glands in the skin.

Photoaging

The damaging of skin due to sunlight exposure.

Langerhans' cells

A type of dendritic immune cell found in high concentrations in the epidermis.

The Basics

Table 1   Aging Skin

Epidermal Changes
• Melanocytes Approximately 15% decline per decade Density doubles on sun-exposed skin Increased lentigines • Langerhans cells Decreased density Decreased responsiveness

Dermal Changes
Decreased collagen—1% annual decline, altered fibers Decreased density Progressive loss of elastic tissue in the papillary dermis

Table 2   Skin Changes in Aging

Loss of Elasticity and Thinning of the Skin
Clinical results—xerosis, laxity, wrinkling, uneven pigmentation, easy tearing, traumatic pupura, neoplasia
Photoaging
Clinical results—actinic keratoses, fine and coarse wrinkling, telangiectasia, blotchiness and pigmentary changes, elastotic skin with giant comedones

Many skin changes occur during the aging process, including decreased elasticity, decreased skin surface lipids and hydration, and decreased skin density and responsiveness. These skin changes can be divided into intrinsic skin changes and extrinsic changes, as explained previously.

Although intrinsic changes usually begin in our 20s, the signs are typically not visible for decades. These include the following:

- Fine wrinkles
- Thin and transparent skin
- A loss of underlying fat, leading to hollowed cheeks and eye sockets, as well as noticeable loss of firmness on the hands and neck
- An inability to sweat sufficiently to cool the skin
- Bones that shrink away from the skin because of bone loss, which causes sagging skin
- Dry skin that may itch
- Graying hair that eventually turns white
- Hair loss
- Unwanted hair
- A nail plate that thins, the half moons that disappear, and ridges that develop

4. Many changes on the cellular level occur with aging. Can you explain these further?

The dermis (middle layer of the skin) suffers a loss of elastic tissue, becomes less vascular, and decreases its ability to withstand minor trauma. The result is easier bruising (purpura), less ability to "rebound," and more wrinkles. The nerves, microcirculation, and sweat glands undergo a gradual decline, predisposing to decreased temperature regulation. Nails undergo a slow decline in growth, with thinning of the nail plate, ridging, and splitting.

5. What are some examples of chronic disease that affect the skin?

Atherosclerosis, diabetes mellitus, obesity, HIV, nicotine abuse, and congestive heart failure are examples of disease processes that can be detrimental to skin. They are known to impede vascular efficiency and decrease immune responses, thereby reducing the body's ability to heal.

6. What is photoaging?

Photoaging refers to the damage that is done to the skin from prolonged exposure (over a person's lifetime) to ultraviolet radiation. Most of the skin changes that occur as we get older are accelerated by sun exposure. Examples include hyperpigmentation, wrinkles, poor elasticity, broken blood vessels, leathery skin, and skin cancers.

The visible effects of photoaging are changes that are usually associated with chronologic aging (calendar years); however, photoaging is not a good indicator of chronologic age because it may make a person look older than his or her chronologic age.

The three approaches to counter photoaging are as follows:

1. Avoid the midday sun.
2. Practice prevention by using photoprotective agents such as sunscreen and clothing.
3. Use skin rejuvenation treatments.

Atherosclerosis, diabetes mellitus, obesity, HIV, nicotine abuse, and congestive heart failure are examples of disease processes that can be detrimental to skin.

Immune system

Comprised of multiple organs and tissues working together to provide chemical and physical barriers to prevent disease. These barriers include the skin, saliva, and white blood cells.

Lupus

An autoimmune disease in which the body attacks is own tissues.

7. What is the immune system, and how does it work?

The **immune system** helps to monitor and fight infection and prevent cancer. It includes specialized white blood cells—T cells, B cells, and neutrophils—that are always on call to help. Your body's immune system is like an army with millions of soldiers, ready to fight foreign substances such as germs and viruses in the body.

As we age, certain parts of the system diminish in vitality, and we have to be more alert to help boost the system to work at full capacity. In autoimmune diseases, such as **lupus**, the immune system is out of control and attacks healthy tissues.

8. Someone told me that gravity is one of the biggest problems for our skin. Is that true?

Yes, gravity is a law of nature and of facial skin. By the time we reach our 50s, our skin's elasticity declines, and gravity's effects show: the eyelids fall, jowls form, the tip of the nose droops, the ears elongate, the upper lip decreases, and the lower lip becomes more prominent. Later we discuss ways to help with this.

9. I am overweight. How does this affect my skin?

Many skin diseases are shown to be worse with obesity, including psoriasis and stasis dermatitis. Losing weight is one of the more important ways to improve your health and help your skin.

Obesity is another extremely preventable disorder that if untreated can lead to medical complications, including orthopedic problems, metabolic disorders, disrupted sleep, a poorly functioning immune system, impaired mobility, increased blood pressure, hypertension, and psychosocial consequences from low self-esteem to depression. Long-term consequences

Cutaneous sensation

The sensory ability of the skin. This is more commonly referred to as the sense of touch.

Adiposis dolorosa

A condition also known as Dercum's disease that is characterized by the formation of tumors in the fatty tissue of the body.

Lymphedema

Swelling of the extremities due to an obstruction in the lymph system that prevents the return of the lymph fluid to the body's core.

Chronic venous insufficiency

A condition in which the valves of the veins do not function properly, causing the pooling of blood in the lower extremities.

Hidradenitis suppurativa

This condition occurs in areas with a high density of apocrine sweat glands and around hair follicles in the groin and armpit.

include cardiovascular disease, insulin resistance, type 2 diabetes, hyperlipidemia, gall bladder disease, osteoarthritis, and certain cancers.

Skin complications related to obesity include:

- a decrease in **cutaneous sensation**
- acanthosis nigricans
- acrochordons
- **adiposis dolorosa** and fat redistribution
- **lymphedema**
- candidiasis
- cellulitis
- **chronic venous insufficiency**
- erythrasma
- folliculitis
- gas gangrene
- **hidradenitis suppurativa**
- hyperandrogenism and hirsutism
- insulin-resistance syndrome
- intertrigo
- leg ulcerations
- necrotizing fasciitis
- **pilaris**
- **plantar hyperkeratosis**
- psoriasis skin infections
- **striae distensae**
- **tophaceous gout**

The Basics

Pilaris

A condition in which the skin of the arms and legs have small, hard, reddish pimples.

Plantar hyperkeratosis

The thickening of the bottom or sides of the feet.

Striae distensae

The condition commonly known as stretch marks occurs when the connective tissue of the skin cannot grow as rapidly as the underlying tissues.

Tophaceous gout

A chronic condition in which there are uric acid deposits throughout the body.

PART TWO

Dryness, Itches, and Allergies

What causes dry skin?

What about dry skin and itch?

What can you do about dry skin?

More . . .

10. What causes dry skin?

Xerotic eczema

A skin condition in which the skin is extremely dry and cracked.

Xerosis (dry skin) is a common dermatological skin condition. Dry skin, or **xerotic eczema**, can be labeled as xerosis, eczema craquele (like a pattern of cracked porcelain), or asteatotic eczema (**Plate 2**). The incidence increases with age and is common in older individuals.

The reduced production of sebum also may play a role in dry skin. Sebum contains wax esters, triglycerides, and squalene, all of which protect the skin from the environment. Certain individuals receiving cholesterol-reducing drugs exhibit dry skin.

Natural moisturizing factor, a substance that retains water inside keratinocytes and renders them plump, also plays an important role in the pathophysiology of dry skin.

Stratum corneum

The outermost layer of the epidermis that acts as a barrier to prevent the exchange of chemicals between the body and its surroundings.

Defects in the **stratum corneum** or barrier can result in transepidermal water loss, which dehydrates the skin and imparts a dry appearance. An impaired barrier may also make skin more susceptible to damage from exogenous sources such as plants, chemicals, and even water.

11. What about dry skin and itch?

One of the most common complaints in my patients over 65 years old is itchy, dry skin.

Does your skin sometimes get dry and itchy? Ever have a persistent itch? Do you ever wonder what you can do about it? Here are some clues. One of the most common complaints in my patients over 65 years old is itchy, dry skin. Because each adult is covered by about 20 square feet (2 square meters) of skin and is constantly exposed to possible irritants, you'll get an itch now and then.

Senile pruritus

The itching of skin that occurs due to the breakdown and aging of skin of the elderly.

Senile pruritus refers to the dry skin of aging. This term dates back to a time when the term *senile* had a more benign connotation, perhaps like misplacing your keys instead of feeling your mind slip into the shadows. Dry skin occurs most often on the legs of older patients but may also be present on the hands and trunk.

12. What can you do about dry skin?

Mild itch may respond to nonpharmacologic measures, which include avoiding hot water and irritants, maintaining proper humidity, using cool water compresses, frequently applying moisturizers, trimming the nails, and applying behavior therapy.

Treatment of moderate dry skin and itch includes ammonium lactate 12% lotion, moisturizers, and topical corticosteroids, as well as certain behavioral-management tactics. The keratolytic (topical agents that remove the dead, flaky portions of skin) effect of ammonium lactate 12% lotion is effective in reducing the severity of dry skin.

Creams that contain keratolytic agents such as urea are not as hydrolyzing but can rid the skin of the abnormally thickened layer. In individuals with sensitive skin, sensitive-skin variant formulation should be substituted for alpha-hydroxy acids; the latter can cause stinging and irritation. Liberal use of moisturizers reduces scaling and enhances the desquamation process. In moderate to severe cases, treatment with application of prescription topical steroids and oral medications may be added.

Secondary treatment consists of increasing hydration and moisturizing the skin. It may be helpful to apply nonscented emollients, such as white petrolatum, liberally and frequently on the skin immediately after bathing and frequently throughout the day. Emollients are creams or lotions that can be applied to the affected area to prevent water from evaporating from the skin's surface. They also smooth over the scaly edges that can flake off and cause intense itching.

Management suggestions include the following:

- Reduce the frequency of bathing with lukewarm (not hot) water

- Use a nonirritant soap such as Cetaphil®, Olay®, Aveeno®, or Dove®
- Avoid harsh skin cleansers
- Apply moisturizer directly on unsightly skin
- Limit friction from washcloths, rough clothing, and abrasives
- Use air humidification in dry environments

With dry skin and itching, you have now learned some important ways to make you and your skin more satisfied.

13. I feel like I need to scratch my skin all of the time and that I may have bugs. What do I do?

It is estimated that at least one third of individuals presenting to a dermatologist have a skin condition primarily due to a psychologic factor. Authors use many different names to refer to skin conditions that are psychologically related, including **neurodermatitis**, psychocutaneous diseases, psychodermatologic disorders, psychosomatic dermatology, and psychocutaneous medicine. Neurodermatitis includes delusions of parasitosis, dermatitis artefacta, lichen simplex chronicus, neurotic excoriations, prurigo nodularis, and trichotillomania.

Signs and symptoms include often intense itching and perception of bugs in the skin. You may show multiple excoriations at all different stages of healing. Often you will have clear areas on the central back that cannot be reached by scratching.

Certain other diseases, such as scabies, eczema, generalized pruritus, **bullous** disorders, and systemic disease, must be eliminated from consideration first. Treatment may include topical antipruritic creams and ointments, oral psychiatric medicines, and counseling.

Lichen simplex chronicus (**Plate 3**) is a Latin term that means "skin that thickens and scales due to long-term scratching."

Neurodermatitis

The cycle of chronic itching and scratching that can cause the affected skin to become thick and leathery. It is also known as lichen simplex chronicus or scratch dermatitis.

Bullous

A large blister (a thin-walled sac filled with clear fluid).

It may start as a minor itching place; however, scratching the spot damages the skin, thus making it heal slightly thicker than before. The skin tries to protect itself by thickening. As the healing progresses, the itch fibers in the skin are activated by slight scar contraction in the damaged area, and the new itching causes more scratching. What is the result? More damage, thickening, healing, and itching—the *itch–scratch cycle*—and it can continue incessantly unless interrupted. A cortisone ointment or cream may help end the vicious itch–scratch cycle, but you also must keep the nails short to eliminate the scratching tools at hand. By rubbing the topical medicine into the itchy area with the flat of your finger pad, you avoid triggering the nasty cycle again.

14. What about an itch that persists?

"Scratching is one of the sweetest gratifications of nature, and as ready at hand as any," Montaigne wrote. "But repentance follows too annoyingly close at its heels."

> *There was a young belle of old Natchez*
> *Whose garments were always in patchez.*
> *When comment arose*
> *On the state of her clothes,*
> *She replied, "When Ah itchez, Ah scratchez."*
>
> —Ogden Nash

Every time I have a patient with an itch, I do a "mind google" search and think of my patient's differential diagnosis. The real Google has over 12,200,000 links to itch.

Not all itches are benign. Itch is a common condition that may be associated with a plethora of various medical conditions, and therefore, examination of the skin may be misleading. Without proper diagnosis and treatment of the underlying disorder, itch may become severe enough to affect your sleeping habits and overall quality of life. Underlying metabolic conditions that produce itch might include renal failure, HIV, diabetes mellitus, thyroid disease, iron-deficiency anemia, neuropathy, hepatic disease, malignancy, and drugs. If you have a persistent itch, work with your health practitioner to find out what can help you. If you do not have an obvious explanation for the itch, you should undergo a physical examination to look for evidence of a systemic disease.

Itch starts with an external stimuli—dust, touch, a mosquito landing on your arm—and is a built-in defense mechanism that alerts your body to the potential of being harmed. Dermal skin receptors will send an immediate signal through fibers in the skin to your spinal cord and then up to the cerebral cortex in your brain that tells you to scratch. You may feel some relief when this itch response is temporarily interrupted, but a persistent itch may result in chronic itch–scratch. Scratching can cause excoriations, which then may progress to secondary eczema or may become infected.

The itch–scratch cycle is the dermatologic equivalent of chronic pain syndrome and should be treated as such.

The itch–scratch cycle is the dermatologic equivalent of chronic pain syndrome and should be treated as such. Just as with chronic pain, there is a reduced threshold phenomenon that occurs in patients with chronic itch. Chronicity not only lowers the threshold for the sensation of itch, but it also increases the intensity of itch. Also, as with chronic pain, short bursts of spontaneous itch may occur, even when the skin is clear.

The term *itch* has evolved into many connotations in our society. Researchers have found that songs get stuck in our heads because they create a "brain itch" or "cognitive itch," analogous to histamines that make our brain itch, and can only be scratched by repeating the tune over and over.

15. What about allergic reactions in the skin?

Allergic skin disorders in older individuals, which may arise from contact with or ingestion of offending allergens, must be distinguished from other causes, such as dry skin.

Discontinue the use of products, such as topical alcohol and strongly scented soaps, that may further dry the skin. It is also helpful to limit bathing to every other day, up to a maximum of once a day (because too much water can actually cause the skin to dry out), using tepid or cool water; therefore, showering or bathing more than once a day should be avoided to prevent dry skin. Control of the environment is also important. Dry skin is often a problem in cooler climates, especially during winter months, when home heating systems are regularly used. This dry heat draws moisture from the skin. Outdoors, cold winter air causes the body to protect itself by drawing blood away from the skin. When this occurs, the skin is not well nourished, and dry skin and itching can result. Consequently, the indoor environment should be cool and vapor humidified, and your exposure to cold temperatures and wind should be limited.

Temperature regulation is a major concern. People need to sense hot and cold and other changes in order to take appropriate preventive measures to maintain homeostasis. Being able to detect when you are cold is essential for survival! Nails undergo a slow decline in growth, with thinning of the nail plate and ridging and splitting.

16. What about allergic reactions to the sun?

Sometimes even after only a short time of sun exposure, allergies to the sun can develop and may present in several different ways. Some people have problems with rashes, bumps, hives, blisters, or red splotchy areas. This is more common in people who are more sensitive to allergies in general, but it may happen to anyone. Certain beauty products and soaps may also make you more sensitive to the sun, including perfumes, cosmetics, and hair dyes.

Chemicals, including those found in certain plants, vegetables, and fruits, can make the skin much more vulnerable to the sun in a process called **photosensitization**.

Many drugs may make you more prone to sun sensitivity; some of the more common ones include birth control pills,

Photosensitization

A condition in which the skin becomes susceptible to damage from the sun.

15

antibiotics such as tetracyclines, thiazide diuretics, sulfon-amides, chlorpromazine, depression medications, arthritis medications, and blood pressure medications. You should always check with your doctor and pharmacist when you receive any new medication to see how it may interact with what you're already taking and whether you should be extra careful when in the sun or if you should avoid it completely.

17. What is contact dermatitis?

Allergic contact dermatitis (**Plate 4**) is an itchy skin condition that is caused by an allergic reaction to material in contact with the skin. The dermatitis is generally confined to the site of contact with the allergen, although severe cases may extend outside the contact area or may become generalized. It occurs hours after contact with the responsible material and will dissipate when the skin is no longer in contact with it. An example is a localized irritation underlying a watch strap because of contact allergy to nickel.

Other common allergens include formalin in cosmetics and insecticides, paraben in cosmetics, rubber, fragrances in hair and clothing dyes, cosmetics, and household chemicals. Plants encountered during gardening or hiking may result in irritations.

Patch testing involves placing patches of various substances on the skin to identify whether a substance that comes into contact with the skin causes inflammation. Patch test reactions tend to increase with age because of the accumulation of allergens acquired over a lifetime. Often an occupational sensitization may occur only after decades of contact.

The most common reason for allergic contact dermatitis in older persons is topical medications applied to venous stasis ulcers or wounds, including lanolin, neomycin, paraben preservatives, and vitamin E creams.

18. I'm itching at night and can't seem to stop. What can I do?

Helen said this:

I visited a friend in a nursing home and now I have an awful itch that is worse at night. I've tried a bunch of medications, and nothing seems to help. What do I do?

Human scabies is almost always caught from another person as a result of close contact. It is not uncommon to treat a whole family that has been infected, along with their friends. The parasite *Sarcoptes scabiei* is a tiny skin mite that brings on a nasty, itchy rash and can spread to others by contact. The disease is very common—more than 300 million cases of scabies occur worldwide every year—and can strike anyone of any race, age, or socioeconomic status.

The microscopic mite burrows, and the body develops an intense reaction that results in severe itching that can lead to a skin infection. An infected person may not notice the itching or swelling until 4 to 6 weeks after the initial infestation.

Scabies may appear as little hive-like red bumps, tiny bites, or pimples and may be crusty or scaly in more severe cases. It usually begins in skin folds and crevices—between the fingers and on the wrists in younger people and around the nipples for women and on the penis for men. The head and face are usually free of infestation, except in those that are immunocompromised.

Treatment must be complete and prompt once the diagnosis is made. Topical treatment with Elimite® Cream on the entire skin from the neck to the soles of the feet should be thorough and left on overnight. Clip your nails short to clear any scabies mites hiding under the fingernails and to decrease the likelihood of further irritation when scratching. Clean your sheets

Dryness, Itches, and Allergies

and clothes that were used within the previous 3 days. Do not use pesticides or fumigate the affected areas—the scabies mite requires human skin contact to survive. An alternative treatment is with Ivermectin®, a pill taken twice and then repeated in a week. Medications for itch may also be prescribed, including antihistamines and oral or topical steroids.

19. What are hives?

Urticaria

The condition, commonly referred to as hives, is caused by the body's natural reaction to an allergen.

Angioedema

Characterized by the rapid swelling of skin.

Urticaria is the medical name for hives, which are welts (pink swellings) that usually last a few hours and then fade away. New hives appear as old areas fade. Hives can be quite small or cover broad areas of the body. The itch of hives can be intense and sometimes burn or sting. If hives occur in deeper tissues of the eyes, mouth, hands, or genitals, the swelling is called **angioedema**.

Hives can be due to a variety of underlying problems, including infections. Repeated and chronic episodes often occur as an allergic reaction to foods (most commonly nuts), chocolate, milk, insect stings, or medications and usually break out within a few hours of the exposure. Hives that come out as a result of sunlight, cold, pressure, or exercise are called the physical urticarias. Pressure urticaria is manifested as a deep welt in an area of prolonged pressure.

Chronic urticaria is defined as hives lasting longer than six weeks. In the overwhelming majority of cases, the hives are *idiopathic*, a term meaning there is no discernible cause. But it is certainly worth finding out if you are in the 5% of cases with a cause. Thyroid or liver problems, herpes, skin diseases, dental infections, sinusitis, or allergic causes can be discovered with a thorough history and physical, along with blood and urine tests and sometimes a skin biopsy. In chronic idiopathic hives, many researchers feel that the body's overactive immune system is the culprit.

Hives are treated mainly with antihistamines, including nonsedating antihistamines such as Claritin® or Zyrtec®. If needed, a sedating type of antihistamine (hydroxyzine, cyproheptadine, or doxepin) is added at night. If the hives continue, a short course of cortisone (steroids) may clear the hives completely.

20. I itch around my anus. It drives me crazy. Can you help?

Perianal itching can be very uncomfortable and can interfere with daily activities and sleep. Keep the anal area clean and dry, and avoid injury to the skin from excessive wiping or abrasion. Eliminate items in the diet such as citrus fruits and juices, coffee and tea (including decaf in excess of 2 cups a day), beer and alcoholic beverages, colas, nuts and popcorn, milk, chocolate, and spices (especially peppers) that produce gas, indigestion, or loose bowel. Foods that produce mucus or aggravate drainage will result in irritation of the bowel and possible anal itching.

If your itch (and scratching) is severe, wear cotton gloves during the night and consider taking antihistamine pills. Avoid the use of perfumed soap and vigorous rubbing with a washcloth. Most soap is highly alkaline, and the residues may collect in the folds of the skin and alter the normal acidity of the skin. Use Cetaphil or other mild cleansers for the shower to avoid irritation.

After bowel movements, wash the anal area with water or a wet cotton or tissue. Hypoallergenic unscented baby wipes can be used for cleaning. Use nonscented toilet paper to pat dry, and avoid rubbing with the toilet tissue. Wear a thin cotton strip directly on the anus during the day. Use one that is so thin that you are not conscious of its presence. Change

Dryness, Itches, and Allergies

the cotton strip frequently, and wear cotton underwear. Each morning and/or night, take a bath in lukewarm water. Apply a mild prescribed or over-the-counter lotion, cream, or ointment after your cleaning and drying routine.

See a dermatologist if the itching continues, and consult a proctologist to rule out rectal disease.

PART THREE

Skin and Pathogens

Can I get HIV now that I am older?

What is shingles?

What can I do to prevent shingles?

More . . .

21. Can I get HIV now that I am older?

Over 10% of all new AIDS cases in the United States occur in people over the age of 50 years. New AIDS cases in the past several years rose faster in middle age and older people than in people less than 40 years old. Although many of these AIDS cases are the result of HIV infection at a younger age, many are due to becoming infected after age 50. Because very few persons over the age of 50 at risk for HIV routinely get tested, it is difficult to determine rates of HIV infection among older adults. Older adults are often first diagnosed with HIV at a late stage of infection when they seek treatment for an HIV-related illness.

HIV cases among older people may be underreported because HIV symptoms and infections may coincide with other age-related diseases and are therefore overlooked. Fatigue, weight loss, and other early HIV symptoms may be dismissed as a normal part of aging. AIDS-related dementia is often misdiagnosed as Alzheimer's disease.

Many characteristics of HIV are specific for older persons. Older individuals with AIDS get sick and die sooner than younger persons because of a late diagnosis as well as co-infection with other diseases that may speed the progression of AIDS. In addition, new drugs for HIV treatment may interact with medications the older person is taking to treat preexisting chronic conditions.

A common stereotype exists in the United States: Older people don't have sex or use drugs. Few HIV-prevention efforts are aimed at people older than 50 years, and most educational ad campaigns rarely show older adults, making them an invisible at-risk population. Older people, therefore, are generally less knowledgeable about HIV/AIDS than younger people and are less aware of how to protect themselves against infection. This lack of awareness is especially true for older injecting drug users, who comprise over 16% of AIDS cases in persons older than 50 years.

Men who have sex with men form the largest group of AIDS cases among adults older than 50 years. Older gay men tend to be "invisible" and ignored both in the gay community and in prevention efforts. The HIV risk factors for older gay men include internalized homophobia, denial of risk, alcohol and other substance use, and anonymous sexual encounters.

Skin **lesions** occur in virtually all patients during the unfolding evolution of their HIV infection—usually a succession of conditions reflecting the gradual decline of immunity. A transient rash may accompany the initial HIV seroconversion illness but may go unnoticed. During the following weeks or years, the gradually declining immunity may be documented only by decreasing numbers of CD4-positive lymphocytes with the emergence of inflammatory skin conditions (e.g., seborrheic dermatitis or psoriasis), as well as autoimmune conditions (e.g., thrombocytopenia, morphea, or alopecia areata). As immunity itself declines, skin infections emerge. **Shingles** affects over 25% of HIV-positive patients and may be followed by postherpetic neuralgia. Molluscum contagiosum, warts, and dry skin may appear. In severe cases, the person may develop purplish nodules on the face and extremities and other locations, which are Kaposi's sarcomas, a form of skin cancer.

Lesion

A vague term meaning "the thing that is wrong with the patient." A lesion may be a tumor or an area of inflammation.

Shingles

An extremely painful rash that is caused by a viral infection known as herpes zoster.

Practice safe sex and use precautions!

22. What is shingles?

Herpes zoster, also known as shingles, is chickenpox the second time around. It is a varicella virus, not herpes—the term herpes is used to describe the herpetic (small blisters) pattern of the infection. Zoster is a viral infection dormant in a dorsal root ganglion and is reactivated in an immuno-compromised person.

Herpes zoster, also known as shingles, is chickenpox the second time around.

Symptoms include pain and/or paresthesias followed by eruption of red plaques that become vesicles, usually along a single dermatome or area of the skin (**Plate 5**). The vesicles later become covered by crusts. The pain may be felt before, during, and after (postherpetic neuralgia) the vesicular eruption.

Although unlikely, it is possible for a person who has never been exposed to the virus to catch chickenpox from someone who has an outbreak of shingles. In severe cases, you should be suspicious of an underlying lymphoma, leukemia, or AIDS.

Cellulitis

An infection of the deeper layers of the skin characterized by redness, swelling, and pain.

Zoster can mimic herpes simplex, poison ivy, or **cellulitis**, and thus, it is important to get a biopsy or blood test if in doubt. Treatment includes oral and topical prednisone, oral antivirals, nerve blocks, topical lidocaine patch, or lidocaine cream.

23. What can I do to prevent shingles?

A vaccine that is now available for shingles has been shown to prevent shingles in approximately half of people 60 years of age and older and also reduce the pain associated with shingles.

Certain people should not get the shingles vaccine, including those who have ever had a life-threatening allergic reaction to gelatin, the antibiotic neomycin, or any other component of shingles vaccine; have a weakened immune system because of HIV/AIDS or another disease that affects the immune system; are on treatment with drugs that affect the immune system, such as steroids; are using cancer treatment such as radiation or chemotherapy; have a history of cancer affecting the bone marrow or lymphatic system, such as leukemia or lymphoma; or have active, untreated tuberculosis. Otherwise, a single dose of shingles vaccine is indicated for adults 60 years of age and older.

24. I still get eczema. What can I do?

Flare-ups and hard-to-control chronic eczema are often due to a coexisting bacterial, fungus, or viral infection. If your eczema is weeping or oozing or crusted, your doctor will probably take a swab and treat for bacterial infection. We are greatly concerned with MRSA infections (see Question 25).

Many patients with eczema have staph bacteria on their skin, which may require systemic antibiotics to limit the infection. If you develop infections repeatedly, long-term antibiotics may be used in maintenance doses.

25. What is MRSA, and what do I need to watch for?

Ron said this:

I've got these abscesses on my left jaw line and left upper thigh. I've had them for over a month. A few weeks back I tried to clear them up. I used some penicillin that I had from an infection last year, and I put on some topical antibiotics; however, these keep coming and I can't get them to stop, and they hurt.

The pus-filled **abscesses** were lanced, cleaned, and packed to prevent another reinfection of the wound area. Cultures of the areas were then sent to a reference laboratory for identification and sensitivity.

Abscesses
Closed pockets containing pus.

The culture of the abscess revealed colonies of methicillin-resistant *Staphylococcus aureus* (MRSA), and Ron was put on the appropriate antibiotic. He was instructed to return at a later date to determine the efficiency of the antibiotics and to monitor the healing process. An infection with MRSA is a very serious matter, and prompt treatment saved him the potentially harsh physical discomfort and disfigurement.

S. aureus, discovered in pus from surgical abscesses by the surgeon Sir Alexander Ogston in Aberdeen, Scotland in 1880, is the most virulent of all 33 staphylococcal species. *Staphylococcus aureus* literally translates to "golden cluster seed." When *S. aureus* is grown on blood agar, it takes on a yellow-gold appearance. *S. aureus* produces an enzyme called penicillinase (a beta-lactamase) that is secreted from the bacteria and hydrolyzes the beta-lactam ring on the penicillin, thus inactivating penicillin.

Methicillin is used to treat bacteria that produce penicillinase. This drug is a penicillinase-resistant drug that is used to treat bacteria (such as *S. aureus*) that produce the penicillinase enzyme. An increasing number of strains of *S. aureus* are resistant to methicillin.

MRSA is resistant to many antibiotics, and intravenous vancomycin is one of the few that is useful in treatment. Because Ron came to our clinical office and not to a hospital, intravenous medications would not be practical. Trimethoprim-sulfamethoxazole (TMP-SMX) was found to be effective against Ron's particular MRSA strain. Ron returned in 2 weeks, and his healing reflected that the antibiotic and his immune system had worked effectively.

26. I was told that I have a fungus infection. What can I do?

Fungal skin infection includes tinea pedis (athlete's foot), the most common type of fungal infection. It is spread by direct contact and may infect the sole and sides of the feet. It may result in peeling, scaling, itching, and sometimes blistering. Onychomycosis (tinea unguium, nail fungus) is a toenail infection that is usually associated with tinea pedis; it can be very difficult to eradicate. Tinea cruris (jock itch) is a rash in the groin. It has an itchy spreading red border that is quite common, especially in men who sweat a lot. Tinea corporis (ringworm) may occur on the trunk or other areas. Tinea capitis (scalp ringworm) can result in scaling and patchy, moth-eaten-appearing hair loss and is epidemic in many Black communities. With the correct treatment, the hair will grow back normally and not result in permanent hair loss. Tinea infections can be effectively treated by a variety of over-the-counter prescription creams, shampoos, and oral medications.

27. How can I prevent recurrence of fungal infections?

Fungal infections often recur in many people even after effective clearing with medication. Fungus likes warmth and moisture, making certain parts of the skin more vulnerable. A fungus sheds spores, like tiny seeds, which wait for the right moment to grow into new fungus, and chooses places such as in our shoes. After effective treatment, here are some rules for prevention:

- Finish your medicine completely and as recommended. The fungus may still be present long after it is no longer visible as a rash.
- Keep feet clean, cool, and dry, and change socks frequently. Make sure that your shoes fit correctly and are not too tight. Discard old shoes, boots, slippers, and sneakers, and do not share footwear with others.
- Apply an antifungal cream twice a week to the bottom of the feet and on the nails.
- Apply an antifungal powder such as Zeasorb-AF® inside the shoes every day to keep spores from growing.
- Avoid walking barefoot in bathrooms, locker rooms, gyms, and public areas and on carpeting.
- Keep toenails short, and cut straight across. Avoid ingrown nails. Make sure that you do not use the same clippers on abnormal nails and normal nails. If you go to a salon to get your nails done, consider bringing in your own set of clippers.
- Consider using an antidandruff shampoo, such as Selsun Blue®, twice a month if you have had a body fungus. The most effective way to get the best results is to lather up and leave it on the skin for about 5 minutes (two songs long) and then wash off completely.

PART FOUR

Rashes and Bumps

I have a lot of small, warty growths on my back and other places. Should I be worried that these are cancerous?

I get little yellow bumps on my face. Are these cancerous?

It looks like I have acne on my upper cheeks. What is that?

More . . .

Sebaceous hyperplasia

A condition that affects the sebaceous glands that produce the oily fluid known as sebum.

Basal cell cancer

The most common type of skin cancer. The lesions appear as a flesh-colored papule with blood vessels and a shiny border.

Favre-Racouchot

A condition in which the skin turns yellow and thickens. The skin appears to have cysts or nodules.

28. I have a lot of small, warty growths on my back and other places. Should I be worried that these are cancer?

Those rough, dark colored plaques that have a "stuck-on," mole-like appearance are called seborrheic keratoses. My patients often call them barnacles. They are generally symptom free but occasionally can itch and be bothersome. If they are irritated or cause discomfort, they can be frozen off with liquid nitrogen or removed by a shave procedure.

29. I get little yellow bumps on my face. Are these cancerous?

These are probably **sebaceous hyperplasia**. Clinically, hyperplastic glands look like yellow nodules that may have a central pore. The number of sebaceous glands remains constant as a person ages, but the glands increase in size and become more visible, particularly in chronically sun-exposed skin. Paradoxically, sebum production decreases over time, contributing to the dry skin seen in normally aged as well as photo-aged skin. It is important to distinguish sebaceous hyperplasia from nodular **basal cell cancer** (**Plate 6**). In contrast to nodular basal cell cancer, the sebaceous gland is not translucent and does not have telangiectatic blood vessels. Nevertheless, when in doubt, it is always best to perform a biopsy.

30. It looks like I have acne on my upper cheeks. What is that?

Favre-Racouchot disease includes a variety of primarily sun-induced skin changes and is common on the face, neck, and back. It is technically called nodular elastosis with cysts, comedones, and sebaceous hyperplasia, and shows yellowish thickening of the skin and nodules acne (comedones) and follicular cysts (**Plate 7**), especially around the orbits. It can usually be seen in the 4th or 5th decade in those chronically exposed to sun. The skin becomes less firm because of degeneration of elastic tissue and fills in with cystic material. Superficial vascular changes result in irregular pigmentation and redness.

31. What are those little tags that I get on my neck and other places?

They are called **acrochordons**. These are the fleshy or dark-colored benign pedunculated papules or nodules—skin tags—on the neck, axillae, groin, chest, and abdomen. Usually, the only time they get painful is when they get tangled in necklaces or clothing. The treatment is snip (scissors) excision, cryotherapy, or cautery.

Acrochordons
Commonly known as skin tags.

32. I've got yellow growths on my eyelids. What should I do?

Jane said this:

I was told I had cholesterol deposits on the inside corners of my eyelids. Once I had them removed surgically, but they returned. I changed to a low-cholesterol diet years ago. What can I do to get rid of them?

These represent minor collections of oil below the surface of the eyelid skin. This is called xanthelasma, which is derived from a Greek word meaning "yellow plates." In certain individuals, this reflects high levels of fats in the blood (cholesterol and/or triglycerides). If you have these, you should have your laboratory tests done to detect your lipid levels. If you have high blood fat levels, this can be treated and lower your susceptibility to heart attacks in the future. If you want these removed, there are many alternatives, including the application of dilute trichloroacetic acid or electrosurgery.

33. What are actinic keratoses? My doctor said I that had them and prescribed a cream to get rid of them.

These are also called solar keratoses and are the dry, rough, and scaly lesions in sun-exposed areas. They usually are not too bothersome, although some may become irritated and cause some discomfort. A certain percentage of the crop may evolve

Rashes and Bumps

Squamous cell carcinoma

Squamous cell carcinoma is the second most common cancer of the skin and occurs most commonly in middle-aged and elderly people with fair complexions and frequent sun exposure.

Cryosurgery

Used frequently by dermatologists to treat many skin problems. Liquid nitrogen is sprayed on to an area of skin, thus freezing it.

Keloids

The increase in collagen growth under normal scar tissue.

Inflammation

The result of the immune system reacting to unwanted stimulation.

into **squamous cell carcinoma**, and that is why it is important to treat them. Treatment includes cryotherapy, retinoids, laser, chemical peels, and fluorouracil (5-FU, a cancer-treating drug). The 5-FU in products such as Efudex® has been the mainstay of treatment for many years.

34. A friend of mine said he got spots "frozen." What does that mean?

Cryosurgery or cryotherapy (liquid nitrogen spray) is used frequently by dermatologists to treat many skin problems, including scars, growths, **keloids**, precancers, and some skin cancers. The light freezing causes a peeling, while moderate freezing may result in a blister.

We use it most commonly to treat actinic keratoses (precancers), and it is often combined with other modalities such as 5-fluorouracil (Efudex) to rid the skin of these lesions.

35. I am Black, and I get razor bumps. I'm tired of them but can't seem to get rid of them. Do you have any suggestions?

Pseudofolliculitis barbae (razor bumps) occurs in up to 60% of Black men and other people with curly hair. In this condition, highly curved hairs grow back into the skin and cause **inflammation** and a foreign body reaction. Keloidal scarring and hard bumps can occur on the beard area and neck. Shaving may sharpen the ends of the hairs like spears and aggravate the skin.

The only 100% effective treatment is to let the beard grow. After growing to a certain length, the hairs will not grow back into the skin. Avoid shaving for 3 to 4 weeks, and apply a mild prescription cortisone cream to decrease the inflammation. If you need to shave, do it every other day to improve pseudofolliculitis barbae. Before shaving with a blade, water soften the beard first with a hot, wet washcloth for 5 minutes.

Preshave solutions can help soften the hairs and lubricating shaving gel (Edge®, Aveeno), or prescription-medicated shaving foam (BenzaShave® by Dermik) will often help. Use only one stroke over each area of the beard. Shave with the grain of the beard, and do not stretch the skin. Switching to an electric shaver may also help because it does not cut as close as blades do. Prepare the beard with electric razor preshave, and use the high setting to avoid close shaving.

Consider electrolysis and laser hair removal when all else fails. This can be expensive and take repeated visits, and there is a small risk of scarring. A few insurance companies will cover some or all of the cost. Medications are also prescribed to speed healing of the skin, including glycolic acid lotion, prescription antibiotic gels (Benzamycin®, Cleocin T®), oral antibiotics, and nightly Retin-A.

36. I've got ulcers on my legs. What can I do?

First you have to find out what kind of wound you have—vascular, diabetic, or traumatic—and then take the correct path to healing. Hundreds of different remedies are available for ulcers and wounds. If you have not had a culture (swab) of the wound or biopsy, I would advise it to help make sure you have the proper diagnosis. I have seen many patients treated for a routine wound who actually have lupus or a skin cancer or other problem. Adhesive films can be applied to the surface of the ulcer with a so-called semipermeable membrane that allows oxygen to pass into the healing area. Moisture is held inside to promote faster healing. Wound gels, debridement, irrigation, and other treatment modalities may also be used depending on the stage and depth of the wound.

Chronic ulcers are a very expensive and bothersome problem. Smoking, poor nutrition, and a lack of exercise also contribute to poor wound healing.

Chronic ulcers are a very expensive and bothersome problem. Smoking, poor nutrition, and a lack of exercise also contribute to poor wound healing. I recommend lifestyle changes as needed and referral to a dermatologist or wound care center if you have one available.

37. I have spots on my penis. Is it syphilis?

You may have red spots on your penis that are not sexually transmitted. Psoriasis is not uncommon in this area. Certain skin cancers such as squamous cell carcinoma, as well as other noncontagious skin diseases, may also be seen.

If a penile lesion persists, get it checked. Syphilis is a sexually transmitted infection caused by a spirochete *Treponema pallidum*. Syphilis is known as the great imitator because of its varying clinical signs and symptoms. Infection is characterized by episodes of active disease (primary, secondary, and tertiary) with intervening latent periods. Tertiary syphilis can develop 5 to 20 years after the first exposure and may affect other body systems, such as the brain, blood vessels, and eyes.

If you are concerned that you may have been infected or have symptoms, a blood test that uses antigens can be performed. A doctor may also choose to perform a biopsy of an ulcer or irritated area to distinguish syphilis from other diseases. Penicillin G is the treatment of choice for a patient with syphilis. If you have a penicillin allergy, tetracycline, erythromycin, or ceftriaxone can be used as alternative treatments. While being tested, you also need to be examined for other sexually transmitted infections, including HIV, hepatitis, and chlamydia. Prevention requires safe sex practices.

38. I've had a raised area where I had acne on my chest. It has been there for 20 years. Is there anything I can do?

Keloids are the raised and often reddish nodules that develop at the site of an injury when skin cells and connective tissue cells (fibroblasts) begin multiplying to repair the damage. The fibroblasts continue to multiply even after the wound is filled and project above the surface of the skin—keloids. The upper chest, shoulders, and upper back are especially prone to keloid formation. Although there may be no symptoms, itchiness, redness, unusual sensations, and pain may occur. Keloids occur in about 10% of people. Men and women are equally affected, but darkly pigmented people seem to be more prone to forming keloids. A hypertrophic scar looks like a keloid. Hypertrophic scars are more common and don't get as big as keloids; they may fade with time.

Although keloids are considered a benign tumor, they can be a significant cosmetic nuisance. Although there is not a single cure for keloids, treatments include cryosurgery (freezing), excision, laser, x-rays, and steroid injections.

Injection of a long-acting cortisone (steroid) into the keloid once a month is usually the first choice, even if the keloid has been on the skin for many years. After several injections, the keloid may become less prominent in 3 to 6 months of time. If they are surgically removed, recurrences are common.

PART FIVE

Systemic Diseases

What is psoriasis?

I have several small, scaly red patches on my face and arms. What are these, and what can I do?

What is rosacea?

More . . .

39. What is psoriasis?

Psoriasis

A condition in which the skin of an individual appears to be scaly and inflamed, particularly near the joints.

Psoriasis is a chronic, noncontagious skin condition that causes raised red patches topped with silvery, scaling skin, usually on the knees, elbows, scalp, and back (**Plate 8**). The fingernails, palms, and soles of the feet may also be affected. The patches, called plaques, are made up of dead skin cells that accumulate in thick layers. Normal skin cells are replaced every 30 days. In psoriasis, skin cells are replaced every 3 to 4 days.

Small patches of psoriasis can often be treated with regular use of hydrocortisone cream. Limited exposure to the sun may also help (protect unaffected skin with sunscreen). If psoriasis affects the scalp, mild tar shampoos may help.

Stress may flare your psoriasis, and stress reduction generally helps. If your psoriasis covers much of your body or is very red and itchy, seek a dermatologist's care. We now have biologic therapies for moderate to severe psoriasis; these include injections and infusions with proteins that modify the immune response.

40. I have several small, scaly red patches on my face and arms. What are these, and what can I do?

Seborrheic dermatitis

A disorder of the skin located on the scalp resulting in itchy skin and dandruff.

Impetigo

An infection of the skin caused by bacteria like *Staphylococcus aureus*.

Seborrheic dermatitis can show raised plaques and/or yellow greasy-looking scales found in the hairline, on the face, behind the ears, in the beard, and on the trunk and genitalia (**Plate 9**).

Symptoms can include itch, redness, and scaling and may mimic psoriasis, **impetigo**, fungus, and other irritating problems. When people have neurological problems such as stroke, there is an increased incidence of seborrheic dermatitis. Treatment includes topical steroids, topical and shampoo antifungal agents, and other prescriptions.

41. What is rosacea?

Rosacea (pronounced roh-ZAY-sha) is a common but little-known disorder of the facial skin that affects an estimated 14 million Americans. The disease can present with redness on the cheeks, nose, chin, or forehead; small, visible blood vessels on the face; bumps or pimples on the face; and watery or irritated eyes. Rosacea is becoming increasingly widespread as the baby boom generation enters the most susceptible ages. A Gallup survey found that 78% of Americans have no knowledge of this condition, including how to recognize it and what to do about it.

Because of its redness and acne-like effects on personal appearance, rosacea can cause significant psychological, social, and occupational problems if left untreated. In recent surveys by the National Rosacea Society, more than 76% of rosacea patients said their condition had lowered their self-confidence and self-esteem, and 52% reported that it had caused them to avoid public contact or cancel social engagements. Among rosacea patients with severe symptoms, nearly 70% said that the disorder had adversely affected their professional interactions, and nearly 30% said they had even missed work because of their condition. Some people mistakenly consider those with rosacea as alcohol abusers because of their skin ruddiness.

Although the cause of rosacea is unknown and there is no cure, help is available that can control the signs and symptoms of this disorder. Treatment includes oral antibiotics; the newest is an anti-inflammatory dosage of doxycycline such as Oracea®. Topical metronidazole gel such as MetroGel® 1% can also be used.

42. I have diabetes. What can I do to protect my skin?

Diabetes is a disease that has a huge impact on our culture. It is estimated to account for 15% of all healthcare costs in

Rosacea (pronounced roh-ZAY-sha) is a common but little-known disorder of the facial skin that affects an estimated 14 million Americans.

Rosacea

An inflammatory condition that manifests itself in the face as redness and small lesions.

the United States. It has been implicated as the chief cause of nontraumatic lower-extremity amputations, 35% of new cases of end-stage renal disease, and a significant amount of cardiovascular disease. It has been said that 100% of all diabetic patients have their skin affected in one way or another. When you consider the older population, this effect is even greater.

As many as 11 to 16 million people are affected with diabetes; the tremendous impact of the cutaneous manifestations of diabetes is obvious. The pathogenesis of these skin diseases is becoming clearer as more research is conducted. Even without that knowledge, some disorders are characteristically associated with diabetes. For example, **diabetic bullae**, the syndrome of waxy skin and limited joint mobility, and **diabetic dermopathy** are virtually pathognomonic for diabetes. Other diseases include fungal infections and **acanthosis nigricans**. The feet are often affected, and oftentimes, because of the reduction in arterial supply and reduced sensation and pain awareness with diabetes, a person may get puncture wounds or imbedded foreign objects without noticing it. This can lead to ulceration and infection.

Disorders of the diabetic skin that contribute to its pathology include **microangiopathy**, infection, and metabolic disturbances of the tissue. These problems cause disease in other parts of the body as well. Consequently, it is important to understand the dermal manifestations of diabetes so that one can effectively manage these common comorbidities. Treatment includes proper maintenance of blood sugar, diet, and exercise and carefully watching for signs of skin problems and infections.

Diabetic bullae

A condition in which large blisters are found on the extremities of individuals who are diabetics.

Diabetic dermopathy

A condition that occurs on the legs of an individual who has diabetes. The skin has spots of hyperpigmentation caused by blood vessel leakage.

Acanthosis nigricans

A condition in which the skin becomes dark and thick, usually present in the areas of the body where skin folds.

Microangiopathy

A disease of the small blood vessels, more specifically the capillaries, that leak protein and other chemicals.

PART SIX

Cancer

What is skin cancer?

What about melanoma?

How do you prevent these cancers from growing and killing?

More . . .

43. What is skin cancer?

Three basic types of skin cancer exist. The most common but least likely to spread is basal cell cancer. One third of all basal cells occur around the nose. Other common areas are on and around the ears, upper back, neck, and cheeks. Squamous cell cancers (**Plate 10**) are more likely to spread, and like basal cells, they are generally a result of chronic sun exposure. **Melanomas** (**Plate 11**) are the deadliest cancer. When it has grown to the size of a dime, it already has a 50% chance of having spread. The rate of melanoma in the 1930s was 1 in 1,500, and the rate is now as high as 1 in 75 persons. The four classic warning signs are moles with asymmetrical shape, irregular border, color variation, and a diameter greater than that of a pencil eraser (**Plate 12**).

Melanomas

A type of malignant tumor that arises from the uncontrolled growth of melanocytes found in the epidermis.

44. What about melanoma?

Melanoma is a form of skin cancer that begins in melanocytes (the cells that make the pigment melanin). Although most people have between 10 and 40 benign moles, the melanoma is a different entity.

I remember a patient named Ted, a stock trader, who had a biopsy on his back. When he returned for removal of the sutures, I told him, "You have a melanoma."

"I figured it was something bad because a few people told me to have it seen. Just didn't have time for it," he told me. "You know, I'm on the phone from early morning on, and in the evening, I have to get out and socialize to get more clients. It's endless."

"How long has it been on your back?" I asked.

"As far as I know, about 2 years," Ted said. "Lately it's been itching a lot. Am I gonna die?" he asked, a trace of worry in his voice.

"This is serious," I told him. "You have a chance of survival if you get this taken care of right away."

Even before I sent the sample to the laboratory for diagnosis, I was fairly certain that he had melanoma. In melanoma, there are four basic warning signs, which can be recalled as ABCD: asymmetry (if a line was drawn through the middle, the two sides would not match), border (irregular in shape, with scalloped or notched edges), color (typically brown or black, and sometimes mixes of red, white, and blue), and diameter (larger than a quarter of an inch, the size of a pencil eraser). Ted's tumor was asymmetrical with many areas of pigmentation, ranging from slightly pink to dark blue.

Melanoma arises because of accumulated DNA damage in a skin cell. The damage so deranges the cell's ability to control its growth that it multiplies repeatedly. The early stages are classified by the tumor's thickness and by how many layers of skin the tumor has invaded. The deeper the melanoma has advanced through the layers of skin, a measure known as Clark's level of invasion, the more likely it is to be fatal. Ted had a Clark's level stage III melanoma. That meant the melanoma had grown into the middle layer of the dermis but had not yet reached the deep dermis or subcutaneous fat.

In the past few years, great advances have been made so that the surgery for a safe and thorough melanoma removal requires removing much less tissue. With thin melanomas, outpatient procedures under local anesthesia are sufficient. Healing generally occurs in 1 to 2 weeks, and scars are minimal; however, when the melanoma has progressed beyond stage II, as in Ted's case, the key question becomes this: Has the tumor shed cells and spread beyond the original site? If it has spread, the lymph nodes closest to the tumor are the most likely site of metastases.

I hadn't detected swelling of nodes in Ted's armpits or neck, but that didn't mean the tumor hadn't spread. A new method, called **lymphoscintigraphy**, can precisely map the lymph system using a small amount of a radioactive substance injected at the site of the melanoma. With the help of a scanner, the path of lymphatic fluid draining from the melanoma to the

Lymphoscintigraphy

A diagnostic method used to identify lymphedema, the spread of cutaneous melanoma, and other diseases.

nodes can be traced. The surgeon can examine the results and biopsy only the lymph nodes that are in line to receive lymph fluid from the melanoma. If the cancer is suspected to have spread widely, however, the physician may order more extensive scans, such as computed tomography scans or magnetic resonance imaging scans.

In Ted's case, a preoperative evaluation included a complete blood count, a chest x-ray, and liver function studies to help rule out extensive metastases. A preoperative lymphoscintigraphy showed the presence of a tumor in the nodes in his armpits. Surgery was done to remove the melanoma and the affected nodes.

In stages III and IV disease, additional therapy may follow surgery. Several cancer drugs are used to treat melanoma. In addition, experimental melanoma vaccines are being studied. These vaccines are designed to boost the body's defenses against an existing melanoma, and many are in clinical trials for patients with stages III and IV disease. Another experimental strategy is to treat patients with naturally occurring immune-system factors that discourage the tumor's growth and spread.

I saw Ted 3 months later, and he expressed his appreciation and stated, "I didn't realize what a mess I was in."

"You're getting another chance," I said.

"Do I have a higher chance of another melanoma?"

"Yes, the chances of having another melanoma are greater with a history of melanoma. You need regular checkups every 3 months for 3 years and then yearly for life," I said. "With careful watching, most second melanomas are caught at an early stage and are treated by surgical excision."

"Is there a special melanoma diet?"

"No, but you'll do better keeping a well-balanced diet with folic acid, vitamins B_6, B_{12}, C, and A, and iron and zinc."

"Is it safe to donate blood?"

"In most cases, blood centers will not accept blood from someone who has had cancer," I said.

"Should I avoid the sun?"

I explained that the Skin Cancer Foundation recommends that all people avoid the sun as much as possible, especially during the hours of 10 a.m. to 4 p.m. I told him to use a sunscreen with a sun protection factor of 15 or greater and to always wear a hat and sunglasses outdoors. People with a fair complexion, blue eyes, and blond hair are the most susceptible to melanomas, as are people with a history of blistering sunburns during childhood.

"I have a sister who has some dark moles on her skin. Who should she see?"

"A dermatologist." The studies show that general physicians don't typically have enough experience to diagnose melanoma skin lesions with the same accuracy as dermatologists. Family members of a melanoma victim have a greater chance of getting melanoma and therefore should be checked also on a regular basis.

I have seen Ted now for more than 10 years since his melanoma surgery, and he continues to be melanoma free.

45. How do you prevent these cancers from growing and killing?

Children must be protected from harmful exposure to ultraviolet rays. Studies have shown that the risk of developing skin cancer increases if children have three blistering sunburns

Studies have shown that the risk of developing skin cancer increases if children have three blistering sunburns before the age of 18 years.

before the age of 18 years. The younger a child is when the burns occur, the greater the risk.

Stay out of the sun. Use sunscreens with a sun protection factor of 15 or greater every day, and use mild antibacterial soaps and cleansers. You should wear sunglasses with ultraviolet protective coating and hats with brims wide enough to protect the head, ears, and neck. Special clothing that protects the skin from ultraviolet damage can be purchased. Remember that the ultraviolet light from tanning beds is equally dangerous. There is no such thing as a safe and glowing tan. Self-tanning creams provide an alternative if one feels a need for a tan. Remember that many medicines taken internally, such as tetracycline and estrogens, can increase your sensitivity to ultraviolet light and the chance of you burning your skin.

Many techniques are available for treatment of cancerous and precancerous lesions. Cryosurgery, the use of liquid nitrogen for treatment of abnormal skin lesions, has been used since the early 1900s. Whitehouse had an article published in the *Journal of the American Medical Association* in 1907 entitled "Liquid Air in Dermatology: Its Indications and Limitations." A doctor named Torre came along in the 1960s and developed a practical apparatus to use liquid air in a spray form. It rapidly developed into the preferred method of cryosurgery for treating benign and malignant lesions. When I ask my nurse whether my guns are loaded, she knows that I refer to the canisters that I use to administer my liquid nitrogen therapy. Like many dermatologists, I shoot them all day long.

Liquid nitrogen is truly remarkable—using liquid at subzero temperatures to destroy tissue in a relatively easy manner. Destruction of malignant cells requires a temperature at least as cold as −50° centigrade. Not only does it seem magical to me that the liquid stays liquid at these temperatures, but the results can be amazing. How does it work? Cryosurgery targets the dermal–epidermal junction, providing separation and removal of epidermal lesions. In simple terms, the nasty, unwanted growths usually blister and fall off. Some of the benefits compared with other surgery include very little, if any, bleeding, no additional anesthesia, low rate of wound infection, no sutures, a biopsy that can be done while the lesion is frozen, rapid healing, easiness, and quickness. Not bad.

The skin is an amazing, versatile organ. We have good treatments for your skin ills. My advice, however, is to protect your skin and prevent skin cancers and other problems.

46. How often should I have an exam?

Every year on your birthday you should get your birthday suit checked. In addition to yearly skin exams by a dermatologist, the American Academy of Dermatology recommends self-exams every month as the best way to catch potentially cancerous skin conditions in the early stages.

47. How do I perform the self-exam?

When you examine your skin, look for any changes in moles or freckles, as well as any new spots that are asymmetrical, more than one color, the size of a pencil eraser or larger, or have uneven borders.

To conduct the exam you'll need these items:

- A full-length mirror
- A hand mirror
- A bright light
- Two chairs
- A blow dryer

Start by looking at your face and scalp in the mirror. Use the blow dryer to get a good look at your scalp. Next, focus on your hands, fingernails, elbows, arms, and underarms. Now examine your neck, chest, torso, and under your breasts, and then use the hand mirror to look at your back, shoulders, back of your neck, buttocks, and legs in the full-length mirror. Finally, sit down and closely look at your legs and feet, especially the soles, heels, and toenails. Use the hand mirror to examine your genitals.

If you find *any* abnormalities, see your doctor as soon as possible.

48. What if I think I have a skin cancer but the doctor does not appear concerned?

It is very important that you explain to your dermatologist what you want. The ability to negotiate is a good skill, and if you feel that you want a lesion removed, make your point clear. Many times a patient felt that he or she had a problem and the doctor refused to biopsy it; later it was discovered to be cancer. Almost every week I see someone with a skin cancer who was told by a previous physician to "not worry about it." Your intuition about your own body can be a very powerful tool.

It is impossible to know 100% of the time what a lesion is without a biopsy diagnosis. I have seen many lesions that look like a melanoma but later turn out to be a pigmented basal cell carcinoma or other less severe problems and not the more harmful melanoma. Providing reassurance and a clear diagnosis is one of the most rewarding parts of my job.

You can be a prevention advocate for your family. Because we know that the bulk of sun damage occurs during childhood, this period of life is a vital time for parents to be good role models and to teach their children effective sun-protection habits.

More than 80% of skin damage happens before the age of 18 years. Skin cancer lags behind about 10 to 20 years later, after the major damage has already been done; therefore, it is especially important to protect children and infants from the sun. Even if you are over 18 years old, you are not out of the danger zone. Sun damage is cumulative. Each time your skin is burnt it keeps a diary and adds it to all the old damage that you've accumulated. With each sunburn, your risk for melanoma doubles.

49. What is Mohs surgery?

Mohs micrographic surgery uses histologically prepared frozen tissue sections to evaluate the surgical margins of excisions performed to remove skin cancers. The use of microscopic control and horizontal excisions and sectioning of cutaneous **neoplasms** should maximally conserve the greatest amount of normal tissue and also provide the highest cure rate possible. Mohs surgery is also very good for recurrent tumors that have failed to respond to previous treatment and for certain types of basal cell carcinomas.

Mohs micrographic surgery

A surgical method that removes skin cancers while simultaneously analyzing the cancerous tissue.

Neoplasm

A new growth of the body's own cells no longer under normal physiologic control.

Cancer

PART SEVEN

Discoloration

Why does my skin seem to bruise easily?

Are liver spots a sign of liver disease?

I have brown patches on my face where it looks like my skin is stained. What are these?

More . . .

50. Why does my skin seem to bruise easily?

As you age, your skin gets thinner, and the underlying blood vessels are less protected from injury.

As you age, your skin gets thinner, and the underlying blood vessels are less protected from injury. The resultant extravasation of blood into the surrounding tissue, commonly seen on the dorsal forearm and hands, is referred to as purpura or ecchymosis. An injury from even a mild trauma may result in a sizable bruise.

Bruising may be an indication of an underlying condition. If bruises consistently appear for no apparent reason, it is important to check for a bleeding disorder. A common reason for bruising is the use of anticlotting medications. Protect your skin against trauma and friction. Long-sleeved shirts reduce shear and friction.

51. Are liver spots a sign of liver disease?

Lentigines

Commonly called liver spots. They occur when portions of the skin become sun damaged. They present with darkening of the skin in a specific region, commonly on the back of the hands, face, and neck.

Liver spots have nothing to do with the liver, nor are they an indication of liver disease. They are more correctly called age spots or photoaging spots and are not cancerous or precancerous. In medical terminology, they are called **lentigines**, lentigos, or solar lentigines. They are usually light to dark brown (nearly black) flat patches on the hands, face, legs, or feet (**Plate 13**). The edges of the spots are rounded, giving them a resemblance to a large freckle. One may appear by itself, or several may cluster together. The causes of these spots are (1) an inherited tendency to form them and (2) chronic sun exposure.

You can help prevent more solar lentigines by avoiding excessive sun exposure and using effective sunscreen. Pigmented lesions that may be similar in appearance but have uneven rather than rounded edges could be melanoma and should be evaluated by a dermatologist.

52. I have brown patches on my face where it looks like my skin is stained. What are these?

The signs of **melasma** are dark, irregular patches commonly found on the upper cheek, nose, lips, upper lip, and forehead that often develop gradually over time. Melasma often occurs after giving birth or after stopping oral contraceptives or hormone replacement therapy.

Melasma is thought to be the stimulation of melanocytes or pigment-producing cells by the female sex hormones estrogen and progesterone to produce more melanin pigments when the skin is exposed to sun. Women with a light brown skin type who are living in regions with intense sun exposure are particularly susceptible to developing this condition.

Genetic predisposition is also a major factor in determining whether someone will develop melasma. The incidence of melasma also increases in patients with thyroid disease. Uncommon causes of melasma include allergic reaction to medications and cosmetics and as a symptom of Addison's disease. Melasma does not cause any other conditions beyond the cosmetic discoloration.

Treatments to help fade the discolored patches include the following:

- Tretinoin, which is an acid that increases skin cell (keratinocyte) turnover. This treatment cannot be used during pregnancy.
- Topical depigmenting agents, such as hydroquinone, which are either in over-the-counter (2%) or prescription (4%) strength. Hydroquinone is a chemical that inhibits tyrosinase, an enzyme involved in the production of melanin. Combination products such as Tri-Luma® can also be used.

Melasma

A condition that usually occurs from various effects of hormones present during times of pregnancy. The manifestation is the presence of a darkened color of the face due to increased melanin production.

Discoloration

- Azelaic acid (20%), which is thought to decrease the activity of melanocytes.
- Facial peel with alpha hydroxy acids or chemical peels with glycolic acid.
- Laser or red light treatment.

All of these treatments and effects are gradual. A strict avoidance of sunlight is required, along with the use of broad-spectrum sunscreens with physical blockers because ultraviolet A, ultraviolet B, and visible lights are all capable of stimulating pigment production. Cosmetic coverups can also be used to lighten the appearance of melasma. More information about these treatments is discussed later in this book.

53. I have this reddish brown patch on my neck. What is this, and can I do anything about it?

Poikiloderma of Civatte

Often occurs in middle-aged women on the sides of their neck resulting in appearance of tangled or leaky blood vessels and pigmentation. The condition is not serious, but its onset is believed to be due to hormonal changes.

You may have **poikiloderma of Civatte**. Poikiloderma refers to a change in the skin where there is thinning, increased pigmentation, and dilation of the fine blood vessels (telangiectasia). Civatte, a French dermatologist, first described this pattern that affects the skin of the sides and front of the neck. Poikiloderma of Civatte characteristically spares the shaded area under the chin.

Most people with poikiloderma of Civatte are usually asymptomatic, although occasionally patients report mild burning and itching and increased sensitivity of the affected skin. Many contributing factors have been identified, including chronic exposure to ultraviolet light, photosensitizing chemicals in perfumes and cosmetics, and a genetic predisposition.

Diagnosis is made on biopsy, laboratory tests, and clinical findings. Treatments include topical retinoids, hydroquinone, and alpha-hydroxy acids, as well as protecting the skin from the sun to prevent further damage. By reducing pigmentation changes, intense pulse light has been beneficial in the treatment of poikiloderma of Civatte.

PART EIGHT

Skin and the Circulatory System

My leg veins stick out, and I don't like them.
What can I do?

I get little cherry-colored bumps on my skin.
What are they?

If I get a dark blue bump on my lip, is it skin cancer?

More . . .

54. My leg veins stick out, and I don't like them. What can I do?

Join the crowd—about 80 million adults in the United States have varicose veins and their smaller cousins known as spider veins.

Varicose veins usually occur in the legs, where their knotted bluish appearance can be a substantial problem. Complications can develop such as venous stasis ulcers, inflammation of veins (phlebitis), or, in severe cases, blood clots that come loose and become emboli to distant organs such as the lungs.

Spider veins are formed by the dilation of small blood vessels and become visible because they live near the surface of the skin. Although not a threat to health, they can be disfiguring. Spider veins are commonly found on the face and legs and appear as a "sunburst" pattern of reddish to purplish small veins.

The incidence of both varicose veins and spider veins increases with age and may be an inherited trait. Pregnancy and hormonal changes may contribute to the development of enlarged veins. Although there is no sure method of preventing varicose veins and spider veins, protection against forming varicose veins may be provided by wearing support hose and maintaining a normal weight.

Treatment for varicose veins and spider veins include:

- Sclerotherapy: a chemical solution is injected into veins to cause them to collapse and close up. It may require multiple treatments to clear all affected veins and more treatments may be needed from time to time as new enlarged veins appear. Side effects can include slight bruising and swelling at injection sites.
- Phlebectomy: an enlarged vein is removed through tiny incisions along its course. The procedure is done in an outpatient setting and is particularly useful for large varicose veins.

- Electrodessication: an electrical current is used to seal off enlarged veins.
- Laser surgery: pulses from a laser selectively destroy enlarged veins and spider veins.
- Surgical ligation and stripping: a procedure usually reserved for larger varicose veins, often done by a vascular surgeon in a hospital. The varicose vein is tied off (ligated) or completely removed.

55. I get little cherry-colored bumps on my skin. What are they?

These are **angiomas**, benign growths that consist of small blood vessels that can be located anywhere on the body. Different types include spider angiomas, cherry angiomas, and angiokeratomas. Although the cause of most types of angiomas is not known, cherry angiomas are due to aging and do not have any known significance. Spider angiomas are more common in childhood and during pregnancy, but when present in large numbers, they may warn of liver damage. Angiokeratomas are an overgrowth of blood vessels and skin cells.

Treatment of angiomas is not necessary unless they bleed or are bothersome. If treatment is required, the dermatologist will recommend the most appropriate method. **Electrodesiccation**, which is touching the skin with an electric needle to destroy the blood vessels, is one of the treatments. We also occasionally use this treatment to eliminate the unwanted facial veins of rosacea. Liquid nitrogen is a cold gas that is sprayed on the skin with a spray gun to destroy the angiomas and is also used in treatment of lesions such as seborrheic keratoses and warts. Laser uses a beam of concentrated light to destroy the lesion and is also used at times to destroy unwanted leg veins or the facial veins of rosacea. All of these common treatment modalities usually give a good cosmetic result, although angiomas sometimes recur after treatment.

Angiomas

These are benign tumors that are comprised of lymph tissue and blood vessels. These tumors are red in color and not usually life-threatening.

Electrodesiccation

Scraping or burning off skin growths (also known as electrodesiccation and curettage). It can be used for less serious skin cancers, precancers, and benign growths.

56. If I get a dark blue bump on my lip, is it skin cancer?

Venous lake

A lesion that appears purple and raised. It is generally located on the lip, and is caused by the leakage of capillaries or due to the inability of blood to flow out freely.

This is most likely a **venous lake**—an asymptomatic, solitary, soft, compressible, dark blue to violaceous, 0.2- to 1-cm papule commonly found on sun-exposed surfaces of the vermilion border of the lip (**Plate 14**), face, and ears. Lesions generally occur among older individuals. If it persists, itches, bleeds, or gets larger and more irregular, get a biopsy.

57. What can I do about dark circles under my eyes?

Do you look into the mirror and seeing a raccoon staring back at you? What causes dark circles under the eyes? Working late, allergies, too little sleep, increasing age, and poor nutrition all can contribute. These are not the physiological reason for the dark circles, however.

The same kind of chemical reaction that produces bruises hits around your eyes. This area is the thinnest and most delicate skin of your face and is populated by with tiny capillaries. Blood sometimes leaks from these capillaries, and your body tries to mop up the loose blood by breaking it down in an oxidization process known as hemoglobin degradation. As the hemoglobin degrades, it turns a dark bluish red. Guess what? You get dark circles under the eyes, but you don't have to get hit in the face!

Certain eye circle creams speed up the rate of the hemoglobin degradation and strengthen the capillaries in your skin to help fade the dark pigmentation and prevent more damage.

What can you do to get rid of the circles? Certain eye circle creams speed up the rate of the hemoglobin degradation and strengthen the capillaries in your skin to help fade the dark pigmentation and prevent more damage. Some of the bleaching creams containing hydroquinone also help the darkness diminish but should be used with caution near the eyes. Tanning can make dark under-eye circles even worse by bringing the melanin to the surface of the skin, making it darker.

What else?

Allergies can contribute to dark under-eye circles. The allergic reaction can elicit allergic shiners that can reflect under the eye. If the allergies cause you to rub or scratch your eyes, the fragility of the skin can break down the capillaries and darken the skin. Fatigue or inadequate rest can make your skin paler, and this makes dark circles look darker. During pregnancy and/or menstruation, skin becomes pale, and thus, the dark circles look darker. Too much sun can make the circles appear darker. As you get older, the skin around your eyes becomes thinner, and the dark under-eye circles can become more pronounced. Eating a balanced and healthy diet allows you to take in essential nutrients that inhibit dark under-eye circles.

A patient of mine named Lisa had tried everything.

Lisa said this:

I put drops of lemon juice under my eyes, but it got in my eyes. So in addition to my dark circles, I also had bloodshot eyes. I used creams, slices of cucumber, slices of potato, tea bags, and everything else.

Then I found what worked for me. I took a vitamin E capsule and pierced it with a pin. Then I dabbed a bit of it on the skin under my eyes. It helped cut down my dark eye circles and puffiness as well. Then I swallowed the rest of the capsule. In the evening before going to sleep I put on a small amount of a prescription bleaching cream, and that also helped my skin. Until I got better, I used a concealer.

Cold washcloth compresses can help constrict the blood vessels and decrease the under-eye darkness. Drinking more water (at least 8 to 10 glasses per day) can help to cleanse your body of impurities that can contribute to dark eye circles. Don't get discouraged, as there are many ways to improve your looks.

58. What about my tiny bruises?

Susan said this:

I am 62 years old, and for many years, I have had tiny bruises about the size of a pinpoint all over my body. I keep getting more all the time, and some have gotten a little bigger. Should I be concerned?

Petechiae

Small red spots under the top layer of skin due to the leaking of nearby blood vessels.

The spots may represent **petechiae**, tiny blood hemorrhages in the uppermost layer of the skin. Petechiae can erupt from variety of causes—from just being normal to having leukemia or lymphoma. Your doctor needs to rule out serious medical diseases and may choose to take a skin biopsy to check your skin on a microscopic level. Other conditions include vasculitis and Shamberg's disease. The cause for petechiae should be explored.

59. What about stasis dermatitis?

Sam, age 71, said this:

I have a scaly, dark colored spots on my ankle. I have been told it is poor circulation and to keep moisturizers on it. What else do you suggest?

Stasis dermatitis

A condition of the skin due to the pooling of blood in the lower legs; leaky valves in the veins prevent the proper return of the blood to the trunk of the body.

Most likely you have **stasis dermatitis,** an extremely common rash that is caused by slowing circulation. Stasis dermatitis occurs from slowed blood flow to the legs caused by atherosclerosis (hardening of the arteries), vein disease, or chronic heart failure.

Leg elevation while at rest is a crucial part of treatment. If you have stasis dermatitis, elevate your heels to a point slightly higher than your hips without bending your knees.

60. What if I wear support hose?

A support-hose prescription such as T.E.D.® or Jobst® brands will help the blood flow in your legs. Heredity, age, surgery, occupation, and other issues are important factors in leg health.

You can improve your circulation through exercise, good posture, choosing proper fitting clothing and footwear, and wearing gradient compression hosiery that does the job for you. These types of hose are particularly important if you are recovering from surgery and need to prevent an embolism.

61. Will the dark color from stasis dermatitis ever disappear?

The brownish tan stain in the skin of your legs is caused by the deposition of iron in the skin from blood that has leaked out previously and by melanin. Although this dark skin color can lighten over time, it usually takes a long time.

Skin and the Circulatory System

61

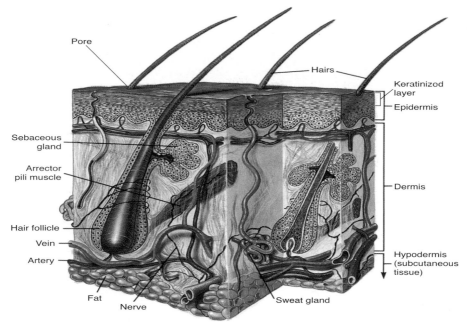

Plate 1   The structure of human skin
Source: Reproduced from Alters S, Biology: Understanding Life. © 2000 by Jones and Bartlett Publishers, Inc., Sudbury, MA.

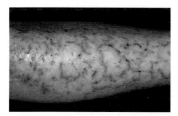

Plate 2   Asteatotic eczema

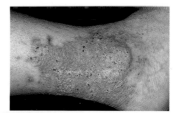

Plate 3   Lichen simplex chronicus

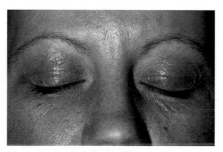

Plate 4   Contact dermatitis

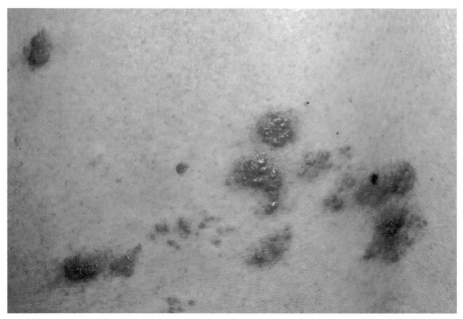

Plate 5   Herpes zoster (shingles)
Source: © Stephen VanHorn/ShutterStock, Inc.

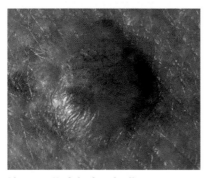

Plate 6   Nodular basal cell cancer

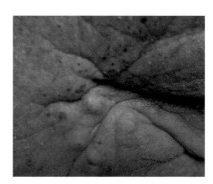

Plate 7   Favre-Racouchot

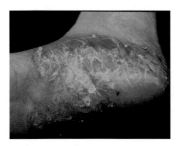

Plate 8   Psoriasis

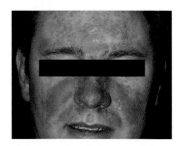

Plate 9   Seborrheic dermatitis

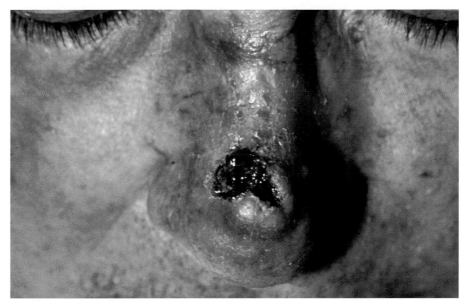

Plate 10   Squamous cell cancer
Source: Courtesy of National Cancer Institute

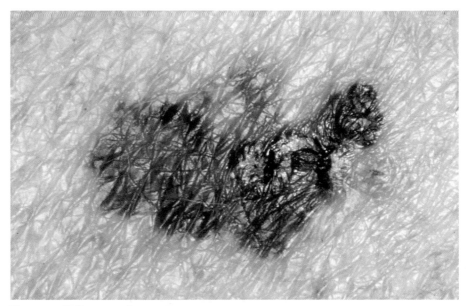

Plate 11   Malignant melanoma
Source: Courtesy of National Cancer Institute

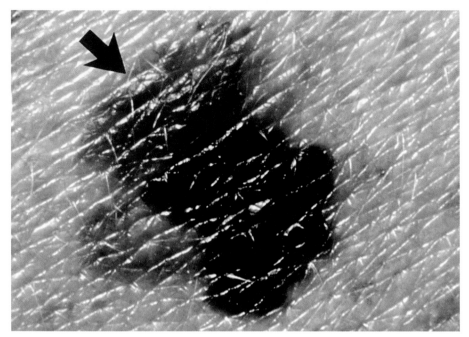

Plate 12   Distinct color variation: warning sign of melanoma
Source: Courtesy of National Cancer Institute

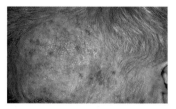

Plate 13   Lentigines (photoaging or liver spots)

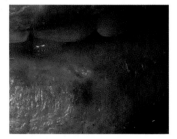

Plate 14   Venous lake

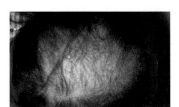

Plate 15   Telogen effluvium

PART NINE

Cosmetic Procedures

What can I do for skin rejuvenation?

What is a chemical peel?

What about laser resurfacing?

More . . .

62. What can I do for skin rejuvenation?

*Botox,
chemical peels,
fillers, facial
reconstruction,
and prevention
are all choices
that you can
make to help
freshen your
skin and lessen
the accumulated
effects of aging.*

Botox®, chemical peels, fillers, facial reconstruction, and prevention are all choices that you can make to help freshen your skin and lessen the accumulated effects of aging. Products to treat mildly damaged skin include alpha-hydroxy acids, derived from fruit and dairy products, alone or in combination with tretinoin. Over-the-counter products containing retinols (of the vitamin A family), antioxidants (especially vitamins C and E), and hyaluronic acids may improve the appearance of fine lines and wrinkles. Daily use of moisturizers and sunscreens is a key to overall success.

63. What is a chemical peel?

As the name implies, this process peels the skin and may include one or more chemicals such as alpha-hydroxy acids, trichloroacetic acid, or carbolic acid. Other terms include chemexfoliation or dermapeeling. The treatment is used to repair the skin damage of superficial to moderate photoaging and to reduce acne scars. Discuss the objectives of your treatment with your dermatologist. Based on your decision, the strength of the chemical solution and the depth of the peel will be modified.

A chemical solution causes the skin to blister mildly and to peel off over a period of hours and days. The new skin that forms to take its place is usually smoother and less wrinkled than the old skin. Often a series of mild, light peels in combination with a skin care program, including retinoids and a sunscreen protection program, is used to treat fine lines and wrinkles. If you have moderate skin damage, a medium-depth peel is often more effective to help eliminate solar elastoses, lentignines, and actinic keratoses.

What about after-effects? The redness that follows a chemical peel is similar to a sunburn and may last 3 to 5 days. If a medium-depth or deep peeling is done, the redness, swelling, blistering, and peeling may last for 7 to 14 days. Medications are generally prescribed to alleviate discomfort. Avoid over-exposure to the sun.

64. What about laser resurfacing?

The laser is a light "pump" that narrowly segregates light of selected wavelength and "pumps" the light radiation to high intensity and varied durations depending on the required task.

"Resurfacing" the skin with laser allows for a reduction or removal of wrinkles, lines, and other effects of aging and photoaging. Other treatments with the laser include removal of superficial brown pigmented lesions and deep pigmented lesions such as port wine stains and birthmarks and removal or improvement of scars, some skin cancers, vascular moles, tattoos, warts, and unwanted hair.

Included in the benefits of laser skin resurfacing are bloodlessness, precise effects, and 1-day outpatient treatment. A medium-depth chemical peel may be combined with laser resurfacing to achieve maximum effectiveness.

65. What about soft-tissue augmentation and fillers?

To achieve soft-tissue augmentation, a substance that is compatible with your body tissues is injected under the skin to eliminate irregularities such as wrinkles, pits, and scars. Collagen is a fibrous protein substance in all human and animal tissue. Injections are usually given in a series of treatments to fill out a wrinkle or depression. The effects of collagen injection may last for 3 to 12 months.

In microlipoinjection, self-donated body fat is harvested from your own body and prepared for this fat-transfer procedure. The fat is used to replace fat lost from under the skin in the aging process. The newest products, including Restylane®, Juvederm®, Radiesse®, and others, show persistent effects for up to 2 years and have replaced many of the former products.

66. What is Botox, and is it right for me?

Purified botulinum toxin in very tiny amounts is injected into a targeted facial muscle, and the resulting nerve blockade of that muscle causes a local immobilization of muscle movement that prevents crinkling and wrinkle lines from forming when you frown or squint. The potent biological effects of botulinum toxin can be used to diminish temporarily frown lines, crow's-feet, and facial wrinkles. Although botulinum toxin is the powerful agent of botulism food poisoning, you cannot contract botulism from the cosmetic use of botulinum toxin.

Although cosmetic procedures have become less invasive and require less downtime, you should know what to expect after the procedure. What are the risks and side effects of the procedure? Although the risks involved in most cosmetic procedures are minimal, any potential complication should be discussed before the cosmetic procedure is performed. Botox rejuvenation can result in temporary swelling, redness, or bruising.

How long will the results last? Most cosmetic results are not permanent, and if you smoke or have other complications when healing, it may take more time to see results. Botox rejuvenation usually lasts about 3 to 4 months. For maximum effectiveness, treatment with botulinum toxin is repeated over several sessions.

Dermabrasion

A surgical procedure used for cosmetic reasons to improve the appearance of the skin.

Dermabrasion is very useful for removal or reduction of acne and chickenpox scars and for facial skin rejuvenation.

67. I have heard that dermabrasion might be great for me. What can I expect from it?

Dermabrasion is very useful for removal or reduction of acne and chickenpox scars and for facial skin rejuvenation. The procedure planes off the surface layer of skin with a rapidly rotating brush and removes the skin surface. A new layer of skin grows to replace the removed skin. Redness of the skin similar to a severe sunburn may occur afterward, and healing usually is complete in about 10 days. Sunlight restriction for several months after treatment is recommended.

Dermabrasion may be combined with other procedures such as soft-tissue augmentation to maximize effectiveness.

At our office, we use a technique that removes less surface skin and is called microdermabrasion. It is quite useful for superficial skin defects and is repeated at intervals.

68. I have bumps on my nose from rosacea. What surgical alternative methods are available?

The electrosurgical resurfacing technique may be used to treat various raised surface areas. I have had several patients with the large bulbous bumps of rosacea, called rhinophymas (think of W.C. Fields' nose), that responded well to a sculpting process using an electrosurgical technique. I smooth out the rough terrain, and the patients generally recover with few side effects. Treating the underlying rosacea also helps to prevent recurrence.

69. What is liposuction?

Unwanted fat deposits are one of the visible signs of aging. Despite diet and exercise to keep looking young and trim, you may still have unwanted fatty deposits. Common areas of concern are on the face, chin, neck, breast, abdomen, hips, thighs, buttocks, knees, and ankles.

Tumescent liposuction is a procedure that removes these localized fat deposits and is performed only after a full medical evaluation. It is important to be in good health and have realistic expectations of liposuction before having the procedure.

An incision is made in the skin, and the fat is removed with a vacuum tube into a collection system. This procedure is performed in an outpatient setting with local anesthesia and antibleeding medication. Fat cells that are removed by liposuction do not grow back. The postoperative pain and need for medication vary in each person. Because of the slow resolution of postsurgical swelling, the final results after liposuction are not seen for 12 to 16 weeks, although most people see improvements within 4 weeks. Liposuction is not a substitute for diet, exercise, or weight reduction but can be used as an adjunct method of improving your looks.

70. What is Retin-A, and should I use it?

Retin-A (tretinoin) is used to reduce fine wrinkles, blotchy pigmentation, and rough skin associated with chronic sun exposure. This is a topical vitamin A derivative and has been used quite effectively for many years to help reverse sun damage. Retin-A is one of the products that we include for the majority of patients who want to maintain more youthful skin and reverse sun damage.

71. What about exfoliators for my face?

The skin constantly renews itself by sloughing its top (horny) layer. At times, because of either overproduction or inadequate removal, these cells build up. This makes the skin appear scaly and can be rough to the touch. Removing this excess scale with exfoliators makes the skin feel better and might make other agents such as moisturizers work better.

72. How can my skin be like Cleopatra's?

Alpha-hydroxy acids (AHA) are compounds that can now be found in over 200 skin treatment products. Mild exfoliation, wrinkle effacement, nail rejuvenation, and overall improved skin and hair comes in the form of shampoos, moisturizers, cleansers, toners, and cosmetics that contain alpha-hydroxy acids. In higher concentration, physicians and others use alpha-hydroxy acids as superficial or mid-depth peeling agents.

To maintain her beauty, Cleopatra used red wine, which contains alpha-hydroxy acid, on her face. This may have been the secret of success for one of antiquity's most attractive women. Alpha-hydroxy acids comprise a group of organic compounds derived from sources such as fruit juices (thus the name *fruit acids*), sugar cane, milk, and grapes. How do they work? Although still not completely understood, they may weaken the bonds between cells and facilitate sloughing and may also be mild irritants that stimulate the skin to renew itself faster by losing its horny layer more efficiently.

Alpha-hydroxy acid is primarily used as a mild exfoliant. A few of the currently available brands include these:

- Eucerin® Plus (5% AHA)
- Lac-Hydrin® Five (5% AHA)
- Alpha Hydrox® (8% AHA)
- Dermalogica® Skin Smoothing Cream (8% AHA)
- Aqua Glycolic® Face Cream (12% AHA)
- MD Formulations® Facial Lotion (12% AHA)

Alpha-hydroxy acids are easy to use after cleansing and drying your skin. Apply a thin layer of the product as you would a moisturizer. You might have a few seconds of mild burning, but if this is too intense or if it lasts for a long time, use a lower concentration of the alpha-hydroxy acid.

Do not use other potential irritants, such as alcohol or harsh soaps. Your skin may seem flakier than usual for the first few weeks of use, and that is okay, as the alpha-hydroxy acid is doing its job.

73. What else works to improve my face?

Blepharoplasty (eyelid surgery) can be used to correct droopy eyelids by removing excess fat pads and skin. A brow lift may reduce lines in the forehead and raise the eyebrows. **Rhytidectomy** (face lift) tightens and trims excess skin on the cheeks, chin, and neck and around the mouth. This procedure works quite well for those with Favre-Racouchot.

Blepharoplasty

A procedure in which the extra skin of either the upper or lower eyelids are surgically removed.

Rhytidectomy

A plastic surgery procedure more commonly called a face lift.

Blepharoplasty (eyelid surgery) can be used to correct droopy eyelids by removing excess fat pads and skin.

PART TEN

Hair and Nails

My nails are getting yellow and brittle.
What can I do?

My hair is gray and feels thinner. What should I do?

Why do some older people grow excess body hair
in places they don't want, especially the ears, nose,
and eyebrows?

More . . .

74. My nails are getting yellow and brittle. What can I do?

Over 90% of older people have nail dystrophies; nails that have been compromised by trauma are more prone to fungal infection. If you suspect that you have a fungal infection, a biopsy (nail clipping) will identify a fungus such as *Trychophyton rubrum*. The treatment is not always benign, and oral medications can be costly and interfere with other drugs you may be taking. Toenails decrease their growth rate over time, and if also thickened, the effectiveness of antifungal drugs is reduced. Many topical treatments have shown limited results. You have to decide how much the discoloration bothers you and whether you are willing to take the risks associated with therapy.

As we age, our nail plates thin, the half moons disappear, and ridges develops. When you moisturize your skin, be sure to include your nails. Biotin in oral supplementation has shown to be effective in some studies.

75. My hair is gray and feels thinner. What should I do?

Gray hair is a characteristic of normal aging—we tend to develop gray hair because the pigment in the hair is lost and the hair becomes colorless. In men, graying takes place earlier and more often than in women—hereditary factors and hormonal situations as well as age are of importance.

The average human head has about 100,000 hair follicles. Growth hormone levels peak at puberty and decrease thereafter—skin thickness and skin total collagen are reduced with aging. Advancing age brings on a gradual decrease in the number of hair follicles over the entire body. Androgenetic alopecia (balding) results primarily from the androgen-dependent conversion of relatively dark thick scalp hairs to lightly pigmented short, fine, villous hairs (like that of the ventral forearm).

76. Why do some older people grow excess body hair in places they don't want, especially the ears, nose, and eyebrows?

Men in old age will develop increased hair growth on the tip of the nose, vibrissae of the nasal entrance, eyebrow area, and hypertrichosis of the pinnae (ears). These conditions may have a genetic basis.

In women, hair on the chin, over the upper lip, or on arms and legs can create an appearance of older age or masculinization and can be quite bothersome. **Hirsutism** is the medical term for excess hair on a woman in the places only adult men should grow hair. For most women, the tendency toward hirsutism is inherited, although excess hair growth may be present in both the female and male family members. Although hirsutism usually begins around puberty, mild hirsutism can start at any age. As women age, they gradually develop more facial or body hair. Hypertrichosis (as opposed to hirsutism) is an excessive quantity of hair in a normal location such as the calf of the leg.

Hirsutism is usually caused by an increased sensitivity or production of the skin to a group of hormones called androgens (testosterone and androstenedione). Androgen disorders (**hyperandrogenism**—increased levels of male hormone production in women) affect between 5% and 10% of all women and most commonly bring on irregular menstrual cycles.

Tests to see whether this is caused by a treatable condition usually include testosterone (T) levels, dehydroepiandrosterone sulfate (DHEAS), 17-hydroxyprogesterone, prolactin, T4, and TSH. A breast exam and an endometrial biopsy may be indicated.

Hair and Nails

Hirsutism

This condition usually affects women. The condition presents itself with large amounts of dark hair growth in the areas on the body where hair is usually not present.

Hyperandrogenism

This condition occurs with the overexpression of male hormones in either females or males.

77. What can I do to get rid of excess hair?

Traditional methods of removal of superfluous hair include these:

1. Shaving
2. Bleaching
3. Waxing
4. Plucking
5. Chemical depilatory
6. Electrolysis or electrothermolysis

An available prescription cream that stops facial hair growth, Vaniqa® (pronounced Van-ih-KA), helps many women and has no major side effects.

In recent years, laser hair removal has been proven effective in removal of unwanted hair, with hair loss for 2 or more years.

In recent years, laser hair removal has been proven effective in removal of unwanted hair, with hair loss for 2 or more years. This is accomplished by photothermolysis—using a laser to generate heat in hair follicles and render them incapable of growing new hair. Many factors, including skin and hair color, are considered in determining the type of laser to use, duration of treatment, and number of treatments.

Be careful about who and where you choose to do your treatments. With medi-spas popping up everywhere, make sure that you find out the treating person's qualifications and experience in the use of lasers.

78. What are the effects of laser hair removal?

All medical treatments have potential side effects, and laser hair removal is no exception. Side effects are considered either temporary or permanent. Local anesthetic may be used during the procedure to decrease pain.

Hyperpigmentation

The darkening of the epidermis due to an increase in the presence of melanin.

Posttreatment pain, swelling, and redness can last for a few hours to a few days. Blistering may be the most painful and noticeable side effect. **Hyperpigmentation** (temporary darkening of the skin) can occur. Medicine to alleviate these side effects should be offered.

Permanent side effects can include skin discoloration, most often permanent lightening of the skin on the treated area. The laser is designed to decrease the pigmentation in darker colored hair and can sometimes affect darker colored skin as well. Scarring and burns are uncommon.

Laser hair removal may or may not be the right decision for you, but the risk of possible side effects must be considered. To minimize risks:

1. Choose a qualified practitioner with a good track record doing laser therapy.
2. Tell your practitioner whether you have any family medical or hormonal conditions.
3. Let your practitioner know whether you have any form of the herpes virus in the intended treatment area. Take any antibiotic or antiviral medications that may be prescribed.
4. Avoid unprotected sun exposure or tanning for several weeks before your procedure. Your lightest skin tone for the treatment will maximize results and minimize side effects.
5. Avoid waxing or plucking the treatment area for several weeks before the procedure. Clean the treatment area on the day of the procedure. Do not wear makeup if your face is being treated.
6. Follow any preprocedure or postprocedure instructions given.

79. What can I do about hair loss?

Hair loss in men or women can contribute to the appearance of looking older than chronologic age. One of the hair-restoration procedures may be used alone or in combination with a procedure for facial skin rejuvenation to take years off your apparent age. Any person who feels that hair loss is a problem should consult a dermatologist. The first step in treating hair loss is diagnosing its causes. These can include heredity, various acute and chronic diseases, nutritional deficiency, medications, radiation, and improper hair treatments.

The most common cause of hair loss in men is male-pattern baldness, a condition with a hereditary basis. In women, the most common conditions are androgenetic alopecia baldness and **telogen effluvium**, which causes thinning of scalp hair but not bald patches (**Plate 15**). A condition of unknown causes called alopecia areata occurs in both men and women, causing hair loss in small circular patches.

Based on medical evaluation, a dermatologist will recommend the procedure that is right for the individual patient. Male-pattern baldness may be medically treated with topical minoxidil or oral finasteride, drugs that can restart hair growth or at least maintain the hair they have in some patients.

Telogen effluvium

A common condition in which the body undergoes alopecia, otherwise known as hair shedding or balding.

80. Is a hair transplant painful?

Most patients report only a small amount of discomfort associated with a hair transplant procedure. All patients are given a relaxing medication before the procedure, and local anesthetic is used. The hair transplant takes place in the doctor's office and is safe and simple in the hands of an experienced staff.

Will you need more than one procedure? The number of procedures will depend on the extent of your hair loss and the number of implants per surgery. It may take 4 months to see the new growth. Further evaluation will help to determine whether more transplant sessions are indicated.

81. What does the healing process involve?

Redness and swelling may go on for a few days after your procedure and are usually mild. If your existing hair is long enough, it may be combed over the grafted area to hide the grafts while they are healing. With the newest techniques, your new hair should look and feel natural.

82. What is the cost of a hair transplant?

Save those pennies. Most physicians charge between $1,500 and $3,000. Compare this, however, with months and years of paying for medicines to stimulate hair growth that may not work well.

83. Is it appropriate for a woman to have a hair restoration procedure? Isn't this something usually done for men only?

Hair loss is a problem that affects about 35 million men and also about 22 million women in the United States. Women have increasingly turned to dermatologists for help in restoring a full-head-of-hair look. Hair loss in women, just as in men, is often the result of the genetic lottery. Along with inheritance, hormonal changes of pregnancy as well as stress and nutritional deficiencies can lead to hair loss.

Hair loss is a problem that affects about 35 million men and also about 22 million women in the United States.

Changes in the hair can be tricky. Thus, the age and condition of the patient are important. For example, when a woman is pregnant, more of her hairs will be growing. After a woman delivers her baby, many hairs enter the resting phase of the hair cycle. Within 2 to 3 months, some women will notice large amounts of hair coming out in their brushes and combs. This common problem is called telogen effluvium, which can also occur after major stress such as trauma or surgery. Do not jump the gun and go wild with surgeries or other techniques, however, because telogen effluvium may last only 1 to 6 months and resolves completely in most cases. Before you consider a hair restoration program, see a dermatologist to evaluate the reason for your hair loss and recommend the most effective hair restoration plan.

PART ELEVEN

Feet

How can I maintain healthy skin on my feet?

I have ugly heels. What can I do?

84. How can I maintain healthy skin on my feet?

By the time you get to old age, you will have clocked over 10,000 miles. The foot is out on a limb—at the end of a neurological and vascular tree—and can be the recipient of trauma and repetitive injuries. The feet may need frequent servicing as we age. Anytime there is a reduction in blood supply and decreased sensation, as with diabetes, the feet can be prone to infection and ulceration. Skin problems such as fungus, stasis dermatitis, and nail dysfunction also increase over time. Range of motion limitations from osteoarthritis and other conditions add to changes in foot pressure and pain. Proper footwear, good nutrition, exercise, and visits to your dermatologist and podiatrist will help prevent problems.

85. I have ugly heels. What can I do?

Alyson said this:

I have really awful, ugly heels. They are always cracked and scaly. I usually soak my feet at night and that helps. What else can I do for them?

This is called tylosis and can be a real annoyance, especially for women. With this problem, the heels can crack, bleed, and even run hosiery for those who wear them. A fungus or an allergic contact dermatitis must also be ruled out, but it's usually the result of severe dryness on the feet and thick heels areas. In rare cases, there are inherited cases. Moisturizers, soaks of various kinds, and over-the-counter skin softeners help, but over the years, I've found that if you practice the following advice three times a week, you should get relief.

Soak your feet in warm, clear tap water for about 20 minutes at night. Pat your feet dry, and apply a good layer of Keralyt® gel or Salex™ (or a similar salicylic acid) over the affected areas. A topical salicylate works by causing the skin to swell, soften, and then slough or peel in areas where it is applied.

Cover each of your feet with a plastic bag, followed by a sock over the bag. Do not tape the bag down. Leave this occlusive bandage on all night but don't walk around on them!

In the morning, take off the bags. Wipe the dead skin cells and remaining medicine off your feet, and apply a good layer of Lac-Hydrin or AmLactin® lotion (or a similar salicylic acid). Ammonium lactate is a combination of lactic acid and ammonium hydroxide. It is a moisturizer that is used to treat dry, scaly, itchy skin and acts as a boost to the overnight occlusion.

Feet

PART TWELVE

Prevention

What role does diet play in skin health?

How does sun protection do me any good now?

What are ways to improve sun protection and prevent skin cancer?

More . . .

86. *What role does diet play in skin health?*

Replenishing the three key components of the stratum corneum—ceramides, fatty acids, and cholesterol—is the aim of some skin care formulations. Diet also plays an important role in maintaining a healthy skin barrier; fatty acids and cholesterol are derived from the diet.

87. *How does sun protection do me any good now?*

Nothing contributes to how a person sees him- or herself more than how his or her skin looks in the mirror. Protecting one's skin from damage early in life can vastly improve how one looks and feels during later years. The three preventable high-risk behaviors that can damage the skin in the later years are smoking, being overweight, and having high exposure to ultraviolet rays.

88. *What are ways to improve sun protection and prevent skin cancer?*

If you play tennis or participate in any outdoor sports, one of your most important strokes may be a backhand across your arms with a dollop of sunscreen. Spread it all over your arms and then proceed to put it on all the parts of your body that you'll be exposing to the sun. Wear a wide-brimmed hat. Drink lots of water, and reapply your sunscreen as needed. Now get out and play!

An overwhelming majority of patients fail to take the topic of sun protection seriously.

An overwhelming majority of patients fail to take the topic of sun protection seriously. Some continue to admire the glowing tan of youth and yet want to be free of wrinkles and blemishes; however, the two can rarely coexist. Others would rather spend bundles of dollars on expensive treatments to reverse sun damage rather than prevent it in the first place. Those with skin cancers wish that they could reverse their poor fortune. Many victims of skin cancer must go through complicated surgery with skin grafts and disfigurements, and others even die. Although the sun brings us life and light, we must respect it and be aware of its power to harm.

Now that you know you are at risk, it's time to learn how to protect yourself from the sun. One in five Americans will develop skin cancer during his or her lifetime. Of all newly diagnosed cancers, skin cancers comprise 40%. That works out to more than 1,000,000 new cases annually and more than 10,000 deaths. Epidemic increases are being seen in all types of skin cancer. In the majority of cases, the cause is exposure to the sun. As the ozone layer continues to thin, we are exposed to higher doses of ultraviolet radiation, increasing the amount of damage and risk for skin cancer. It's time to protect yourself from the sun. The sun is to skin cancers as cigarettes are to lung cancer.

Although skin cancer is a serious threat on its own, it's not the only unpleasant consequence the sun's ultraviolet rays have to offer. Did you know the sun is harmful to your eyes and immune system as well as to your skin? It is also detrimental to those with allergies.

89. There are so many sunscreens on the market. How do I choose?

A broad-spectrum product provides protection against both the A and B wavelengths of ultraviolet (UV), both of which can cause skin damage. UVB wavelengths are the principal cause of sunburn, and UVA can penetrate to deeper layers of the skin. A mixture of UVA- and UVB-absorbing chemicals, including oxybenzone, cinnamates (octylmethyl cinnamate and cinoxate), sulisobenzone, salicylates, titanium oxide, zinc oxide, and avobenzone (Parsol 1789) is important. Using sunscreens can prevent photoaging, actinic keratoses, basal cell carcinomas, and the development of melanoma, the most deadly skin cancer.

Prevention

For maximum sunscreen effectiveness, do the following:

- Use a broad-spectrum, nonirritating sunscreen with an SPF of 15 or higher and both UVA and UVB protection.
- Apply sunscreen 20 minutes before you go outdoors.
- Use about 1 ounce (enough to fill a shot glass) to cover the entire body. Cover all exposed areas liberally. Pay special attention to face, ears, nose, arms and legs. Remember that lips can burn, too; thus, cover lips with a lip balm sunscreen of SPF 15 or higher.
- Reapply every 2 hours or after swimming or heavy sweating to keep the SPF at its maximum level.
- Use a product that does not worsen an existing skin condition.
- Use clothing for photoprotection.

90. I can't seem to find a sunscreen that doesn't bother me. What can I do?

If side effects occur, they are usually a contact irritant reaction to a chemical in the sunscreen, and thus, it should be avoided. Other possible side effects include phototoxicity or photoallergy caused by interactions of chemicals in the sunscreen with sunlight. If you have an existing skin condition such as acne, eczema or other dermatitis, actinic keratoses, or rosacea, you should consult a dermatologist regarding selection of an appropriate sunscreen. With careful consideration and selection, you should be able to find and use an excellent sunblock.

By adding clothing with a high SPF, you can block nearly 98% of UVA and UVB radiation. This is particularly important if you burn easily and are at high risk for photoaging, skin cancer, and other sun-induced skin conditions. If you spend a lot of time in the sun while hiking, fishing, gardening, and working outdoors, you must use extra precautions.

91. I have always gone to tanning beds. Should I continue?

Remember that there is no such thing as a safe tan. Tanning booths with high-energy UVA bulbs are a major promoter of skin cancer and contribute to premature skin aging. You do not need to live in a sunny climate to wreck your skin—just go in a tanning booth! It's your choice—look withered like a raisin or stay clear! For a safe alternative, try sunless tanning with self-tanners, which are lotions that give you the tan without the risk of UVA and UVB exposure.

92. What about smoking and the skin?

The dangers of smoking cigarettes have become well known, although the damage to the skin is less studied. The smoke released from burning cigarettes at temperatures of 830°C to 900°C contains some 5,000 chemicals, many of which are hydrophobic agents that can diffuse through many cell membranes, reaching to the far ends of the body's precious organs, including the skin. Many of the dangerous chemicals are in the form of free radicals and oxidants, which can cause the malfunction of many biological processes, creating cell damage. Smoking has been shown to increase many symptoms associated with aging, altered hormone production, reduced fertility, cancer, cardiovascular and respiratory disease, and lung, esophagus, pharynx, larynx, stomach, pancreas, bladder, uterine, cervix, and skin disease.

Today there are around 1.25 billion smokers who will die an average of 7 years earlier than their nonsmoking counterparts. Quit today.

93. What about hormones? Should I take these to improve my skin?

Growth hormone injections and other supplements are a matter of controversy. Studies published in the *New England Journal of Medicine* and other journals that analyzed older

The smoke released from burning cigarettes at temperatures of 830°C to 900°C contains some 5,000 chemicals, many of which are hydrophobic agents that can diffuse through many cell membranes, reaching to the far ends of the body's precious organs, including the skin.

Prevention

persons who were given growth hormone confirmed that there was no change in muscle strength or maximal oxygen uptake during exercise. Other studies involved those who underwent progressive strength training for 14 weeks, followed by an additional 10 weeks of strength training plus either growth hormone or placebo. Resistance exercise training was shown to increase muscle strength significantly, and the addition of growth hormone did not result in any further improvement. In other words, hitting the gym helps and is less expensive than growth hormone.

It is not known whether the long-term effect of administration of growth hormone is harmful. Because older age is associated with an increased incidence of cancer, it may be wise to look at the research. In one study of 152 healthy men, prostate cancer was increased among men who had serum concentrations of insulin-like growth factor I in the highest quartile compared with those whose concentrations were in the lowest quartile. Growth hormone increases serum concentrations of insulin-like growth factor, and although this does not demonstrate causality, it certainly raises concern about growth hormone use in older men. Studies have shown that it can lead certain susceptible people down the path to diabetes.

Although it is not known precisely how much growth hormone is prescribed for off-label uses, estimates suggest that one third of prescriptions for growth hormone in the United States are for indications that are not approved by the Food and Drug Administration. Problems include potential misuse of healthcare funds and general high costs of the drug without evidence of benefit. Acceptable use of growth hormone is to replace deficiencies in certain disease states.

94. What about facial exercises to improve my skin?

You want to maintain a youthful look; however, facial exercises are repetitive facial movements and can actually lead to fine lines and wrinkles. A groove forms just beneath the surface of the skin each time we use a facial muscle. Facial expression equals lines. As we age, the bounce in our skin (elasticity) diminishes. The skin stops returning to its line-free state, and the wrinkles and grooves stay. Thus, cut out the facial exercises and look for better alternatives.

95. How does my sleeping position affect my face?

Sleeping on your pillow the same way every night for years can lead to wrinkles. These wrinkles are called sleep lines and can eventually become etched on the surface of the skin. Men often notice these lines on the forehead because they often sleep with their face pressed face down on the pillow. Women tend to sleep on their sides and are most likely to see these lines appear on their chin and cheeks. What should you do? Sleep on your back so that you do not develop these wrinkles. Whatever you do, however, get enough sleep so that you are rested and feel good.

96. Can I use topical steroids safely?

You may need prescription-strength corticosteroids to control your skin disease. Keep in mind not to overuse it, and choose the right product for the area of skin being treated. The generic preparation, called triamcinolone, is very effective and economical (about ten bucks for a big tube), but I do not recommend any steroid use for prolonged periods, especially on the face. I recommend 2 weeks of use, and then use moisturizers or other alternatives such as Protopic®. Overuse of topical steroids can lead to striae (stretch marks), atrophy (irreversible thinning of the skin), rash, tearing, bruising, and telangiectasia (enlarged blood vessels in the skin).

97. What if I cannot afford my medications?

Ask your physician about samples and discount plans and coupons. Try Partnership for Prescription Assistance at 888-477-2669, or go to www.pparx.org. The Consumers Union has many downloadable savings guides. Many pharmacies are offering major discounts, especially for antibiotics and generic drugs. For cosmetic procedures, payment plans are often available.

98. What about exercise?

Be heart and skin smart—exercise regularly. Good circulation is one of the keys to good skin health. There are three basic types of exercise: stretching, strengthening, and aerobic. Stretching exercises lengthen muscles and improve flexibility. Strengthening exercises tone muscles and improve strength. Aerobic exercises strengthen the heart muscle specifically, making it the most beneficial type of exercise for preventing heart disease and improving your skin health.

Doing aerobic exercises, such as walking, jogging, or low-impact aerobics will improve your circulation and breathing and lower blood pressure and help your body use oxygen more efficiently. You can also combine aerobic exercises with stretching and strengthening exercises to create a well-rounded workout routine. Following a regular exercise routine will make you feel healthier and more energetic, while combating the factors that put your health and skin at risk. Check with your doctor before doing a vigorous exercise program.

Exercising will help you to look and feel better!

99. What can I do now?

Charlie said this:

I'm 67. I've already had lots of sun damage. I used baby oil out in the sun when I was a kid. My skin is a mess. I've had three skin cancers taken off. I don't think it makes much difference what I do now.

The memory of your skin is cumulative. Every time you expose yourself to high levels of ultraviolet radiation without the necessary and available protection from clothing and

The memory of your skin is cumulative. Every time you expose yourself to high levels of ultraviolet radiation without the necessary and available protection from clothing and sunscreens, you can add on more sun damage.

sunscreens, you can add on more sun damage. Each person varies in the amount of sun that he or she can safely receive yearly, depending on factors such as ozone levels, cloud cover, latitude, season, and atmospheric pollution. Sun-protecting behaviors will help counter tendencies toward genetic skin pigmentation changes and damage based on your inherent skin type. Ultraviolet radiation damage can suppress cell-mediated immunity in the body and have an adverse affect on the eyes and skin and increase the risk of cancer. Why add to your troubles?

100. How can I maintain what I have gained from reading this book?

PPP—practice persistent prevention. Prevention is still the best medicine. Use these suggestions to prevent illness:

Prevention programs must promote exercise, good nutrition, and protect against obesity, smoking, alcohol, and sun abuse. The most effective prevention plans must be effective, sustainable, and not harm the participants. A crucial way to protect your skin health is to detect an illness early, while it is still easy to treat. You can do this in two ways: by getting periodic medical exams from dermatologists and by becoming a good observer of your own body and health. If you have one of the problems included in this book or any other health problem, get it treated as soon as possible.

Appendix

American Osteopathic Association (AOA)
The AOA urges men and women to contact them for information on preserving good health and coping with chronic conditions.
1-800-621-1773
www.osteopathic.org

American Osteopathic College of Dermatology (AOCD)
www.aocd.org

American Cancer Society (ACS)
1-800-227-2345
www.cancer.org

AAD Free Public Newsletter
www.aad.org/forms/NewsletterPublicSignUp

National Institute of Arthritis and Musculoskeletal and Skin Diseases (NIAMS)
1 AMS Circle
Bethesda, MD 20892-3675
1-301-495-4484 or 1-877-22-NIAMS (226-4267) (free of charge)
TTY: 1-301-565-2966
Fax: 1-301-718-6366
www.niams.nih.gov

National Psoriasis Foundation
www.psoriasis.org

American Society of Dermatologic Surgery (ASDS)
www.asds.net

Glossary

A

Abscesses: Closed pockets containing pus. Some abscesses are easily diagnosed clinically, as they are painful. Some may come to a head such that the pus becomes visible. Deep and chronic abscesses may look like a tumor clinically and require biopsy to distinguish them from a neoplasm.

Acanthosis nigricans: A condition in which the skin becomes dark and thick, usually present in the areas of the body where skin folds. Areas commonly affected are the back of the neck and groin.

Acne surgery: The removing of acne lesions, usually by opening up comedones (blackheads) and pimples by using a needle or small pointed blade and expressing the lesions with an extractor.

Acrochordons: Commonly known as skin tags. They are small, benign tumors protruding from the skin via a small stalk with a large, round-shaped end. Oftentimes these growths are removed for cosmetic reasons.

Adiposis dolorosa: A condition also known as Dercum's disease that is characterized by the formation of tumors in the fatty tissue of the body. The tumors cause large amounts of pain due to the pressure they can place on nearby nerve fibers. The tumors themselves are not life-threatening, unless the proper functioning of the nearby organs is affected.

Angioedema: Characterized by the rapid swelling of skin. This condition is usually a result of vascular leakage and the buildup of fluid from the blood. Such a condition can be fatal if swelling occurs in the pulmonary air passageways.

Angiomas: These are benign tumors that are comprised of lymph tissue and blood vessels. These tumors are red in color and not usually life-threatening.

Atypical: The simple, straightforward definition would be *unusual*, but *atypical* means much more than that. In a diagnosis, the use of the term *atypical* is a vague warning to the physician that the pathologist is worried about something, but not worried enough to say that the patient has cancer.

B

Basal cell cancer: The most common type of skin cancer. The lesions appear as a flesh-colored papule with blood vessels and a shiny border. These lesions often appear on the head and neck and can at times bleed if irritated. Treatment involves basic removal via surgical methods.

Blepharoplasty: A procedure in which the extra skin of either the upper or lower eyelids are surgically removed. It is often times used for cosmetic reasons to treat droopy or baggy eyes. The procedure is also used to improve peripheral vision if excess skin blocks external light from reaching the cornea.

Bullous: A large blister (a thin-walled sac filled with clear fluid).

C

Carcinoma: A malignant neoplasm in which cells appear to be derived from epithelium. This word can be used by itself or as a suffix. Cancers composed of columnar epithelial cells are often called *adenocarcinomas*. Those of squamous cells are called squamous cell carcinomas and those of basal cells are called basal cell carcinomas.

Cellulitis: An infection of the deeper layers of the skin characterized by redness, swelling, and pain. It is usually caused by a group A *streptococcus* or *Staphylococcus aureus*.

Chronic venous insufficiency: A condition in which the valves of the veins do not function properly, causing the pooling of blood in the lower extremities. Properly functioning valves prevent the backflow of blood through the veins; without this function the blood cannot efficiently return to the heart due to the opposing effect of gravity. This condition is the underlying reason for varicose veins.

Cryosurgery (cryotherapy): Used frequently by dermatologists to treat many skin problems. Liquid nitrogen is sprayed on to an area of skin, thus freezing it. Light freezing causes peeling, moderate freezing blistering, and hard freezing scabbing. It is used for acne, scars, warts, keratoses, some skin cancers, and other growths.

Cutaneous sensation: The sensory ability of the skin. This is more commonly referred to as the sense of touch.

D

Dermabrasion: A surgical procedure used for cosmetic reasons to improve the appearance of the skin. A small spinning diamond wheel or similar device is used to remove the uppermost layers of the dermis resulting in a refinished or smoothed appearance.

Dermatographism: An allergic reaction that causes the skin to be raised or inflamed when an image is drawn using a writing instrument like a pen. This can be used to determine the severity of various allergic responses on an individual.

Dermis: The layer of skin found between the epidermis and the subcutaneous tissue. This region contains blood vessels, nerves, hair follicles, and exocrine glands.

Diabetic bullae: A condition in which large blisters are found on the extremities of individuals who are diabetics. The blisters spontaneously form, but are usually treatable and nonscarring.

Diabetic dermopathy: A condition that occurs on the legs of an individual who has diabetes. The skin has spots of hyperpigmentation caused by blood vessel leakage. The color is believed to occur due to the presence of the protein hemoglobin found in the blood. Hemoglobin is brownish red in color due to its iron content.

Dysplasia: An atypical proliferation of cells. This may be loosely thought of as an intermediate category between hyperplasia and neoplasia. It occurs when the epithelium proliferates and develops the microscopic appearance of cancerous tissue, but otherwise tends to behave itself and stays on the body surface without actually invading it. Not all doctors accept dysplasia as a concept or as a precancerous growth, but generally lesions diagnosed as dysplastic should be considered for removal.

E

Electrodesiccation: Scraping or burning off skin growths (also known as electrodesiccation and curettage). It can be used for less serious skin cancers, precancers, and benign growths. A local anesthetic is injected, and then the abnormal tissue is scraped off with a curette. The area is then cauterized until bleeding stops. This may be repeated if the growth is cancerous. The wound will need to be dressed until it heals, and it usually leaves a small white mark.

Epidermis: The outmost layer of the skin. It is visible to the naked eye and is comprised of stratified squamous epithelium. This outermost layer is constantly shedding and regenerated by the lower layers of the skin. The epidermis provides protection from microbes and the environment.

Epithelium A specialized type of tissue that normally lines the surfaces and cavities of the body.

F

Favre-Racouchot: A condition in which the skin turns yellow and thickens. The skin appears to have cysts or nodules. The condition is usually present on the head, neck, and face.

G

Granuloma: A special type of inflammation characterized by accumulations of macrophages, some of which coalesce into "giant" cells. Granulomatous inflammation is especially characteristic of tuberculosis, some deep fungal infections, sarcoidosis, reaction to foreign bodies, and several skin diseases of unknown cause.

H

Hidradenitis suppurativa: This condition occurs in areas with a high density of apocrine sweat glands and around hair follicles in the groin and armpit. Painful boils or lesions can occur and become very large if not treated. These lesions can burst and leak pus.

Hirsutism: This condition usually affects women. The condition presents itself with large amounts of dark hair growth in the areas on the body where hair is usually not present. The growth is found in the places where hair is normally only found on men. The condition is not life-threatening and is usually treated for cosmetic reasons.

Hyperandrogenism: This condition occurs with the overexpression of male hormones in either females or males. This overexpression results in the appearance of male features such as deep voice, facial hair, and acne.

Hyperpigmentation: The darkening of the epidermis due to an increase in the presence of melanin. This condition can be caused by acne, inflammation, overexposure to the sun, and following pregnancy or hormone use such as birth control pills. Examples of hyperpigmentation include melasma and postinflammatory changes.

Hyperplasia: A proliferation of cells that is reactive and not neoplastic. In some cases, this may be a result of the body's normal reaction to an imbalance or other stimulus, whereas in other cases, the physiologic cause of the proliferation is not apparent. An example of the former process is the enlargement of lymph nodes in the neck as a result of reaction to a bacterial throat infection.

I

Immune system: Comprised of multiple organs and tissues working together to provide chemical and physical barriers to prevent disease. These barriers include the skin, saliva, and white blood cells. The body relies on these mechanisms and pathways to repair damage or infected cells. Improper regulation of these mechanisms can cause autoimmune diseases.

Impetigo: An infection of the skin caused by bacteria like *Staphylococcus aureus*. Impetigo presents itself with the formation of light-colored blisters or irritated areas on the skin. Many older individuals are affected due to lack of proper hygiene.

Inflammation: The result of the immune system reacting to unwanted stimulation. It shows as swelling, pain, tenderness, redness, and/or heat. Immune system cells are seen in the specimen being examined. These inflammatory cells include: (1) neutrophils, which are the white blood cells that make up pus and are seen in acute or early inflammations; (2) lymphocytes, which are typically seen in more chronic or longstanding inflammations; and (3) macrophages (histiocytes), which are also seen in chronic inflammation. Some types of inflammation are readily diagnosable, such as infected skin wounds; others require a biopsy to show the cause and prove that they are not neoplasms. The suffix *-itis* is appended to a root word to indicate *inflammation of*.

Intralesional injections: The direct placement of a medication into a problem skin area through a very fine needle. Most often, a dilute solution of triamcinolone is used. Acne cysts, psoriasis, keloids, and areas of alopecia are treated this way. If too much medication is used, a white spot or dent develops but eventually goes away.

K

Keloids: The increase in collagen growth under normal scar tissue. These growths expand over the boundaries of the scar and begin to cover normal healthy tissue. Individuals may have symptoms of pain and intense itchiness. If not treated, these growths can hinder movement and cause discomfort during everyday activity.

Keratinocytes: The cell type that comprises a majority of the epidermis. The cells provide a tough outer layer when dead and replace themselves by dividing from the lower layers of the skin and moving up to the visible layer.

L

Langerhans' cells: A type of dendritic immune cell found in high concentrations in the epidermis. When a microbe or antigen is present, the cell signals the rest of the body to prepare the immune system mechanisms to fight off the microbe and prevent the microbe from causing an infection.

Lentigines: Commonly called liver spots. They occur when portions of the skin become sun damaged. They present with darkening of the skin in a specific region, commonly on the back of the hands, face, and neck. Changes in such spots should be monitored to prevent cancerous growth.

Lesion: A vague term meaning "the thing that is wrong with the patient." A lesion may be a tumor or an area of inflammation.

Lupus: An autoimmune disease in which the body attacks its own tissues. The skin of an individual with lupus can show signs of sun damage, hair loss, decreased circulation, and a rash that may cover the mid-face in a butterfly pattern.

Lymphedema: Swelling of the extremities due to an obstruction in the lymph system that prevents the return of the lymph fluid to the body's core. Individuals with this condition may suffer from decreased mobility and hardening of the arm and leg. There are often underlying causes such as injuries or tumors that have placed pressure on the lymph vessels.

Lymphoscintigraphy: A diagnostic method used to identify lymphedema, the spread of cutaneous melanoma, and other diseases. A radioactive fluid is injected into the lymph vessels. The radiation given off is then monitored to see if the radioactive fluid remains in the original location via a blockage or if it returns to the core body via normal lymph flow.

M

Melanocytes: Cells in the basal layer of epidermis that are involved in the production of dark colored pigment known as melanin. The level of activity in melanocytes determines the difference in skin color between fair-skinned people and dark-skinned people, not the number (quantity) of melanocytes in their skin.

Melanomas: A type of malignant tumor that arises from the uncontrolled growth of melanocytes found in the epidermis. Risk factors include exposure to mutagens such as ultraviolet rays found in sunlight. Melanoma is the most dangerous type of skin cancer, causing the majority of skin illness deaths due to the cancer's ability to metastasize through the bloodstream or lymph system. Early detection along with a biopsy and surgical removal increase survival rate dramatically.

Melasma: A condition that usually occurs from various effects of hormones present during times of pregnancy. The manifestation is the presence of a darkened color of the face due to increased melanin production.

Metastatic: When cells that can travel through the lymph vessels or blood vessels lodge in some distant organ and grow into tumors. There are two major routes of metastasis: (1) hematogenous, in which the cells travel through the blood vessels, and (2) lymphogenous, in which the lymphatic vessels conduct the cancer cells. In the case of lymphogenous metastasis, the metastatic tumors can grow from cancer cells entrapped in the lymph nodes that collect the lymph draining from the organ where the original cancer has developed. Most malignant tumors spread both ways but prefer to spread one way more often.

Microangiopathy: A disease of the small blood vessels, more specifically the capillaries, that leak protein and other chemicals. This condition is oftentimes present in individuals who suffer from diabetes.

Mohs micrographic surgery: A surgical method that removes skin cancers while simultaneously analyzing the cancerous tissue. This allows for a reduction in the amount of noncancerous tissue removed and also reduces the chance of cancerous cells being left in the body. Before the surgery begins, the tumor is marked in regions so that each piece of the tissue removed can be cataloged and analyzed under a microscope. With this method, more cancerous tissue and less noncancerous tissue can be removed for improved tissue recovery.

N

Necrosis: Death of tissue. Necrosis may be seen in inflammation, as well as in neoplasms.

Neoplasm: A new growth of the body's own cells no longer under normal physiologic control. These may be benign or malignant. Benign neoplasms are typically tumors (lumps or masses) that, if removed, never bother the patient again. Even if they are not removed, they are not capable of destroying adjacent organs or seeding out to other parts of the body. Malignant neoplasms, or cancers, are those in which the natural history (i.e., behavior if untreated) is to cause the death of the patient. Malignancy is expressed by (1) local invasion, in which the neoplasm extends into vital organs and interferes with their function, and/or (2) metastasis, in which cells from the tumor seed out to other parts of the body and then grow into tumors themselves.

Neurodermatitis: The cycle of chronic itching and scratching that can cause the affected skin to become thick and leathery. It is also known as lichen simplex chronicus or scratch dermatitis. Continued scratching leads to greater irritation and prevents healing. Stress and anxiety tend to worsen the condition. Application of soothing agents and psychological intervention can help reduce the urge to scratch.

P

Petechiae: Small red spots under the top layer of skin due to the leaking of nearby blood vessels. The presence of such spots are strong indicators of other health issues that are related to the cardiovascular system, such as diabetes.

Photoaging: The damaging of skin due to sunlight exposure. Such damage appears visually as discoloration or browning of the skin and formation of wrinkles. Thickening of the skin is another result of photoaging; severe photoaging is a risk factor for skin cancer.

Photosensitization: A condition in which the skin becomes susceptible to damage from the sun.

Pilaris: A condition in which the skin of the arms and legs have small, hard, reddish pimples. For many the skin may appear to be dry and inflamed, but there is no pain associated with the condition. The skin has a rough feeling, but there are no severe detrimental effects.

Plantar hyperkeratosis: The thickening of the bottom or sides of the feet. The skin condition is caused by an abnormality of the protein keratin located in the epidermis. The presence of the thicker skin is for protection as a result of friction and irritation of the feet.

Poikiloderma of Civatte: Often occurs in middle-aged women on the sides of their neck resulting in appearance of tangled or leaky blood vessels and pigmentation. The condition is not serious, but its onset is believed to be due to hormonal changes.

Polyp: A structure consisting of a rounded head attached to a surface by a mushroom-like stalk. The typical skin polyps that develop (skin tags) are benign.

Psoriasis: A condition in which the skin of an individual appears to be scaly and inflamed, particularly near the joints. The cause is not completely known, but the relationship between the skin and the immune system is critical. For individuals with this condition, the body produces skin cells faster than they can be removed; as a result, there is a buildup that leads to its characteristic appearance. The underlying cause is believed to coincide with inflammatory chemicals, which trigger the accelerated division of skin keratinocytes.

Punch biopsy: Typically used by dermatologists to sample certain pigmented growths to rule out melanoma. Other times an entire lesion can be easily removed with a punch biopsy, which is the tool of choice. The punch biopsy is also used to drain some cysts and eliminate the need for a wide excision. After a local anesthetic is injected, a biopsy punch, which is basically a small (1 to 4 mm in diameter) version of a cookie cutter, is used to cut out a cylindrical piece of skin. The hole may be closed with a suture and heals with minimal scarring.

PUVA: A combination of psoralen (P) and long-wave ultraviolet radiation (UVA) that is used to treat several severe skin conditions. Psoralen is a drug that makes the skin disease more sensitive to ultraviolet light. This allows the deeply penetrating UVA band of light to work on the skin.

R

Rhytidectomy: A plastic surgery procedure more commonly called a face lift. The procedure gives individuals a more youthful appearance. The procedure involves making an incision near the ear and hairline. Then excess skin is removed while the remaining skin is tightened to reduce the appearance of wrinkles and other imperfections.

Rosacea: An inflammatory condition that manifests itself in the face as redness and small lesions. Often times the condition begins during adulthood and continues to worsen with age. Individuals should try to avoid activities that increase blood flow to the face and increase its red appearance. Such activities include hot showers, saunas, and sunlight.

S

Sebaceous hyperplasia: A condition that affects the sebaceous glands that produce the oily fluid known as sebum. These glands increase in size and shape to give an abnormal appearance. The condition generally affects older individuals of both genders. The location of the condition is usually on the forehead, and manifestation is the appearance of white raised bumps that are unusually shaped.

Seborrheic dermatitis: A disorder of the skin located on the scalp resulting in itchy skin and dandruff. The condition can be extremely uncomfortable and embarrassing for many individuals. Severity increases during times of stress and colder months. The condition is treatable in a mild state with over-the-counter medications; prescription medications are also available.

Sebum: The oily substance produced by glands in the skin. It contains not only oil, but also proteins and lipids. It helps keeps skin moist and keeps hair waterproof. Overproduction of this fluid can lead to diseases such as acne.

Senile pruritus: The itching of skin that occurs due to the breakdown and aging of skin of the elderly. It appears to be related to the drying of skin and can be treated by using soothing creams.

Shave biopsy (tangential excision): Slices off a surface growth using a blade. A curette does a similar task with a special scraping tool. These are often done to remove a small growth and confirm its nature at the same time.

Shingles: An extremely painful rash that is caused by a viral infection known as herpes zoster. Rash often extends from the back to the chest in individuals over the age of 60. Infection is due to the dormant chickenpox virus that can be reactivated during an immune compromised state.

Squamous cell carcinoma: Squamous cell carcinoma is the second most common cancer of the skin and occurs most commonly in middle-aged and elderly people with fair complexions and frequent sun exposure. The cancer develops in the outer layer of the skin (the epithelium), sometimes from small sandpaper-like lesions called solar (sun) or actinic keratoses. Although it is possible for squamous cell carcinoma to spread to other areas of the body, early treatment generally prevents it.

Stasis dermatitis: A condition of the skin due to the pooling of blood in the lower legs; leaky valves in the veins prevent the proper return of the blood to the trunk of the body. The skin appears to be discolored due to the leaking of blood and the breakdown of the molecules in the blood such as iron.

Stratum corneum: The outermost layer of the epidermis that acts as a barrier to prevent the exchange of chemicals between the body and its surroundings. This layer is comprised completely of dead cells with large concentrations of keratin. The layer is continually replaced; about every 2 weeks, the cells are shed and replaced from the lower layers of the skin.

Striae distensae: The condition commonly known as stretch marks occurs when the connective tissue of the skin cannot grow as rapidly as the underlying tissues. Due to the constant tension of the increased volume of tissue, the skin appears to have tears or scars. The condition is often found on the abdomen of pregnant individuals and the arms or chest of bodybuilders.

Subcutaneous layer: The tissue that separates the dermis from the underlying connective tissue. This layer is important in anchoring the skin; it contains fatty tissue that helps to provide insulation and energy storage. All of the blood vessels and nerves that supply the superficial layers of the skin run though this layer of tissue.

Suppuration, suppurative inflammation: A type of acute inflammation characterized by infiltration of neutrophils at the microscopic level and formation of pus at the gross level. An abscess is a special type of suppurative inflammation.

T

Telogen effluvium: A common condition in which the body undergoes alopecia, otherwise known as hair shedding or balding. This condition occurs during times of stress; the hair of the body sheds and does not begin growing again in a normal cycle. The condition can last for months or years, but normal growth can begin again.

Tophaceous gout: A chronic condition in which there are uric acid deposits throughout the body. The enzyme that breaks down the uric acid causes intense pain and discomfort. Uric acid is a byproduct produced naturally from many of the foods we eat, such as meats. Areas that are commonly affected are the joints, fingers, and toes.

Tumor: A mass or lump that can be felt with the hand or seen with the naked eye. This may be a neoplasm, hyperplasia, distention, swelling, or anything that causes a local increase in volume. Not all tumors are cancers, and not all cancers are tumors.

U

Urticaria: A condition, commonly referred to as hives, that is caused by the body's natural reaction to an allergen. The body releases cytokines and histamines that cause the blood vessels to leak. This leakage results in the formation of red spots and swelling. The formation of hives is an important sign that an allergic response

has occurred; other areas of the body may be experiencing the same effects, such as the airway and throat.

UVB phototherapy: A treatment for skin eruptions using artificial ultraviolet light. The initials UVB stand for the type B ultraviolet, the part of sunlight that causes sunburn. Carefully controlled, it is an extremely effective therapy tool for significant skin diseases such as severe psoriasis.

V

Venous lake: A lesion that appears purple and raised. It is generally located on the lip and is caused by the leakage of capillaries or due to the inability of blood to flow out freely. The elderly often suffer from these lesions, which are usually about half a millimeter in size; these lesions are not usually deleterious.

X

Xerotic eczema: A skin condition in which the skin is extremely dry and cracked. Symptoms include itchiness and general discomfort.

Index

Index

Index

Date Due

BRODART, CO.   Cat. No. 23-233   Printed in U.S.A.

The
Distinguished
Guest

also by SUE MILLER

Inventing the Abbotts
The Good Mother
Family Pictures
For Love

The
Distinguished
Guest

Sue Miller

▟ HarperCollins*Publishers*

HarperCollins books may be purchased for educational, business, or sales promotional use. For information please write: Special Markets Department, HarperCollins Publishers, Inc., 10 East 53rd Street, New York, NY 10022.

FIRST EDITION

Designed by Nancy Singer

Library of Congress Cataloging-in-Publication Data

Miller, Sue
  The distinguished guest / Sue Miller. — 1st ed.
   p. cm.
  ISBN 0-06-017673-3
  I. Title.
  PS3563.I421444D57 1995
  813'.54—dc20   95-2951

95 96 97 98 99 ❖/HC 10 9 8 7 6 5 4 3 2 1

for Doug

In 1982, when she was seventy-two years old, Lily Roberts
Maynard published her first book. It was put out by Tabor
Press, a small feminist publishing house in Chicago. Tabor Press
was named for and funded by the estate of Judith Tabor, whose
husband had made a fortune in refrigerated transport vehicles.
Though their names, Judith and Gabriel Tabor, appeared linked
on plaques here and there in Chicago—in public libraries and
museums and hospital wings—Tabor Press had been Judith
Tabor's own project, endowed by her after her husband's death,
and run exclusively by women.

The first printing of Lily Maynard's book was only five
hundred copies, but they were beautiful books, carefully
designed and produced, with marbled endpapers, and a wood-
cut reproduced at the start of each chapter, a church with a narrow spire. Lily loved to hold her book, loved to turn the thick,
cream-colored pages slowly, to read her own words, so transformed by the authority—the heaviness, as she felt it—of print,
that she was often startled by them, by their power. The book
was called *The Integrationist: A Spiritual Memoir*.

Tabor Press was at that time run by a committee of four
women who rotated being chair. As it happened, the woman in
charge of the watch on which Lily Maynard's book was published, a thin, energetic person named Betsy Leaming, was also

the person in the house most interested in commercial success, and the only one who understood anything about publicity. She sent Lily's book, with a cover letter, to the editors of women's pages for a number of major newspapers in the Midwest. The letter summarized Lily's life, quickly: the cloistered, wealthy Minneapolis background, her forced removal from college by her father after she voted for Roosevelt in the 1932 election, her marriage and transformed life in Chicago with Paul Maynard, a radical young Protestant minister called to an inner-city church. It told of their bitter struggle and eventual divorce over religious and ideological issues, centering on integration and the black power movement; and then, in Lily's own words, "the slow learning about what was left." The letter laid out some of the various angles an interviewer might take with this material. Perhaps best of all, it enclosed a photograph of Lily with her pure-white hair sculpted back into a bun, and the piercing dark eyes. She had been a remarkably handsome younger woman in her unsmiling, sober way, but age had softened her face to a melancholy and gentler beauty.

Lily was a good interview, it turned out, by turns elegant and cantankerous. Quotable. She discovered she liked to talk. She liked the sense of public weight her opinions began to acquire, and this made her yet more quotable. Often as she sat back and made a pronouncement, a nearly mischievous smile would lighten her somber face. Speaking about the appeal Saul Alinsky's radical brand of community organizing held for the Protestant leaders in her Chicago neighborhood, she shook her head and sighed: "Those old church boys were just tired of being thought of as do-gooders. The idea of hanging around with tough guys appealed to them. Alinsky restored their sense of masculinity." On the radicalism of the sixties: "It was mostly a call for street theater, a cheap yearning for more drama in political and public life. Everyone let himself forget that the processes of true change are always long and slow and effortful, and probably for the most part pretty boring."

Orders picked up and Tabor went to press again. Betsy

Leaming followed her early letter with a copy of an interview with Lily in the *Tribune*. There were glowing and positive reviews. There began to be other interviews and more orders. Tabor found itself unable to keep up with the demand. Eventually they sold the contract to a much larger house in New York, which, in essence, published the book anew. This time there were reviews in the daily and Sunday *New York Times*. Suddenly Lily was invited to read at colleges, to lecture at feminist conventions, to speak to women's church groups. The galleys of other writers' books thunked through her mail slot regularly, with requests for any comments she might have. There were more interviews, and she was featured prominently in an uplifting article in *Newsweek* on aging in America. She'd become a public personage.

Her children were bemused by the transformation, by encountering their mother, who'd always been formidable and remote, more intimately in her work and in interviews than they'd known her themselves in what they laughingly began to call "real life."

Clary wrote to her brother, Alan: "I have to confess to you some bitterness at Mother's success, at her parlaying (oh, oh! here comes the accusation) our whole family's misery into her own triumph. Her spiritual triumph, at that. And oddly, I resent too, the skill with which it's been done, the points she gets for that."

Though Alan had his own differences with his mother, he thought of himself as more forgiving of her public achievement, and of her transformation. This in spite of the fact that it was he of the three children who had perhaps suffered most on account of his mother's spiritual crisis. He was the youngest in the family, five years younger than the middle child, Clary, and he was the one who lived alone with Lily after his parents' marriage ended, since the two girls had already left for college. He could still remember the silent dinners with Lily before he escaped to his room to do his homework—the steady, and to him revolting, sound of his mother's chewing and swallowing sharpening his awareness of her physical being. Whenever he heard her footsteps pass in the hallway, he stopped still in the fear that she might knock on his door, might want to talk to him.

But Alan was happily married now. He had put his own uncomfortable teenage years behind him. When he opened the *Times Book Review* and, for the first time without anticipating it, encountered his mother's startled and imperious gaze across space and time, he felt safe.

What Rebecca might feel, no one knew. She'd disappeared in 1971 when a bomb she was helping to build was accidentally detonated. Two of her friends had died in the explosion, and the FBI had declared her complicit in their deaths. The last time Clary and Alan had heard from her was in 1989. Clary had stood in her sunny gravel driveway in California under the branching live oak and opened an envelope with no return address, postmarked Pittsburgh, Pennsylvania. Inside there was an old-fashioned, thick postcard with scalloped edges, stamped in Guatemala. On its front was a faded travel photo of a town square dominated by an ornate white church. On the other side, in cramped handwriting, Rebecca expressed the hope that Clary and her children were well, that Alan was happy. She said she had work to do that she felt was important, and that her life was full of shared sacrifice and deep rewards. Clary had wept reading the card on the telephone to Alan. She remembered her so clearly, she said: all the times Rebecca had let Clary come into bed with her and they'd whispered and laughed about boys, about teachers, about their mother. The window in the basement that Rebecca left unlocked to climb in and out of after her curfew. Their excursions together downtown on the IC, when they'd pretend to be Italian, or German, making an inflected vocabulary out of the names of artists and foods: "Caravaggio prego, tintoretto manicotti pesto olio olivo. Si, si." In German they used philosophers, guttural gibberish.

In her book, Lily had said that one of the hardest things for her about Rebecca's disappearance was the way it brought back to her her conflict with her husband—Paul—about the role of confrontation and violence in changing the world. Under Rebecca's photograph in the book, the caption read, "Rebecca at age eighteen, before I lost her." It was one of the things Clary hated most about the book, this implicit claim by her mother ever to have "had" her sister.

Alan and Gaby live on the bank of a river. In the field alongside their house they have planted young apple trees— Duchess, Gravenstein, Yellow Newton, Jonathan. It is Gaby's idea that one day these trees will resemble the gnarled fruit trees she remembers from the countryside near her grand- mother's house in France. The little leafy sticks will thicken and bend, and she will make cider and pies with their fruit. She and Alan will grow old watching their grandchildren play among them. She is comfortable thinking of her life in these terms.

Tonight they have friends over for dinner, a meal Gaby has prepared with care and skill. On the round table, among the guttering candles and the odd, brightly colored crumpled nap- kins, sit their thick white dishes with the remaining crumbs of a lemon tart they've eaten for dessert. They have all had a lot to drink by now, and they are talking animatedly about the crazi- ness in their families. When Alan jumped into this conversa- tion—and he jumped in eagerly—he was sure no one could compete with him: the divorced parents, the chilly, famous mother, the new-age sister in California, the vanished one in Central America. But he was wrong; Tim Garner has a sister in jail for manslaughter, Melanie Mercer a father who went out for a half-gallon of milk and never came back. There's a brother who believes the CIA can read his thoughts, another who's a Hare Krishna, another who's been married six times. They laugh harder with each additional detail in the candlelight, it all seems so unbelievable. Tears sparkle in their eyes.

"These are all such *American* stories," Gaby says with a wonderment only Alan hears as carrying judgment.

Before he can feel defensive, Tim says, "You're absolutely right. There's nothing to be ashamed of here. It's the American way." They laugh.

If they chose to look up now from the cluttered table, from the circle of familiar faces in the yellow, warm light, they might see around them through the reflection of the dinner table in the glass walls of the house, the toss of dark trees, the moon's slow slide over the opposite bank of the river. Alan does this. He relaxes and feels himself lapse momentarily into a state he's familiar with: he seems to be floating away from this group of his closest friends—from his dearest friend, his wife. He seems to be watching them all from slightly above, watching them in the setting he has imagined and created for them, thinking of minor adjustments he might like to make.

Alan designed this house. He is an architect, and he teaches design at a small arts college in Massachusetts. The house stands on the banks of one of the many rivers that feed into Buzzard's Bay in Massachusetts and Rhode Island. It won a small award two years before and was featured in a design magazine. He and Gaby have lived in it for six years, though for a decade before that, while they lived in awkward rented places and then a cramped house they bought in the village nearby, they spoke of the house as though it were already a reality, as though it existed somewhere else and it was only a matter of getting there. "My God, I can't wait to get into my own kitchen and have a little counter space," Gaby would say. Or a place for the children to put their sports equipment. Or a guest suite for when her mother or sister came from France and stayed.

And yet, now that they are here, Alan finds himself still thinking of this as temporary. He still imagines the improvements that could be made, he still drifts away, as he is doing now, and corrects this or that aspect of the design for things he didn't foresee or take into account. He still imagines that something is missing. "Where we live now," he sometimes begins in talking about the house. Recently Gaby has noticed this, has taken to correcting him: "Where we *live*, Alan, if it pleases you."

Perhaps it's a mistake, he thinks abruptly, for an architect ever to build his own house.

Gaby has begun to talk now, in her deep, unevenly accented voice, about Clara, about his sister Clary, adding the details of her life—her many divorces and remarriages and children by different fathers, her belief in past lives—to the list of family eccentricities. How she and Alan joke that she has, in fact, so many versions of her own earthly life, it's no wonder she believes there might be even more.

Alan is thinking of his life, his one life here, where he lives now. The house he has made, the woman he has married. He watches Gaby's mobile, animated face, the square, strong hands speaking too, accompanying her story. Gaby is a cook, she has her own gourmet shop and catering business in the expensive little village nearby. At home they eat well, they drink good wines. Their children, although they are in college now and graduate school, like to come back to visit. Often they are present at an evening like this, helping with the meal, talking comfortably with people twice their age and more.

His friends are laughing again now as Gaby finishes. Laughing at Clary, at poor beautiful Clary who has used such gaudy, foolish tricks to hold herself together, to keep herself going: crystals, past lives, psychics. The stepwise movement through drugs, then vegetarianism, then analysis, then drink, and now the recovery movement. He feels a pang of loyalty to her.

"Of course," he says, "Clary'd have her own riff on us, I suppose."

"Oh come on," Wade London says. "You lead exemplary lives. Irreproachable."

"No, no. Much could be made of certain elements here."

Gaby's gaze is steady on him, wary. She knows she shouldn't have talked about Clary that way. He's too protective of her.

"A certain, perhaps . . . yuppie? obsessiveness about detail.

Do you know how long it took me, for example, to choose these knobs?" He gestures behind himself at a low storage wall of cherry, its doors and drawers studded with square brass knobs. "Or Gaby to plan this meal? To cook it?"

"It *was* a great meal," Melanie offers. "That couscous, yikes. And the *shrimp!*" Gaby is pleased, even if it is a dutiful comment. She curtsies her head at Melanie, who is slender and nervous, and always the conciliator.

"Fine. I agree," says Alan. "But that's what we're about, to my sister. Appetites and greed. Comfort. Materialism."

Gaby's face lights in delighted recognition. "Oh Alan, that's not Clara talking. That's your *mother.*" She has learned to say this exactly as midwestern Americans do, giving it the doubled or tripled consonant at the end, and everyone laughs with her, even, after a beat, Alan. Pronounced this way, the word itself becomes a kind of joke.

And then Wade says, "I saw that story of hers a couple of months ago in *The Atlantic.* I liked it, actually."

Alan nods. Stories are what Lily turned to after the memoir. "After all, you can't do *two* of them," she'd said. She's published perhaps ten or twelve stories. Several in *Ms,* three or four in little magazines, and within the last few years, two in *The Atlantic,* one in *The New Yorker.* They're fiction, but everything in them, even the most alien details, seems as familiar as toothache to Lily's children. ("Of course I use my life," Lily had said in the one interview Alan had read, "What else do I have?" *Waspish,* the interviewer had called her. Actually, she'd written, "Alternately waspish and flirtatious." That was a side Alan knew less well.)

What had made Lily turn to fiction? "I was fed up with being so damned discreet," she told the interviewer. And it was true that in the stories, more disturbing, more psychologically violent things happened, as though Lily were acknowledging the dangerous emotions that had been held in check in her life and only hinted at in her memoir. In one, a middle-aged woman flees her husband and allows herself to be used by a younger man she meets at a cheap resort to reinvigorate his own failing marriage. In another, an older woman discovers, years after the event, that a beloved, difficult son—a radical—killed, she believed, while building a bomb, was instead present by coincidence when it went off, an accidental victim only, drunk and drugged and asleep in a corner of the room. In yet another, a young, idealistic minister of an inner-city church is duped and exploited in an outreach to the gangs around him, the church transformed to a warehouse for guns and drugs—but he's so thrilled by the romantic turn his life has taken, so moved by the rhetoric of action and violence, that he consents even to this.

Still, neither Alan nor Clary had thought the memoir could have been called discreet. Lily had written:

In those summer Sundays of our new marriage, I could sometimes experience the hour or so in church as a kind of drug, a near-aphrodisiac really. All my senses were dilated by it, by the gradual and powerful accumulation of layers of physical awareness combined with my own spiritual hunger, my greed, really. The Midwest heat outside was always intense by eleven o'clock, and the dark little church was cool and damp by contrast. When you entered the doors, there was a long, dizzying moment of welcome blindness, accompanied, for me, by a near-sexual weakening in my legs. The air inside smelled deliciously of mildew, a mushroomy, earthy odor that changed slowly as the space filled up with people. The odor of soap was added first, and talc, then perfume, and finally, as the service wore on, a basic but not unpleasant smell of sweat. And, of course, there was always, floating above them all, the erotic smell of the flowers. Summer flowers, plucked from their gardens by the church ladies on this committee.

I always arrived early because I couldn't bear the idea of the eyes of the congregation on me as I walked to my place alone. *The young minister's new wife*: it was how I thought of myself too. I thought of our sexual delight in each other as being visible in my every gesture, even in my carriage, and I know I myself would have stared with prurient curiosity. Instead I always tried to be there ahead of the congregation. Except of course for the odd old woman or two, up since dawn, no doubt, chores long since accomplished, and in need of a way to fill the time. We all dipped our heads—our hats, I should say—at each other. (Of course we all wore hats, and gloves too, which we hoped matched our shoes, or "went with" our hats somehow.) When I bowed my head to pray after I sat down, I was aware of the brim of my hat—it was a wide-brimmed hat that first summer of my marriage, a beautiful hat I'd bought to make my young husband love me more—shutting the world out, blocking my view of these ladies. The hat was straw, and it had a faint straw smell, a clean, farm odor.

The music played by the plump, elderly organist during this interval of sitting was like an odor too: never sharply defined, always meandering, soothing. Occasionally you could hear through it the leaky wheeze of air from the old pump-organ. It made me catch my breath too when I heard it, it made my sleepy pulse blossom irregularly.

Behind me, I could hear the room slowly filling up, the footsteps, the whispered greetings. And then there was the sudden thump! thump! thump! of the stops being thrown open, the music would peal out, and Paul would enter, coming down the aisle like a bride. But more determined, more sure of himself by far than I'd been on the day of our wedding, than any bride ever was. He would disappear around the side of the pulpit, and then appear again in it, above the flowers, transformed by his black robe, his gravity, and magnificent to me: my messenger from God, my bridegroom. I felt in danger of weeping as I lifted my eyes to look at him.

We had stood by now. Everywhere in the room was the constant rustling sound of shifting feet, of moving flesh, of clothing redraping—the sound people make simply standing still. The Paul looming above us was and was not my Paul. His face was and was not the face I'd studied from almost the same angle as he rose above me the night before, his lips as they began to speak were and were not the lips that had sought mine. His voice was and was not the voice that had cried out my name then, over and over. "Let us pray," he would say, and I would become, at his command, a prayer.

There were two baptisms that summer, and both times, watching the placid baby lie across my husband's arm, the yards of sheer white cloth, hemstitched or embroidered, spilling down over the yards of dull black of Paul's robe, looking at his face bent over the child's, pronouncing the holy words—his wet fingertips moving over the child's eggshell skull, blessing it—I experienced the purest envy. I was able to conjure it away partially by reassuring myself that we would have a child too, that it too would lie just this way in Paul's safe arms as he bent over it. Yet I knew I wasn't confronting the heart of my feeling, which was that I wanted somehow, too, to *be* that child, to lie just that still in his arms, to have him hold me as I lay open before him and consecrate me in the name of the Lord.

Could this be called discretion?

Of course, it wasn't so much for passages like these that Tabor Press was drawn to the book, or to Lily. It was rather the later passages, where she moved away from her husband and from the notion of a male, commanding God with what seemed in the book a slow but inevitable, triumphal turn.

(What Alan remembers of that time are the anguished, intense talks between his parents that trailed off at his appearance, the excruciating family meeting called to explain the separation, and after that, for what seemed like years, the sound of weeping from behind closed doors. He was tormented after his father left by his sense of solitary responsibility for Lily. Hearing her weep, he knew he should knock and offer comfort. She was, after all, his mother. She was, after all, human, and in pain. The one time he finally mustered the courage to do it, there was a long pause before the door was opened, a pause she clearly used to pull herself together. Because when she stood before him, she was composed, her reddened, swollen eyes the only giveaway. "Yes Alan?" she had said coolly, as though he had asked a question. "Is there something you need?")

Now, at the table, they have moved on. They are arguing about an article in the same issue of *The Atlantic* as Lily's story, an article that proposed a new basis for immigration laws, connected to maximum feasible populations which would be absolutely set for various areas of the country.

"It's ridiculous," Tim is saying. "As long as we measure the health of our economy by housing starts, it just ain't gonna happen that way."

"*Is* there such a thing as health without housing starts, without population growth?" his wife, Susan, asks.

"It's been done. Look at western Europe in the eighties."

"Yes," Gaby says. She's behind Alan, and he can't see her. She's getting glasses and bottles of brandy and liqueurs from the storage cabinet. "France had it for many years."

"But France is a mess now. And so is Sweden and all those socialist countries."

"Well, and it's partly immigration that did it," Gaby answers.

"Oh horseshit, Gaby," Tim says. "They *needed* those workers to come from Africa and so forth, because no French people would do those jobs."

"Yes, but they came and they came and they came," Gaby says. "That is precisely my point."

She is angry, Alan can tell as she sets the glasses down just slightly too hard, and he is startled by this, as he often is by her politics as they apply to France. He doesn't understand the line she draws—and he's heard her father and brothers draw it too. They are repulsed by a character like Le Pen, by anything so openly racist, but they speak in a way no educated American would dream of speaking about the blacks and the foreigners among them—their laziness, their slack morals, their drugs, their smells, their peculiar food.

"Here's the thing," Melanie says quickly. "No society should import people to do the dirty work. Ever. Not slaves. Not guest workers. It's morally reprehensible. And it leads to big trouble. Like France," she says to Gaby. She smiles nervously. "Like us. Instead there should be some mandatory, like, dirty-work service. Like the army, or the Peace Corps. But everyone should have to do a stint."

"And how would you define dirty work?" Wade asks. "*Who* would define it?"

"Well, it's obviously those jobs that go unfilled when there's high employment. Service jobs. Micky D's."

"Housework!" Susan says.

Alan looks again at Gaby. She is sitting in her place at the table. Her face has relaxed, she is smiling at Susan. The moment has gone by.

They begin to argue about the implementation of Melanie's plan. Teenagers, they agree, should be the dirty-workers. They exchange a few stories about their teenagers, their children. They talk about the pear brandy Gaby has served. Alan is watching Gaby, feeling a sense of her difference, her Frenchness, which he isn't conscious of most of the time.

And then he is thinking of the story Lily published in *The Atlantic*. A story about an elderly woman who had abandoned her husband and children in middle age to run off with an alcoholic painter. Now, old and alone and sensing her approaching death, she imagines the lives her children might have led. She calls information in the cities she thinks they might have landed in, and when there is someone with one of her children's names, dials the number and listens without speaking. In each case, she is able to argue herself out of the possibility that it is her child whose voice she hears, and so—Alan felt, reading the story—is also able somehow, magically, to forestall her death another day.

Was it, in some sense, an apology for Lily's own life? Was it her fictional speculation about the life his father might have led after the divorce? Was it only invention?

Alan couldn't tell, and he'd felt the same sense of disquiet he felt whenever he read Lily's work. More her fiction, he realizes now, than the memoir. (Although the stories have recently been published in a collection Lily had had sent to him—the enclosed card said, "Compliments of the author" and was signed, "Mother"—he hasn't read it yet.)

The evening winds down, and when the first couple rises apologetically to go, the others get up too. They have busy days the next day, they have children, yards, boats, cars, tennis games, golf games to play—possessions and connections which need tending.

After the guests are gone, Alan comes outside to fetch the glasses they left on the deck. They had been sitting here earlier in the evening, watching the sun's red deepen in the cirrused clouds in the western sky, and then the mosquitoes descended on them in a faintly whining cloud and they rose almost as one, slapping themselves and laughing, and fled inside.

The air now is cool and smells briny. The river makes a gentle lapping noise below him though he can't see it, it's just an energetic blackness out there below the trees. Inside the house, Gaby is at work in the kitchen, moving with her darting efficiency on the lighted stage he's made for her life. Watching her, he thinks of a moment earlier in the week when they lay in bed together in the afternoon, looking out over the other end of this deck into the trees and talking lazily of their two sons, speculating on how they were changing, on what life would hold for them. (They have spent hours this way over the years, lying here and in other bedrooms of their marriage, talking about their children, always seeing them as in progress—as people who both are, and yet are still becoming who they are.)

He feels far away from that moment now, and he has doubly the feeling of spying on Gaby. First, because he is: watching her when she doesn't know she's being watched. And second, because he has a secret he's been keeping from her. That isn't, of course, how he's framed it to himself. He feels he's waiting for the right moment to talk about it with her. But it's on this account that he has a sense of being uncomfortably distant from her, aware that even the physical world she's immediately conscious of—the bright hot kitchen, the sound of water running from the tap, the clash and gong of dishes and pots as she handles them—is utterly different from his.

And how odd, he thinks, that his mother appeared at their table tonight, unbidden—consciously anyhow—by him. For that is the secret, that's what it is: that Lily is going to have to come and stay with them for a while.

chapter **2**

Thomas wasn't home. Alan rang three times, then sat down to wait on the stoop. Then he got up, and although he knew this was futile (but maybe Thomas had fallen asleep, was deep in that late-adolescent sleep), he rang again. He was picturing his son as he'd so often seen him, the long body angled across a bed or a couch, sometimes just slouched back in a comfortable chair—mouth open, dark hair wildly matted—gone, gone in exhaustion. From the open window to the first-floor apartment, he could hear voices raised in argument over the music playing on the stereo. He shaded his face and peered through the glass of the outer doorway to the inner door and the darkened hallway beyond that. No one.

He sat down again. The stoop was in sunlight. The stone touched his buttocks with warmth. He bent his knees up and rested his elbows on them. Alan was a tall man, tall and fair, as his father had been. As he'd aged, he'd gotten almost gaunt. Sitting on the stoop this way, he looked awkward, ill-at-ease in his body, all angles and bones. The music on the first floor throbbed, a pulsing adagio. Baroque, Alan thought. He could hear the voices too, the slapping venom in them, but not what they were saying. For this he was grateful.

He surveyed the sunstruck street. Boston itself seemed breathless and exhausted today in the heat. Not a car moved on this street, though every parking place was full. Alan had had to park more than a block away, even then illegally, in a spot designated for residents only. In fact, there didn't seem to be a legal place for a visitor to park in Thomas's neighborhood, and this annoyed him with its unreasonableness. If he got a ticket, he'd give it to Thomas for making him wait.

No, he wouldn't. He could hear Thomas's voice: "I mean, I know you're pissed, Dad, but does this seem logical to you?" Logic, logic. Thomas thought he owned it. He thought of Alan, and maybe even Gaby, as old and arbitrary creatures.

Two students walked by, carrying instrument cases. Flat, rectangular. Alan thought horns maybe. Clarinet? Oboe? They were dressed the way Thomas dressed, with an unerring instinct for the homely. As though they were farmers, or carpenters. The girl wore no makeup, and her stringy hair was only slightly longer than the boy's. Both wore clunky work shoes. Or maybe she wasn't a girl. Alan watched their backs moving away. Was that a girl's walk? Da *dump*, da *dump*. No, in Alan's book. As he was watching them, the boy tossed a cigarette into the street.

The street was littered with junk, in fact. This neighborhood was on the edge of the ghetto. It had been infiltrated by students from the conservatory and from Northeastern, and maybe as a result no one group seemed to care about it or to think it was worth the effort to maintain. There was new junk blowing around—food wrappers, cups, leftover trash—and old junk too, grayish, cottony pieces of unnameable stuff flattened in the gutters. And when the breeze stirred, you heard, in addition to the leaves' motion, the whispery rattle of plastic shopping bags snagged here and there in the trees and bushes.

Alan had grown up on the south side of Chicago and he knew that this was far from squalor, but it bothered him anyway. It bothered him, he thought, because Thomas romanticized it, held it up against Alan's life, Alan's home. Thomas saw this, his own home, as ... what? real, true, gritty. Authentic. When he came to visit Alan and Gaby, he sometimes asked how things were in the burbs. In burbsville. The stix. The boonies.

Alan remembered 63rd Street abruptly, their walks across it—Rebecca, Clary, himself—on the way to Sunday school. Lily would still be home, getting Sunday dinner ready, waiting until the last minute to go to the eleven o'clock service. Paul would have gone over to the church much earlier. The three children went alone, walking through the heart of the ghetto. Rebecca was in charge, and she drove Clary and the foot-dragging Alan along with terror of the streets, of the people still lingering in front of bars under the elevated tracks after Saturday night: "He *saw* you," she'd whisper with vicious energy. "He's going to *get* you. Run! Run!" It was still sometimes the terrain of Alan's nightmares—a blasted urban street, glass glittering in the gutters, buildings derelict and stinking, and a black person, a man usually, hunting him. (Though the one time something really threatening did happen, it was a black woman, waked suddenly from her stuporous sleep in a doorway to see Alan in his Sunday best strolling past. A black woman who cried, "Thas my baby! My chile!" and started to struggle up, her voice rising in pitch. "You taking my baby. Thas *my* baby!" They did run that time, and Rebecca, perhaps terrified that her tactics would be uncovered, made them promise never, ever to tell.) From time to time when he thought of Rebecca now, doing her radical good works wherever she was, Alan wondered what she'd say if he could tell her she had shaped the racist night-mares that pursued him for years afterward.

Thomas came up out of nowhere on a bicycle and squealed to a halt, resting one foot on the curb. He was panting. "Hey," he said, and grinned at Alan. Alan couldn't help it, he grinned back. Thomas's curly black hair was wet, as though he'd just showered, and pushed back from his face by the wind. The face itself was bony and angular—it had thinned out this way sud-denly four or five years ago and somehow Thomas hadn't grown into it yet. He also hadn't shaved in a few days. He swung himself off the bike and lifted it to his shoulder.

Alan stood up and moved out of his way. "I'll state the obvious," he said. "You're late."

"Sorry I'm late, Dad." Thomas looked over his shoulder at his father as he fumbled one-handed with the key in the lock. "I got carried away." He went in. "Nah. That sounds like I was doing something maybe responsible. I just didn't watch the time. I was at a friend's for breakfast." Alan grabbed the inner door from Thomas's hand and followed him up the wide, dirty stairs. The cracked linoleum formed a shallow scoop of each step. In the hallway, there was the noise of life behind the doors: a TV, a baby wailing loudly, music—jazz—and then they were in front of Thomas's apartment. The door was battered and scratched. Thomas unlocked three different locks. He pushed inside, set his bike down, and yelled, "Hello?" No one answered.

Alan headed down the long narrow hall to the bathroom. In the dim light, he tried not to see how dirty it was, not to look at the scarred toilet bowl, the wisped, dusty hairs curling along the baseboards, the scummy sink. The toilet's flush was wheezy.

When he came back, Thomas was standing over the message machine and an adult voice was telling him to make an appointment with someone. A beep off, then on, and a breathless girl left a long message, mostly preface: "Hello, ducks. If you get this message before Saturday, okay, go ahead, pay attention to it. If you don't, you're out of luck, you're a loser, what can I say, why aren't you *ever* home, you should check this machine more often, and the message is . . . " and she announced a party, gave the place and time.

Alan was standing by the open front door. "Can we go, Thomas? I don't want to be late."

"Just a sec."

Another voice came on, wanting Thomas to join him at Wally's for a beer. "Miss you, pal," it said, and clicked off. How long since he'd been home, Alan wondered. And if he wasn't sleeping at home, where, with whom, was he sleeping?

None of my business, he reminded himself.

Now there was someone else announcing his name, calling for Thomas's roommate. Thomas fast-forwarded the machine.

"Thomas, I'd like to go. You can do this when you get back. We're late, in case you didn't hear me earlier."

Thomas flicked the machine off. His face was closed. The child, scolded. "Right. Let's hit the road."

On the way to the airport, Alan asked Thomas about the trio. He had stayed in Boston this summer specifically to work in it, with an elderly professor who was retired except for this annual effort. As Thomas had told Gaby and Alan earlier—they had wanted him to get a job this summer—people killed each other to get into this group.

"It's good," he said now. "It's interesting." And he talked, for a few minutes openly and with enthusiasm, about the music they were working on, about the old man, about the differences in musicianship among the three players.

A silence fell. Alan looked quickly over at Thomas. His face had fallen into repose, into the brooding gravity that lurked behind what Alan thought of as the Thomas-mask, the smiling, happy-go-lucky good guy.

"Have you talked to Ettie lately?" Thomas asked abruptly.

"Your mother did, a few days ago. He'll try to get home one weekend while Gran is staying."

Thomas nodded, rocking his whole body a little along with his head. "Yeah, he told me. I just wondered if you knew."

"You guys talk often?"

Thomas shrugged. "A medium amount. I mean, what's often?"

This irritated Alan. Everyone knew what *often* meant. He didn't answer.

"How long *is* Gran staying?"

"I can't say. We're waiting, essentially, for some old geezer to die."

"The guy whose apartment she's going to move into?"

"Even further down the line than that. *That* guy is in a nursing bed, and the woman who lives now in what will be Gran's apartment needs that bed. The nursing bed. But she can't move there until the old guy kicks the bucket. So to speak. And he was supposed to—he was in intensive care and on the way out—but a miracle of modern medicine pulled him though." On the still river, just a few boats, their sails sagged and luffing. Alan smiled at Thomas. "So now we're all praying for a different kind of miracle."

"So it'll be like, what? A year?"

"God, no! A couple of months, at the most. They've virtually promised."

"Well, that's not bad, Dad."

"Easy for you to say."

"Come on. She's cool."

"Do people still say *cool*?"

"I don't know. I do, apparently."

They settled into silence. Alan was thinking of Ettie— Etienne, his other son. Although he was two years younger than Thomas, he seemed older. He was short, like Alan's wife, Gaby, and compact like her too, and perhaps that was some of it. Unlike Thomas, Ettie was comfortable in his body, coordinated and graceful and a terrific athlete in those sports where size didn't count for so much—baseball, soccer. Sexually too, he seemed older than Thomas. They'd actually caught him with his girlfriend in his bedroom when he was fourteen, and he'd taken one of Thomas's girlfriends away from him a year or two later. It was this episode Alan was remembering.

She wasn't his girlfriend, Ettie had argued. Thomas had never even asked her out.

"But you knew! I told you how I felt." Thomas had been crying earlier, and now his voice threatened to break again.

They were standing, absurdly, Alan and Thomas, in the hall outside the boys' bedroom, talking to Ettie through the closed, locked door. This was where Alan had found Thomas when he came home from teaching at the college—sitting in the hall, his eyes swollen, waiting for the moment Ettie should emerge.

Because he was going to kill him, he said, when he did.

Alan had to piece the story together from their alternating versions on opposite sides of the door, but about the facts there was basically no disagreement. Thomas had adored this girl, a girl in the class one below his and one above Ettie's. He'd talked about her to Ettie, sought his advice about the way to approach her. He imagined he might ask her to the movies one day. He was getting ready, he felt.

And then Ettie moved in on her.

It wasn't his fault, Ettie said, and he explained all the circumstances, the party, her calling him up, the several times they'd met alone.

While he talked, Thomas had begun to fight tears again, and when Ettie was done, he attacked the door, kicking it, slamming it with his fists. Alan had reached out to restrain him, to embrace him, but he spun away, crying out in alarm, and sat down on the floor again, his back against Ettie's door.

Alan sat down too, and slowly they began to talk about it. Thomas answered Alan's questions in an exhausted, deadened way. Finally Alan persuaded Thomas to come out to dinner with him. As they were leaving, he called this through the door to Ettie.

"I heard you already," Ettie said. "I heard everything you said."

"Tell Mom."

"I *will*," he said furiously, and Alan could hear that he was angry at him, that he felt betrayed that Alan had taken Thomas's side.

When they were driving home after their long, mostly silent meal, Thomas said, "You should know, Dad, that I'm still going to kill him."

Alan looked at Thomas in the lights reflected from the road. His tone was businesslike, perhaps even casual, his posture relaxed.

"That's not going to work, Thomas," Alan said.

"I don't care."

"If it came down to it," Alan said, "you'd be the one to get hurt."

"I don't care."

"You know he's stronger than you are."

Now Thomas stirred, a convulsion of his gangly body. "You don't need to *tell* me that, Dad," he said furiously. "Of course I know that. Jesus."

After a long time, Alan said, "You know I think you're in the right, don't you?"

"It doesn't matter to me."

"Well, it may not matter, but I want you to know it, because I'm not going to let you do it. Hurt him. Or more likely, yourself."

They drove in silence. Alan drove past their turnoff, but it was five minutes or more before Thomas asked, "Where are we going?"

"I'm not sure," Alan said. "Not home."

"Dad, I want you to take me home."

"I think we're going to New Hampshire," Alan said.

After a long time, Thomas said, "Dad."

"We'll just take a trip," Alan said. "We'll just stay away awhile."

"I don't want to," Thomas said.

"Well, I don't either, but that's the story. That's what we're going to do."

And for the next three days, Alan and Thomas wandered northern New England. They bought boots and hiked a little on the lower reaches of the White Mountains, through the wide patches of granular snow held in the shadowed woods. They sought out covered bridges and drove back and forth through them.

They were days of peculiar but real pleasure. They moved from one cheap motel to another, from restaurant to restaurant, from convenience store to convenience store, pretending to be connoisseurs of this trashy world. ("Which do you prefer, Velveeta or Cheez Whiz?") They compared bedding, mattresses, the cleanliness of bathrooms, the number of cigarette scars on the furniture, the number of bugs. And Alan was grateful for nearly every moment of it.

In the end, it was Thomas who suggested it was time to get back. It was a Sunday. His piano lesson was Monday. He needed to practice. They were in what was called a "family-style" restaurant in a mill town in Maine. Alan had been trying to signal the waitress for the bill. Now he lowered his hand and looked at his son.

"It goes without saying, Thomas, so I'll say it, that I won't take you unless you're ready to let go of this thing with Ettie."

"Yeah, yeah."

And that was that. Alan paid the bill, they got in the car and drove back. It got hotter as they moved south, from winter to spring. In their absence, the magnolias on Bowman's town green had come into bloom. When they got home, Thomas went directly to the piano. He played for the remainder of the day, and Ettie moved around the house like a shadow.

For several months after that, there was an uncomfortable formality between the boys, and then somehow it ended, and they were once again what they'd often been: the oddest of friends—Thomas awkward, enthusiastic, too intense; Ettie self-contained and confident.

And still as successful with women as he'd been then. Even when he'd been home earlier this summer, he'd had number-less telephone calls to make, and he confessed to them all at dinner one night that he'd managed the ending with one woman and the beginning with another badly, so that he was having to scramble not to hurt anyone's feelings. "It's a pretty messed-up, bigamous situation at the moment," he'd said glumly.

There were jokes about "overlapping" women, there were Groucho Marx, big-a-me, big-of-you jokes, but they were all aware that this—whatever you'd call it: tendency? ability? failing?—seemed to have become part of who Ettie was.

And of course he was also practical, practical, practical. He was spending this summer in New York, doing a kind of business internship in a bank before he went back to college. And whatever he did in the end, Alan was sure he would be successful. The gods would smile on Ettie.

As for Thomas, who knew? Alan and Gaby had made him go through four years of college, which was perhaps a mistake. Now he was at the conservatory, in a world they didn't understand. Whenever they suggested something for his life, the summer job for instance—Ettie had one after all—he would say, "That's impossible," and they would realize that all their assumptions about what was good for him were irrelevant, maybe even wrongheaded.

Alan's concern and love for both of his sons made him slightly uneasy around either one alone, but his relations with Thomas were perhaps more tense. He felt this was because he was naturally more drawn to Thomas, more sympathetic to him. This made him feel protective and anxious on Ettie's behalf, and made him steel himself against Thomas a little, will himself not to fall for Thomas's sloppy, careless charm. Most of all, not to value Thomas's gifts above Ettie's, though by nature Alan did, of course. At the same time, it was the presence of those gifts and the unknown world they'd opened to his son, that sometimes made him feel shut out of Thomas's life.

What he had noticed, a few moments before, was that Thomas had turned the conversation away from Alan's interest in his own music to Ettie, to his brother. It was the first time Alan had remarked this. Maybe Thomas felt too that he was the more natural son for the family he'd been born into. Maybe he was himself aware of trying to make room for Ettie, of not wanting to claim too much of the attention for himself.

Alan sighed.

"You're just not looking forward to it, are you?" Thomas asked.

Alan looked over quickly at him. Thomas was smiling. He was thinking of another parent, another child: Lily and Alan. Alan smiled back. "It isn't bad, as you say. And it's never dull, having Lily around. I think she's a lot frailer than we remember her, though." Alan usually visited his mother in Chicago once a year or so, but it had been longer this time. Almost two years. Clary, who'd helped Lily empty out and sell her apartment when they thought she could move into the retirement community, had told him she'd failed a lot in this interval.

"Yeah, I haven't seen her for, I dunno, maybe four years," Thomas said. "But actually I've noticed her letters are pretty . . . spidery now. The writing, I mean." He lifted his own hands, held them up flat, fingers spread, as though appreciating their steadiness, their power. Alan glanced over at them. They were huge, though the fingers were long and slender. The tips were slightly spatulate.

He looked at his hands gripping the steering wheel, thinking of how he took their strength, their control for granted. He saw them as extensions, really, of his thinking mind, his brain. He saw them as necessary tools. He'd injured one once, the right hand, in fact. His drawing hand. He'd been angry at Gaby, at her confession of an affair. In his rage, he put his hand through a window. He'd sliced a nerve. It had taken months for the nerve to regenerate, months of not knowing whether it would, whether his ability to draw was gone. He and Gaby had been unusually tender with each other through that time, both stricken with fear and guilt. There was a faint white crescent curving down from the loose skin between thumb and forefinger and across the back of his hand as a reminder of all of that. Alan turned his hand on the wheel so he couldn't see it.

He parked the car in the big central lot. He and Thomas agreed, as they walked through its damp, echoing darkness, that Thomas would stay with Lily, once they'd greeted her, and Alan would go back for the car and swing around to get them and Lily's luggage.

They were about ten minutes early for Lily's plane. They started toward her gate, but the sign by the security barrier said that only ticketed passengers could go past it. Alan went back to the ticket counter to get passes. The line there was long and it was moving slowly. He felt a rush of irritation at Thomas. This was his fault. If he'd been on time, they'd be at the gate now, with the passes. He returned to where his son was standing slouched against the wall, unshaven and scruffy. He looked like a drug dealer, Alan thought.

"There's not going to be time to get passes before the plane comes," he said. His voice was chilly. "We'll just have to hope she can make it by herself."

They leaned silently again the wall for a minute or two. Then Thomas said, "Maybe they'll escort her, the way they do with kids." There was apology in his voice, and Alan instantly forgave him. "Or if she's really out of it, maybe they'll put her in a wheelchair."

Alan shrugged. "Well, let's not worry. Either way, I'm sure Lily will be okay. She'll be running the show. Whatever it is."

Some passengers had begun to file past them now. Alan stepped forward and asked one of them where they were from. Not Chicago. Washington. He and Thomas stepped back against the wall once more.

And then the wave of people redoubled itself. Another plane must have unloaded. Alan and Thomas stepped forward and stood about four feet apart, letting the crowd flow around them, scanning.

"Check it out, Dad," Thomas called suddenly. Alan looked at him. He was laughing. "We're surrounded by Lilys." He gestured. "It's like camouflage."

And it was true. There was what seemed to be a convention suddenly, of old women. Old women in pantsuits and pastel sweatsuits, many with that extraordinary white hair touched to pale blue. There was a powdery floral scent in the air. The women were wearing name tags, most of them. "Hi, I'm Betty." "Hi, I'm Louise Farmer." They moved more slowly than the other passengers, who hurtled through them, grim-faced and determined. They were in clusters of two and three, the unimpeded helping those with walkers and canes. Their bright, thin voices swam around Thomas and Alan.

"I give up," Thomas called over. "I'll never spot her."

"Oh yes you will," Alan answered. "There's no one like Lily. You'll know her when you see her."

But they didn't. Alan didn't. She had to plant herself in front of him, and even then his instinct was to keep looking past this tiny creature teetering on two canes before him, to keep searching for his true mother.

"A fine welcome," she said, and he almost jumped at hearing her voice.

chapter 3

Gaby padded barefoot around the dark kitchen, her hands moving quickly and surely in and out among the familiar shadowy shapes, making coffee. Every time she opened the refrigerator, a knife of light slashed into the room and she had to squint her eyes shut, but she didn't turn the lights on. She never did. She didn't like to at this hour. *Her* hour, of the day. Of the night.

"How do you stand it?" her friends asked her. "God, four A.M., I could never do it." But this was Gaby's routine, she was used to it. Not just used to it—she'd chosen it, she'd shaped it. At work by four-thirty, she was usually home again around two. In mid-afternoon she napped for several hours and then, around five, she got up and returned once more to the shop for an hour or so to close up.

It had been the children who had waked her in the past, returning noisily from their after-school activities, banging the doors of whatever house they were in, thumping and clattering, dropping things—books, musical instruments, sports equipment. Now it was Alan, who came in and gently touched her shoulder. Often they sat and talked in a desultory intimacy as she came slowly awake. This had come to be, too, the time of day they were most likely to make love, with the late sun streaming in the room and lying with a warm, hard light across their aging bodies. And in the last few years, he'd taken to coming back to the shop with her almost every day and helping her with the closing up.

In the winter, yes, sometimes she did mind it. It was especially hard sliding into the frigid embrace of the car in the darkness, her breath pluming smokily from her nose. The car's heater would just have begun to blow tepid air on her legs˚by the time she was pulling up at the shop. The shop itself was cold and hollow-feeling until the oven's heat and the odor of baking made the space seem slowly smaller and more welcoming.

She loved these days though, the pale darkness of summer. The windows were open to the noises of daybreak—the first delicate stirrings of trees in the wind, the fierce, awakened energy of the birds. And she loved to watch the pearly light imperceptibly arriving as she moved alone in her house while Alan still slept. Alan, and Lily today. She'd been there four days.

And had already seemingly made herself perfectly at home. They'd put her in the guest suite and arranged it as she requested, as a kind of bedroom-office. Lily had immediately settled into a routine centered on her work—boxes of papers she'd sent ahead by train and now had Alan set out around her worktable for her. And they had settled into a routine too, centered on her.

It was clear to Gaby that Alan was having more difficulty adjusting to Lily's presence than she was. And it was true that when she was with them, Lily *presided*, in a sense, in spite of having to make her pronouncements in a weakened, whispery voice. She could be biting, she could be sarcastic, and Alan often responded with his own version of the same thing.

Partly for this reason, Gaby has been getting the old woman ready for bed at night. Alan gets her to the bathroom in the morning and leaves her sitting in bed with coffee, awaiting Noreen, the woman they've hired to help out. Since Noreen leaves before dinner each day, Gaby decided quickly that it would be better for both Alan and Lily if she were the one with bedtime duty.

She has surprised herself with the tenderness she sometimes feels for Lily as she performs this service. Just last night,
as Gaby was leading her from the bathroom to the bedroom to
help her get undressed, Lily whispered in that rushed, breathless way, " 'When you shall be old, you shall stretch forth your
hands and another shall gird thee and carry thee whither thou
wouldst not go.' "

"Ah," Gaby had said, for want of anything better to say.
Was this a protest?

"John. The Book of John," Lily whispered.

"Oh yes!" Gaby said, as though she recollected the passage.

Lily sat carefully down on the edge of the bed. She tilted
her head back and her face labored a moment. Then she
incanted softly, " 'When you were young, you girded yourself
and walked whither thou wouldst: but when thou shalt be old,
thou shalt stretch forth thy hands and another shall gird thee
and carry thee whither thou wouldst not.' "

A few moments later, as Gaby knelt down to untie and
remove Lily's shoes, she had a sense, suddenly, of doing something holy, something that made her feel, in some deep way, *of
use.* Holding the shapeless foot in its thick stocking on her lap,
she had felt tears of compassion and love spring to her eyes.

But then there are the other moments, those moments when
Lily seems in one way or another to sneer at Alan. At these
times Alan seems unable to resist carping back, and the two of
them seem then to Gaby not so much like mother and son as
like jealous siblings, each of them resentful of the very air the
other takes in. It reminds her sometimes of the squabbles Ettie
and Thomas got into when they were small; and her irritation
now reminds her, too, of the rage she felt at her sons when they
bickered and teased each other, when they wailed and called to
her to adjudicate. Once, she remembers, wincing, she had
banged their heads together to stop a fight; and then screamed
at them in helpless, high-pitched French that they would drive
her mad.

Of course, with Alan and Lily, Gaby isn't free to distribute her anger evenly, and so it's Alan she feels herself turning away from. Last night, he'd come out from their bedroom to find her skimming through the Bible. "Jesus, Gaby, what are you *doing*?" he asked.

She'd been annoyed instantly, but she held her voice level. "Looking for something your mother just said to me, about being led around by others when you're old."

"It's in the Bible?" He sounded offended by this very idea.

"She said it was John. Do you know it?"

"I know nothing about the Bible. Nothing." His voice was flat and absolute. She watched him. Lanky, barefoot, he crossed to the island, went behind it. She watched him open the refrigerator, stand in front of it for a moment, looking. He shut it without having taken anything out, and left the room. Of course he knew the Bible! Whole passages by heart. How absurd for him to deny this! Gaby had snapped the book closed.

She sat now at the wide kitchen island that separated the cooking and living areas of the house and lifted her oversized white coffee cup. In the dusky light, the room was beginning to take shape, the low sleek forms of the furniture Alan had chosen in their familiar places. Among them now loomed the humps and curves of Lily's furniture, five Victorian pieces come down from her family that she wanted Alan and Gaby to have. In this half-light, they made Gaby think of the hulking beasts, the imaginary monsters of childhood—*wild things*—and she smiled.

They'd arrived before Lily, sent ahead by train too, along with the dozen or so heavy cartons of books and papers. Alan had assumed that Lily would take the furniture with her when she left. Thomas had helped Alan, and they'd crammed everything into the guest room to make Lily feel at home. Gaby had directed the removal of a few of their own things, and the placement of Lily's possessions.

Lily had been astounded when she'd arrived. Didn't they realize her intentions? These chairs and tables were gifts! She'd kept what she wanted, she assured them. It was all in storage at the retirement community until she could move in. These were for Alan and Gaby, to do with as they wished. And she insisted that they be moved right back out into the living room.

Gaby took another swallow of coffee. Odd, she thought. It had taken Lily to add the element that made her feel at home in this house at last. When they'd moved in, they'd discarded most of their old furniture, things they'd acquired cheaply over the years at yard sales or flea markets, or as friends cast them away. Alan had a vision of how he wanted the house to look, and the old stuff didn't fit it. Besides, some of the new furniture was built in, and all of the storage was, so they simply didn't need the bureaus and wooden boxes and chests that had held cookware and towels and clothing in their other homes. The result was a clean, bare elegance that made Gaby feel empty-hearted.

The night after they moved Lily's furniture from the guest room into the living room, she'd lain in bed, excitedly thinking of how she might have it upholstered once the old woman had left, and remembering the profusion of dark objects and bric-a-brac in her family's house outside Paris, walking again in her mind through the maze of tables and chairs and screens and little desks at her grandmother's house in the country.

Now she was thinking of the other architects they knew, of their houses, uncluttered and serene for the most part. Messy lives, though. Gaby had always suspected that this was more true for architects than for other professional groups. It was their lack of schedule, she had often thought. Their working days were fluid, changeable, full of people and the whims of people. Full of women. Look at Alan: what would he do today? He had a house being built, so he'd probably drop over there and make sure it was going well, perhaps be in touch with the clients—the owners—if there were problems to work out. He was hoping for at least two other projects that Gaby knew about, a little church in Vermont (money was the question there), and a big elaborate addition onto one of the old houses in the village. So there would be time in the office, time on the telephone, maybe coffee or lunch or a drink with someone or other, charming them, amusing them, persuading them that this or that detail or surface or type of window was worth the extra cost in terms of what it would give back to them. Persuasion. Aesthetic conversions. Seduction, really. And it was more often the women than the men who cared, who had to be persuaded. Perhaps that was how architects got into trouble.

Gaby sighed. They'd had their share of trouble certainly. And made it through. Though Gaby, not Alan, had been the cause of the last crisis, with her affair. And this house, as she well knew, was a seduction too, meant to win her back. She was to have fallen in love with Alan again.

"*Don't*," she had wanted to say. "You don't need to."

He had needed to though. And she supposed in a certain way it had worked. She did love the house, and he believed in that love. What he might not have believed was that she'd never stopped loving him, though this was true.

It wasn't Gaby's first affair. She'd had one much earlier in their marriage too, before the children were born. Alan had never known about that one. It had happened at a time of difficulty between them anyway, when Alan himself was having multiple lovers—though they carefully spoke of it then as an "open marriage," rather than infidelity.

No, Gaby's real lover, as she thought of him, had come along two years before the house. She hadn't told Alan about it until it was over. And then, foolishly, she had thought she could present it as a kind of fait accompli, a reason for having been withdrawn temporarily, and sad. One day, making dinner, she had simply announced it to Alan, that it had happened and now was done with.

He had been shocked, and then outraged. He had walked away from her, stood with his back to her at the window. Then, abruptly, he'd lifted his arm and the glass exploded.

There'd been blood everywhere. Gaby had grabbed a clean towel and wrapped it tightly around Alan's hand. She'd called to the boys, told them to finish fixing dinner, to clean up, that she didn't know when she and Alan would be back. She'd driven him to the clinic.

After that, there was the wait, not knowing whether Alan's hand would recover. There were Alan's questions too, which Gaby tried not to answer. She didn't want to talk about it, she told him. She didn't want to play twenty questions.

Alan did, of course. And slowly he found out most of what he wanted to know.

The man was much younger than Gaby, someone she'd met in the shop—he stopped in for morning coffee and a roll each day. She had thought they would sleep together perhaps once or twice. She'd supposed because he was younger, "and quite attractive," she told Alan, that all he was interested in her for was a quick affair.

She reminded Alan that he'd been away a good deal right then, that he'd had that project in Dallas.

Dallas. Dallas had been eight months earlier. "So this, this affair, which has fairly recently ended, began eight months ago."

Well, yes, she said. But it ended two months ago. And now, no more questions.

But Alan couldn't let go of it. *Six months!* For six months then, everything had been a lie. Every good moment between him and Gaby. All of it was going on while Gaby thought of someone else, wanted to be with someone else.

It wasn't like that, she said. Not at all.

Then what was it like, he wanted to know. What was it like when she made love with *her friend*? What was it like when she made love with Alan in that time?

And then all the other questions. Who was he? What did he do? Where did they go to be together? How often? Did he come to the shop anymore?

Gaby tried to put him off, but as he discovered, when he asked a question that called for a simple yes or no answer, she felt somehow honor-bound to respond. When he asked what they did together sexually, her lips tightened and she turned away from him, but there was a lot he could find out with another kind of question.

She caught his gaze on her often, appraising, trying to gauge her attractiveness to someone else, she supposed. Someone younger. She had grown a little heavier through the years, though she wasn't plump or fat. She was solid, solid and wide. She had a short, strong body that looked better naked, actually, than it did clothed.

It was early spring when she'd told him about the affair. One day in late summer when it seemed his hand was going to be all right again, she'd come into the house they were living in then, the old, ramshackle house they'd bought in the village. She'd been watering the garden. She was wearing a bikini. She was barefoot, and her feet were wet and flecked with blades of grass. She'd browned everywhere, as she liked to do in summer, and her short, curling hair was damp at her forehead and her neck.

She had a story to tell Alan. A young couple had been walking past the house just now, teenagers. Their neighbor had mowed his field earlier in the day, and the sweet smell of the fresh grass was everywhere. "Christ," the girl had said to the boy, "don't you just *hate* the smell of new-mown hay?"

Gaby was laughing as she repeated this, and Alan laughed too. Then he stopped and looked hard at her, at her body, at her legs and feet, and she knew what he was thinking of. After a long moment, he asked his last question. "So, you're done with him. That's it."

Gaby paused and then sighed. She had wanted to spare him this hurt, and herself the hurt of revealing it. But now she said wearily, "My dear, I would say, on the contrary, that he was quite done with me. But that *is* it."

She heard him inhale sharply, but he turned away before she could see his response. They never talked about the affair again. He had nothing more to ask.

Gaby couldn't have said, exactly why, after that, Alan

turned from what had happened and began to plan their house—holding it, changing it in his mind until his hand healed and he could begin to figure it out on paper. It had startled her, the sudden enthusiasm he had for the project. She was still feeling bruised and tentative. The last thing she would have said she wanted to do was to focus a lot of energy on building a home, on Alan, on windows and countertops and knobs and appliances. Almost immediately she understood, too, that he was wooing her with all this, showing her his value. Though she began with a distracted toleration of it, slowly she was drawn in, she started to enjoy it, planning the place they would live in together for all the long years ahead.

Gaby looks around now at Alan's gift to her, familiar in every detail, and still moving to her when she thinks of how it came to be.

But Gaby also has a picture of the house in her mind that Alan doesn't know about and couldn't imagine, a picture that rises occasionally just as she is taking most pleasure in her surroundings, a cautionary note.

She had gone to the house, alone, two days before they were to have moved in. She was on her way home from the shop, and her decision to turn down their new long drive was pure impulse—to look one last time at the house empty, to walk through its echoing space in solitude, hearing her footsteps in the bare open rooms. To think of her life as *starting over* again, the illusion we all need from time to time, the impulse that probably drove her to the affair in the first place. The affair that had led to this: the house they'd made together. That Alan had made for her. It was strange, she was thinking as she drove under the arching boughs of the driveway, strange how things worked out.

To her surprise, the door stood open, though there were no cars parked in the yard. Gaby felt a tremor of apprehension. A few beer cans had been flung around on the packed dirt. She didn't stop to pick them up, but neither did she rush forward. She walked in rhythm with the sound of her pulse, suddenly throbbing in her ears. She had known of houses vandalized around town. Mostly the houses of summer people, houses at the ends of lanes or long driveways, as theirs was, used for parties or just sport on a weekend night in the off-season when no one would be around to hear it happening. But the summer people were rich, they didn't live here. She and Alan did. They were part of this community. They knew everyone. Gaby regularly served coffee to the fishermen coming off their boats in the morning. She knew their children from Little League, from hockey or soccer or basketball games at the school. Not *us*, she thought. *Not our house.*

She stood in the opened doorway. Whoever had done this had worked quite well within the limited means. There was no furniture to wreck, there were no objects to steal, no dishes to break. But they had poured beer around—the floor was sticky with it and the cans strewn here and there. They'd sprinkled cleanser on it, and Gaby saw the bottle of dishwashing liquid lying on the floor near the kitchen island, so she assumed that was part of the brew. They'd unfurled toilet paper over the mess, and it lay gaily in streamers everywhere, in some places wet and plastered down, in others fluttering or trembling in the breeze from the opened windows. Several windows were smeared and printed with their hands, with the usual unimaginative array of dirty words.

Her first thought—her only thought for a while, besides a kind of abstract rage—was that Alan mustn't see this, mustn't see what someone had done to his house, his gift for her. Moving quickly now, panting, although she didn't notice it, she went back to her car. She drove to the market in the shopping mall, bought plastic trash bags, five rolls of paper towels, a mop, a plastic pail, dishrags, soap, floor wax, ammonia.

When she returned and was lugging the grocery bags in, she noticed what she hadn't seen before: that the key was in the door. Alan had one copy, but they'd left this one under a rock at the side of the house for each other or the workmen as a spare. She came down the steps, went to where it should have been, and turned the rock. Gone. Whoever had done this had known, or been told, where to look for the key.

As she worked through the afternoon, mostly on her hands and knees, scooping up the paste and soggy paper with the paper towels, filling trash bag after trash bag, she pondered it: who could it have been? Why? There was a long list of workmen besides the regular crew—whom she dismissed immediately as possibilities: they loved the house. Unfairly though, the faces of the others—the mason, the tile guy, the plumber, the electrician—all rose up. Their sometimes stupid or sullen helpers, more likely. It wasn't until she was done and thought to look in the other rooms, just to be certain they were all right, that she found the little pile of human excrement stinking in a corner of her bedroom. And thought: *teenagers.* Probably there'd been piss in the soggy mess she'd been kneeling in all afternoon. She checked all the other rooms and found one other heap defiantly deposited next to the toilet on the floor in the guest bathroom. Her sons' faces rose before her. They'd both been out the night before, a Friday. Both were home by their curfews, Ettie at eleven, Thomas at midnight. Thomas had had the car. Ettie had been brought home by a friend who drove.

When Gaby had cleaned up the two piles of shit and scrubbed the floor where each one had been, she carted all the trash bags out to her car. She put the cleaning things away in the storage spaces Alan had carefully designed for them. She locked the door and pocketed the key this time.

The dump was closed by now, so she couldn't take the bags there. She drove back to the shop—only a little earlier than she usually returned to close up anyway—and one by one tossed the bags into the garbage bins around back. She went inside. Carefully she washed her hands and arms up to the elbows. Then her face. Then she sat on the counter and hoisted her legs up and into the deep-welled work sink. Her knees were red and tender-looking. She carefully scrubbed them, bending down to reach her calves and feet, then working up her thighs nearly to her crotch. The water ran freely over her ankles, her broad feet. Gaby rested her elbows on her knees and watched it swirl down into the drain.

When she came home, Alan was in the vegetable garden. He waved to her and she went inside. Both boys were in the kitchen, both eating. The bread was out on the chopping block, and crumbs were scattered over the counter.

"Where *were* you, Mom?" Ettie said. They would have expected her to be home in bed through the afternoon. They would have expected her to fix them a snack before she went back to the shop.

Gaby looked from one of them to the other. Innocent, innocent. Both were chewing, Ettie neatly, his compact, natural grace evident even in this small act. Thomas had a moustache of milk on his upper lip, and he opened his mouth with each swivel of his jaw.

"I had a terrible mess to clean up at the new house," she said, looking back and forth between them.

Both mouths stopped chewing. Thomas's hand stilled with the bread in midair. Ettie looked at Thomas. "See?" he said. "I *told* you you couldn't trust those guys."

"Shut up!" Thomas hissed.

They stood, all three in silence. Neither boy would look at Gaby.

Thomas then, it was clear. Gaby stepped forward quickly, quickly slapped his face twice, two *gifles*.

He stepped back, his eyes opened, liquid and vulnerable.

"No one will speak of this to your father," Gaby said to them both. She turned to Thomas. "And I want you to think of how you shall apologize to me that I've had to pick up the shit of your friends in my hands." She held her hands palms up, as though in offering to him for a moment, and then she left the room.

Of course Thomas did apologize, profusely, and with tears. It was sadder than Gaby had thought it could be. He was so unpopular, so difficult at that age, and he'd thought if he offered a place for a party where there'd be no adults, where no one would know, that somehow he could change his life socially. But they wouldn't leave when he asked them to, and he'd had to come home, he had the curfew. But, he said, they'd promised, he'd made them promise, to clean up before they went. And he'd called one of them the next day, and he'd said of course they had, what did Thomas think? They were complete idiots?

When Gaby thinks of all this now, the vision of the house that day comes to her along with the sight of Thomas's adolescent face streaked with tears, and she's saddened and touched. So she feels moved by the house, yes, by the sense of it as a gift to her; but also weighted by it oddly, by its importance in their marriage, by the feeling of protectiveness of Alan connected to it.

It is strange, then, that it is Lily's gift that has made her feel finally at home. Lily, whom she could have forgiven anything, she thought, except the thing she seemed best at: diminishing Alan, making him seem boyish, unserious, in their almost daily squabbles.

Now in the melting gray light, Gaby sighed, rinsed her cup, put the milk back into the refrigerator. She slipped on her clogs, swung her big bag over her shoulder, and crossed the room. As she passed behind one of Lily's chairs, she let her hand fall on the carved fruit at the center of its rounded back, caressing briefly the smooth shapes—apples and pears and grapes, and the thick-veined wooden leaves.

chapter 4

Violet Roberts, Lily's mother, had, like Lily herself, married late by the standards of her day. And Henry Roberts was forty-two when Violet became his wife. In the first six years of their marriage, Violet had five miscarriages. When Lily was born only slightly prematurely and survived, there was an almost religious caution and hush that surrounded her care and upbringing, that hung like perpetual weather over her cradle, her crib, and then her bed.

There were no more children after Lily. She grew up in a household of adults, most of them two generations older than she was. Henry, who was almost fifty by the time Lily came along, had been born in 1861. Though he was a successful businessman—he was an executive at Pillsbury—he was also a Victorian, and in a Victorian sense, rigid and remote. Whatever energy Violet had had as a younger woman had dissolved in the sorrow of the tiny babies she'd produced, and dressed in their frilled gowns, and buried. She was completely overshadowed by him.

On Sunday afternoons throughout Lily's childhood and youth, while Henry took his ritual after-dinner nap, Lily and her mother dressed again in their church coats and hats and went to the cemetery to help change the flowers or greens in front of the tiny arched headstones—each with a name and a single date on it, birth and death as one. Violet spoke of each grassy hillock and stone as though it constituted the child buried under it ("Henry looked terrible"); and over the years, Lily came to think of the lettering of each name, the particular way the ground rose over each tiny grave as somehow *having personality*. Certainly as much as she felt she did.

The whole household centered on Lily, but in an odd way— without making a single concession to her being a child. The concern was primarily for her physical well-being, a particular obsession of her death-ridden mother. There were liniments and cod-liver oil, there were weekly enemas. The whole family Fletcherized, meals were nearly silent but for the endless required chewing. Glass straws were used to drink with, even at the dinner table, and the light musical clink of these straws falling against the sides of their glasses—only this noise and her father's pronouncements about politics—punctuated the other minimal sounds.

Lily grew up a peculiar child, almost lifeless but for her caution. She dressed in clothes which were simultaneously too fancy—as though every day were Sunday—and strangely dowdy. (Often they were purchased or sewn to match a dress or coat of her mother's, who was now in her mid-forties.) Lily had a strange, elderly way of speaking, too. She called children her own age "tykes" or "little fellows."

These children didn't actively dislike Lily—there wasn't enough there to dislike. They simply ignored her. There were many examples around Lily of the painful alternatives to being ignored, and she was grateful for whatever it was—her own silence, her family's wealth—that allowed her invisibility. And she was invisible in spite of being an extraordinarily pretty child, for other children notice animation long before they can see beauty, and there was very little of that to notice in Lily.

When Lily was stricken with polio at sixteen, it seemed a long spell cast over the house was broken; the thing they'd all been waiting for had happened at last. There was a kind of wild relief in Violet, an energy and resolution in her grief, and a sudden attentiveness in Henry. The months Lily spent in the hospital were the first she'd spent away from her family. The food was different, there were sweet drinks with her meals, always red, in Lily's memory. The other children, if they weren't desperately ill, were encouraged by the nurses to be lively, and Lily for the first time had friends, learned dirty words, heard tales of the interesting, and to her utterly bizarre, ways other households were run.

When Violet visited the hospital, she seemed transformed—dynamic, insistent on Lily's pushing herself, trying harder, moving more. Lily understood that her mother had been rehearsing for this moment all her life, that she was passing her will into Lily. Lily also understood that it was on account of Violet's will, which slowly did become her own too, that she would survive. There was a kind of laxity on the nurses' part about certain children; though they seemed no worse off than some others, it was understood that somehow they weren't what the nurses called "fighters." They wouldn't make it. Lily saw that she was a fighter, at first almost against her own will, and then, as she recognized it in herself, purely on account of it.

She was sent to her grandmother's farm that summer to continue her recuperation. This was her father's mother, ancient and abstracted, who talked to herself wherever she was in the house—talked and laughed, with animation so intense that Lily was certain the first few times she heard her that company had arrived, and she hid in her room. There were three cousins on the farm too, younger children of her father's sister, who lived in another house on the property. Lily was expected to play with them, to stay outdoors, out of her grandmother's way, and she did. She should have been far too old to play in this sense, but she was still so unused to other children that she brought a naive energy to the task, and this let her pass for ten or twelve. At any rate, the others seemed to accept her as a child, in spite of her adult body. They treated her as though they thought of her as damaged, somehow retarded or slow-

witted; but she was of real service in their games. One of the
strongest, clearest memories of her young life originated in
these circumstances. Lily included it in her book.

Maggie and I had gone down into the unmown
meadow to pull up daisies and braid them into
daisy chains for our hair. I'd not done this before, and
Maggie had to show me how, slowing her neat little
fingers so I could see the way she worked the stems
together. Each of us was sitting, lost in the tall grass,
and neither of us had to move to reach what seemed
an infinite number of the flowers. Maggie was perhaps seven or eight feet from me, and I seemed to
see her, my pretty little cousin, through a veil made
of the tall grasses, the daisies and buttercups nodding
above the low strawberry plants. She wore a flowered
pinafore, I remember, over her dress. The sun was
high, and the heat was, for Maine, intense. In our airless universe, I smelled the strawberries, heard the
steady low drone of a thousand bees working in the
ocean of blossoms. Carefully I wove the crisscrossing
plaits of the raw green stems, always imagining this
as a crown which would reveal the true me, magically.

Suddenly, simultaneously, Maggie and I stopped
and sat still, looking at each other. My Aunt Lydia,
Maggie's mother, was calling us. "Lily?" The voice
rose on the second syllable. "Maggie?" Again and
again. We looked at each other, and said nothing. At
one and the same time, we were as if strangers with
no impulse to recognize each other, and conspirators
making a silent pact. Presently the voice moved farther away and we could hear only the plaintive echoing, "Eee?" "Eee?" of the repeated second syllable of
each of our names, like a distant calling bird. Then it
stopped. With one breath we sighed, and each of us

bent to her work again, somehow more intimate with each other in our closed-off world than we'd been before. I think, in fact, that I've never felt more intimate with another person. Even now sometimes on a hot day if I hear bees buzzing, I can shut my eyes and see the grasses and flowers stirring gently around me, smell the rich hot odor of summer, and feel again a yearning for such a sense of union—through my will—with another person. For what I believed was that I had made it happen. I, Lily Roberts, had felt my will move in that place, and announce itself, join itself, to another's.

Why we didn't answer my aunt I don't know precisely. Only it mustn't happen, we knew this. It mustn't, she mustn't be allowed! And so she wasn't, and I knew such a sense of triumph and joy in that moment, such a sense of recognizing myself, myself as *Lily*, that I can never forget it.

Part of what Lily had done in her memoir was to trace the recurrence of that feeling through her life—her own *Lilyness*, as it were. The quick triumph and equally quick defeat of it when she voted for Roosevelt and then was pulled out of Vassar by her father as a result—and she remembered it as that, almost physically that, a pulling. He came unannounced to Poughkeepsie by train after he'd received her letter. (This letter was careful and polite. It put forward in painfully logical terms the reasons Lily had chosen Roosevelt over Hoover. It was signed, "Ever your devoted daughter, Lily.") By the time she knew her father was on campus, he'd already seen the dean, and arranged for her luggage to be packed and sent on after her departure. He gave her twenty minutes to gather an overnight bag, and they walked back immediately to the train station. He didn't speak to her on the long ride home, and she didn't again feel the stirring of her will, her sense of self, until she met Paul Maynard, come to serve as a substitute pastor in their church while Dr. Atherton was ill.

And now, here is Lily in the guest room at Alan's house, arranged the way she likes it, going through the letters Paul wrote her at that time and a little later, before they were married, when he had gone ahead to the church in Ohio. Alan and Gaby have hired a girl for her, Noreen, dumb as a post but good-hearted, Lily will concede, and Noreen has set Lily up for the morning, the box of papers—mostly these letters, but some from her mother too—on the table pushed in front of her, and a bowl of cereal, oatmeal with maple syrup, cold by now, off just to the side of them.

As Lily finishes each letter, reading slowly, thoughtfully one last time, she tears it with trembling precision in two, then four, and drops it into her wastebasket, set close to her chair for this purpose. She is doing this because she is old. She is dying, she feels. It has begun. And she has left the world exactly what she wishes it to know about Paul and herself, about their love and their marriage and the end of all of it. These letters are nobody's business but hers. She wouldn't like anyone, even family, pawing through them after she's gone. (These are the very words she said to Noreen, who agreed with her absolutely. And when she said them, she imagined it just that way: big hands, animal hands connected to no particular body, roughly stirring through her letters—these memories—scattering them through sheer carelessness. *Wounding* them, as Lily thought of it.)

The correspondence is in file folders, ordered in clusters of years, usually three or four years together in one folder, but sometimes only one when there were many letters. Lily arranged it in this fashion when she began to write her memoir. She hasn't gone through it since that time. Oh, occasionally, searching for a certain memory to nourish a story idea, she has tracked down one in particular, or read through a year of her life, but she hasn't read some of these early letters in twenty or more years, and certainly not in order.

When Paul moved to Ohio, they were already engaged, and planning to be married within the year. Paul had gone ahead alone to "establish himself," which meant, as they all understood, to save some money. (Though Lily had come into her trust by then, her money was not to be used for any joint expenses, at his insistence.) Most of the letters contained long accounts of social events in Belvaine, descriptions of people she would meet, especially of the women who had spoken of looking forward to her arrival. Sometimes Paul would be invited by a church family on a day trip or outing to some local historic sight or natural wonder. Lily is struck now, reading the letters, by the energy he had for these encounters and trips, by the care he had for detail in these letters, by his concern to give her a sense of what it was like to be there. He wanted her to feel, already, a part of it, and of his life.

> I have been thinking of you here often, Lily, and often my question as I go through some event centers on what your response might be or how you might be experiencing a certain thing if you were here by me. It is like looking at the world with a new set of eyes on the one hand, and on the other is slightly disorienting, and occasionally makes me feel sorry for myself.
>
> I went on a trip with the Barretts, all seven of us packed into their car on a day when the temperature must have hit ninety degrees! to what constitutes, locally, a "mountain." We climbed it, interminably it seemed, because of the pace of the two youngest children. It is really a large mound, but it's true it had a long and very lovely view over rolling fields, with the property boundaries (or perhaps they were creeks or streams?) marked by thickets of trees. Madam Barrett had outdone herself with the spread. Not just ham, but cold chicken too, a potato salad, pickled onions and beets and cucumbers. Muffins and two kinds of pie. Oh, and cold lemonade and beer, the beer for the gents,

those being Barrett and me. I dug in, trenchermanlike, and felt in Mrs. Barrett's attentiveness that she was probably only too aware of the nature of my bachelor meals in the parish house.

On the way home we took a long detour, ostensibly to show me the Ox River valley. Barrett talked, as he had at lunch, nearly without pause. I felt he was, and had been, politicking, presenting his view of the men's group he heads at church, and of the various factions that settled out as they chose a pastor—a process, dear Lily, that took nearly two years, so you see how very special I am, and also that to become Mrs. Paul Maynard is no small achievement on your part! At any rate, so drowsy was I with the effects of the heat and the sun and the beer, and the incessant accompaniment of Barrett's animated voice, that it occurred to me after a while to try the experiment of not saying a word in reply.

It was true that the river valley was lush and gently beautiful, with an occasional open vista across the dark waters to the fields beyond, but Barrett noticed neither this nor my clamped lips. He talked steadily all the way home, and I took some amusement from my private joke on him.

And then, as we all got out of the car, I to take my leave, and all the Barretts to stretch their legs and change their seating arrangements, Mrs. Barrett spoke quietly to me alone. Had something I'd eaten upset me? Oh no, I assured her, all had been delicious. Good, she said. And then pointedly, but perhaps not without some amusement herself, "I just worried at how quiet you were on the way home."

I was ashamed of my little game then, Lily, and impressed with her kindness and perception. She is, I would think, only a few years older than you, though worn down by the myriad small Barretts, and perhaps by the largest one too. I prayed for more generosity of spirit that night, but felt, as I often do here, that if you were sharing these experiences with me, I would be easily capable of that. I would have your eyes to meet mine over an inedible meal or an endless account of someone's minor illness, and the promise of our shared amusement later. Remember how we laughed together after we got stuck with the Weeds at the church supper? Not unkindly I think, but with a leavening humor. (I loaned you my handkerchief to wipe away your tears, I remember, and got it back several days later pressed into a neat square I kept in my drawer for weeks because it made me think of you, laughing till you cried.) Oh, come soon, Lily! and leaven my life again! Lighten my load.

Your devoted,
Paul

When Lily finishes this, she sets it down. This memory shocks her. So long ago, and in anger and bitterness over what Paul eventually did—as she saw it—to their marriage, to their life together, to the church they shared, she had cast their love in different terms from the ones that have come back to her, reading this letter. She had thought of the Lily who moved out of her father's house to marry Paul as someone moving from one suffocating relationship to another. She had written of her marriage as an ugly chrysalis inside which she was slowly transformed into a being who could emerge only as it was discarded. And that is how she has come to remember it too, with this coloration of embittered hindsight. She had forgotten—how could she have forgotten?—the gladness in her heart when these letters came, the joy of the thought of joining her life to Paul's.

Paul! she is thinking now, and she sees him as he was then; tall and big-boned, but skinny and so fair that from across a room—and it was across a room that she first saw him, in the church hall at a welcoming supper—his eyebrows and lashes disappeared and he looked strangely old and frail. But when he stopped at their table and was introduced, holding a plate of food heaped so high Lily wondered he wasn't embarrassed to admit such hunger (he was always hungry, she discovered later), she saw that he had thick pale eyebrows and lashes. That with his keen gray eyes, his sloping jaw and long nose, he looked, in fact, like a wolf. And hungry indeed! His eyes ate her, and it was she who looked away.

This picture arrives as news to Lily; it shakes her. She is flooded, suddenly too, with the memory of her youthful self— she would have been twenty-five at this point—of her unquestioning love for Paul. He asked . . . no, he didn't even need to ask! She sensed what he wanted and stepped forward in anticipatory offering.

Lily's face, though she doesn't know it, is a mournful mask.

And then it shifts, just slightly. *She will not.* She shakes her head. *This cannot. No.* (There is no need for her to think this thought through, but she feels a kind of door willed shut inside her, and then the welcome sense that she is safe again, that she need not consider any longer the feelings which threatened.)

She snorts and reaches for another small spoonful of the cereal.

Lily will take all morning to eat the cereal. This is what it's come to. Parkinson's. Worst so far in her face, which is frozen in blank, childish expectancy; and in her throat, so that swallowing is a slow, consciously controlled activity. She has been taking the evening meal with Gaby and Alan, but she eats almost nothing, preferring to wait until she's alone again to struggle with solid food (though Gaby, seeing how little Lily manages to get down even then, has recently begun to put her dinner into the blender before she brings it in to Lily). She can drink more easily, and she does, and several times has wound up a little tipsy by the end of the meal. When Alan expressed concern the night before, she said, "It's all calories, dear boy."

Of course, Lily reminds herself ruefully, she is like a child.

It's worth remembering that. Not reduced to diapers yet, but it will come, if she allows it to. The gloppy food has, the purées of what the grown-ups had for dinner. The baby-sitter to make sure she gets to the toilet when she needs to, to help her dress and fix her meals.

She likes Noreen, she reminds herself. She has spent herself lavishly, actually, considering her diminished energy, charming Noreen, because she would find the merest hint of distaste for herself on Noreen's part unbearable. And it has worked, to a degree. Noreen believes herself to be caring for a distinguished guest, a famous author, a *personage*, and Lily has subtly encouraged this.

Though she saw that Noreen was peeved when she mentioned her guest for tea today.

Guests are Lily's vice, the only one now but drink left to her. Writing was a vice, but in the last year, Lily has had trouble indulging it at all anymore. Guests are the residue of that life. She wouldn't have them if she hadn't done the writing, and now she finds life unimaginable without them.

The possibility of feeding in this way on their attention was revealed to her so slowly that she didn't initially appreciate what it might mean. At first there were just a few letters, people wanting to know if they could meet her, have a drink or coffee, or lunch; do an interview for this literary magazine or that newspaper. Lily always said yes; and slowly she discovered that the encounters animated her, renewed her. She felt she was uncovering a version of herself—strong, opinionated—that she hadn't fully understood before. She was playful. She invented things sometimes. Or changed them. Distorted them.

Then the Parkinson's started and it gradually grew harder for her to write. In fact, the last two stories Lily has published were written years earlier. She revised them a little before she sent them off, and pretended to everyone that they were her latest productions. Privately she knew better. And privately too she realized that she had begun to use the visitors as a way of making fiction of her life, since she seemed not to be so easily able to make fiction on the page. Sometimes recently, in the midst of telling a story, she will realize how far from the truth she has strayed, and it thrills her. She will stop, shrug. "Of course, it may be that none of it really happened that way," she'll say, and smile. "Who can tell?" And she'll pour the guest more wine, more tea or coffee, the pitcher or bottle rattling against the cup, the glass, in her trembling hands. *Enigmatic*, she's been called. *Complex*. And even more visitors arrive.

Lily has brought with her to Bowman a list of people she's corresponded with from this area who wish to meet her. And in spite of Noreen's grumpiness—you'd think she entertained every day—she's had only two to call in the two and a half weeks she's been here. This afternoon's will be the third, though she intends to make something different out of this one.

She announced it at dinner the first night she was here. Alan had just finished telling her about Noreen, explaining how none of them could be home through the day, so that hiring someone to help her out had seemed the answer.

"We'll be very sociable then," Lily said. "I'm to have an amanuensis too."

"A what?" Thomas said. "Sounds like a surgical procedure."

"Well it isn't," she said matter-of-factly. "If we had a dictionary, you could look it up." She glanced around the room and then turned to Alan. "In my youth, we had a dictionary in the dining room for just such occasions."

Alan had had to wake Lily from a deep sleep for dinner, and when she'd opened her eyes, she hadn't immediately recognized him. She'd seemed frightened. But the tenderness that this vision of his mother had called up in him had vanished through the course of the meal. "This would be the same dining room, I presume, where the advantages of the class system were so carefully explained? Where you learned, most of all, how to pour tea so expertly?" He could hear the strain of childish defiance in his own voice.

Lily laughed, a laugh that seemed mirthless because her face didn't change. "Touché," she said. "Though if I hadn't written the book, you wouldn't have the ammo, would you?" She turned to Thomas. "A-man-u-en-sis," she said. "She will write for me, since I can't do the job myself anymore, for the most part." And she held up her hand, clawed and trembling. They all felt compelled to look at it.

She loves this, Alan thought. *The drama of this illness, the attention it gets her.*

When Lily is done for the day with the cereal, with 1935's letters (and in the end she has torn up all Paul's letters from that year with what she thinks of as hardly a pause), she lifts the little silver bell Gaby has given her and rings for Noreen. Noreen yells back, something Lily can't quite hear, but after a minute, she understands that she is waiting.

She could get up by herself—at home she had to and she did—but it is a struggle, and she'd just as soon wait. Simply *to be waiting,* though, makes her aware, abruptly, of the tension in her body, of its wish—she sees her illness this way, as having its *own* will—to turn to stone, to become utterly rigid. She is dying, she is freezing, she feels it acutely, and stills, her eyes open. Time stops. She thinks to reach for the bell again. But doesn't. Or call. Or move.

And then Noreen is upon her, talking, sliding the table away, and Lily feels a letting down, her thoughts are flowing again in response to Noreen's chatter. She's been baking, yes, for Lily's visitor, she says. "I had to get the cookies off the pan or they'd stick, and then I thought, well, I might as well get the last batch in. Come on now, upsy daisy, here we go." Her voice is singsong and noisily cheerful.

Lily walks easily on Noreen's arm to the bathroom. Noreen settles her there and leaves. A few seconds after Lily flushes— they've worked this out—Noreen opens the door and offers her arm to Lily again. As they move back into the guest room, Lily says, "It's odd, isn't it Noreen? how well I move with you, when by myself it's stop-start, stop-start. Like a robot. We should try out for the Rockettes, don't you think, dear?"

Lily smiles at Noreen and wins Noreen's smile back. "Not with my legs," Noreen says.

Noreen is a solid, plain woman. A no-color woman, Lily thinks. Dishwater hair she has permed so fiercely it looks like the insubstantial dustballs that move under furniture. Grayish, troubled skin visible under her thick makeup, eyes whose color Lily couldn't tell you, though they're fringed with electric-blue mascara. She wears jeans and sleeveless blouses to work in, sometimes shorts on a hot day. Her flesh is white and soft-looking. But her smile animates her briefly, as it does now.

Once Lily has changed, she sits back in her chair to let Noreen do her makeup. She likes just foundation, a little blush, lipstick, and a touch of pencil to fill in her dark brows. "I feel more authoritative with darker eyebrows," she's told Noreen.

Noreen is smoothing foundation on Lily, and the old woman turns her face greedily to receive the loving stroke. "In my day, you know Noreen," she is saying, "you were thought of as cheap if you wore even the amount of makeup you're putting on me now." Noreen makes an agreeable noise. "Really until the sixties, it was just lipstick and perhaps a little eyebrow pencil or mascara. But *rouge*! Unheard of except for ladies of the night. Or actresses. And eyeliner, no, no, no!"

Lily can feel the words trembling almost out of control in her throat, and her mind is rushing too, remembering that time. Noreen's tongue is protruding slightly in a wet curve between her lips as she lightly pencils in Lily's eyebrows. She's frowning, perhaps not really listening. "When the sixties arrived and my girls began to ring their eyes in black, I felt a band of gypsies had moved in with me. Who were these slatternly creatures?"

Lily rolls on, the words tumbling out, explaining her misjudgments of people in church based on their makeup, her dawning awareness that everything was changing in this way too. "Well, why not? I finally thought. The whole world seemed to be falling apart, why shouldn't it be that young girls chose to look like prostitutes? That they began to wear dresses so short you were meant to see their underpants? Why shouldn't there be a thing known as *hot pants*? Why not?" (The bitterness in her voice comes from her quick memory-glimpse of Paul at this stage, his turning away from their life together—part of this sea-change. Now she clears her throat and tries to move her thoughts away from him. She has put this behind her long since, long since.)

"Do you know, Noreen, it was actually unthinkable, until the sixties, that any woman would wear blue jeans, or even slacks, to go downtown? Or even on a busy street? Much less those neon pajamas the women around here wear!" This is a joke Lily has made to Noreen before about the bright-colored exercise suits which the summer people wear around town. Lily is not above an appeal to class divisions, though she would never allow herself to do anything similar based on race. "How things have changed, wouldn't you say? We were so ruled, so constricted. And yet there was a kind of greater attractiveness to life generally then, and one can't finally say, I think, whether one way is better than the other."

Noreen is nodding, has been nodding and offering an occasional comment. Now she lifts Lily's chin. "Hold your mouth still a minute, dear. That's a girl," she says. Carefully she applies Lily's lipstick.

When Lily stands before the mirror, she's pleased. She looks erect and imposing, she thinks. She's wearing a loose, soft cotton tunic of a very light green with three-quarter sleeves. Her pants are of the same fabric, comfortable. Around her neck are the small gold beads which were her mother's. Earlier this morning, Noreen did her hair, pulling it back into the bun on her neck, and the makeup makes her look cared for and alert. She rests her trembling hands on her canes and calls gaily to Noreen, "Onward! Forward, Noreen. To the living room!"

Noreen is grinning as she takes Lily's arm. She's as pleased with her charge as a little girl with a carefully dressed and coiffed doll. Lily *is* her doll, in a sense. She looks, Noreen thinks, like a sweet little old lady, even though she's clearly having a bad day, jolting from within as though an electric shock were continually passing through her bones.

She settles Lily in a chair, then pushes the coffee table and the other chair around as Lily directs her to. Lily says she's to offer wine as well as coffee and tea, she's to bring the cookies over now, and once things have settled down with her visitor, she can sit on the deck and relax, or go shopping if she needs to.

As Noreen is assembling the tray in the kitchen, she looks over at Lily in the chair on the other side of the room. The sun is lying across the old woman's hands, and they have turned up, as if to grab it. Her canes rest against the chair, her face is blank and open and without intelligence.

Then she sees that Noreen is watching her. Something shifts inside, some chemical change occurs, and she cries out with sudden animation in her rushed, soft voice, "I say bring on the dancing girl, Noreen! Let's see what we shall make of Miss Linnett Baird."

chapter 5

Linnett, actually, had proposed the terms. She wanted to do a long article. She preferred, she'd written Lily, essentially to hang around with a subject for a few weeks rather than do extensive interviews. But she knew this could be burdensome and wondered if there was some service—secretarial perhaps? culinary? chauffeurial? was there such a word as chauffeurial?—she could perform for Lily to make it seem less so. And thank God Lily had chosen secretarial. Because, as it turned out, Linnett was in a cast. She had fallen while she was jogging two weeks earlier.

It was very early in the morning, and she was groggy and angry, and therefore not paying attention to where she was putting her feet. There was a long grassy hill sloping down to the dirt track that ran around the reservoir near her house. She was running down this hill, her body tilted back against its pull, her hands holding her breasts against the jolting of her descent, when her foot caught in a hole, a deep animal hole. She heard the sound of the bone breaking just as she began to fall.

She was angry because she'd slept with a man she hadn't intended to sleep with and certainly didn't want in her life. She'd drunk a little too much—Linnett often drank a little too much—and it had just happened. This is how she would describe it later to her friend, Natalie, who came to pick her up at the hospital. *It just happened.* And then she'd fallen asleep without asking him to leave, so that when she woke, he was there, taking up well more than half the bed, lying on his back, drawing long, stentorian gasps of air. She'd lain and looked at him for perhaps a minute, flooded by shadowed images of their rough, unloving lovemaking the night before. There was a whitish fleck suspended in one of his nostrils which fluttered with his every exhalation.

She swung herself slowly and carefully out of the bed, not wanting to wake him. As she pulled on her running clothes and splashed her face with water, she was aware of a rising self-disgust. And the anger. With satisfaction, she saw how puffy her face looked this morning, how unattractive she was. "Not only is he probably in your life," she said to her reflection, "he's in your *bed*." And then she laughed silently, quickly, at her perverse priorities. "Jerk," she said to her own face.

Ten minutes or so later, as she sat holding her ankle on the cool wet grass, with involuntary tears starting down her face, she had the distant, satisfying thought that at least now she would not have to go home and wake him, or exchange pleasantries over breakfast, or wait for him to leave so that she could begin to work. In her mind's eye, she emptied the three rooms of her little house, she saw only the messy sprawl of her minimal possessions waiting for her in the still, dusty sunlight, she saw her bed a blank tangle of rumpled sheets.

And it was true that when Natalie dropped her off at the house three hours later and she eased up the steps and into the kitchen, he was gone. He'd left a note on her pillow in bed—it crunched under her head as she flopped down. She picked it up, held it high away from her face to read it. "Where'd you go?" it said. "I'll call you later." She groaned aloud. She rocked her head slowly back and forth on the pillow. Her eyes swung around the room, scoured the tongue-in-groove boards of the old ceiling, the cracked glazing, curling away from the casement windows, the array of pictures tacked to the painted, wood walls: John Lennon curled naked around Yoko Ono, Baryshnikov in mid-leap, Linnett herself in another incarnation—her hair permed into an Afro, her baby niece on her hip—and photographs of various people she'd interviewed. She was dizzy from medication, tired, and slightly hung over. She fell quickly into a deep sleep.

The cast ran from mid-calf to her toes. When she woke up, still groggy from the pain pills she'd taken, she lay in bed and thought through the next six weeks in her life, in particular the arrangement she'd made with Lily Maynard. Briefly she hesitated about it. But too much was already in place. She'd gotten an expense advance from *The New Yorker*. She'd rented a little house on an estate a few miles down the road from where Lily was staying. There was no reason, really, not to go ahead with it. She'd be slower getting around, there'd be a certain awkwardness. There wouldn't be the long walks she'd imagined with Lily Maynard, and she'd have to ask for her patience in certain situations. But it wasn't as though she'd need to be waited on, and she could certainly still perform the service she'd arranged to perform for Lily.

No, all this would mean was that she'd have to make a few accommodations. She'd need a backpack or something like it to carry stuff around in. And she wouldn't be able to manage her stick shift for the duration, clearly. Who did she know who had an automatic she could trade for her car?

She got up and made some coffee. While it was brewing, she called her ex-husband at the university.

"Baird here," he said, as though he were still in a newsroom somewhere.

"Baird here too," she answered.

There was a pause. "Can I call you back?" he said neutrally. "I'm with a student."

Some gorgeous young thing, she could tell. "Sure," she said. "Or how 'bout you stop by for a beer this P.M. when you're done?"

"Around five-thirty?"

"Sounds good to me," she said.

"See you then," he said, and hung up.

By the time his car pulled up outside, Linnett had made her bed and done some business telephoning. She'd taken a sponge bath and washed her hair. She'd chopped a salsa and dumped some nacho chips in a bowl. Now she was sitting on her sagging porch couch with a beer in her hand, her legs propped up on the railing. She'd taken a Percocet about half an hour earlier, and had moved into a territory of vague goodwill toward the world.

"Hey," he said, climbing the stairs. "Hey, are you wearing one go-go boot or have you broken your leg?" He had on his summertime teaching uniform—a baggy seersucker jacket, a striped shirt, chinos, and white tennis shoes. No socks. He was a large balding man, just slightly overweight.

"Ankle," she corrected. "But I'm feeling no pain."

He came over and tapped on the cast, gingerly. "When? How?"

"Ah, ever the journalist. Where's your sympathy? That comes first."

He smiled at her. "Where's a beer for me? That comes first."

"Inside. Refrigerator." He started into the house. "Bring out the chips and stuff too," she called to him. "I was trying to resist till you got here."

After he'd settled next to her on the couch, beer in hand and the chips and salsa resting between them, he asked again, "How'd you do it?"

"I fell when I was jogging this morning."

"What a cliché."

"I know. I'm sorry. But at least it wasn't a heart attack. That's a really tired ploy."

He was chewing loudly. "Does it hurt?"

"Yeah, but I got drugs."

"Hey, whad'ja get?"

"You can't have any."

He elbowed her lightly. "Bitch," he said companionably.

They sat in friendly silence for a moment, surveying the weedy scraggle that was Linnett's yard. In the distance down the empty road, where there'd once been a cornfield, there was a soldierly row of raw new houses, the beginnings of what would be a major development. He spoke again. "It's gonna cramp your style a little."

"Not much. but I do have a problem I want your help with."

"Please, no."

"You don't know what it is yet."

"Linnie, I mean it. My own life is all I can manage right now." He was shaking his head. Jowly, she thought. He's getting jowly.

"It's no big deal," she said.

He sighed. "What is it, then? What is it?"

"I want to trade cars. Yours is automatic."

"It's underinsured," he said quickly.

"But I'm a better driver than you are anyway. And my *car's* better than yours. This is a no-loser for you."

"How long?"

"Month. Month and a half."

"What's in it for me?"

"I told you. A better car, a better driver for your car."

"What else?"

She gestured at the bowls between them with her bottle. "All the beer and salsa your heart desires."

"What about my other heart's desires?" He did a Groucho Marx turn with his eyebrows.

"That's not your *heart*, idiot." He smiled. "You're just horny, Franky boy."

He nodded several times. "True. Very true."

"Find someone. You don't even try. You just ogle the under-graduates. Which is now, I hasten to point out, *against* the rules."

"How would you know? That I ogle?"

"I know. I hear things."

"Gossip is odious. You should be above it."

"I also heard you went to a party at Eda and Earl's where there were lots of available, grown-up women, and you sat in the kitchen playing Scrabble the whole time."

He shrugged and ate another chip. When he'd swallowed it, he said, "Wanna play?"

"Scrabble?"

"*Bien sûr.*"

"What about the car?"

"Yeah, you can have the car. Let's play Scrabble."

Over the game, she told him about Lily, about the article she wanted to do. And then she was aware that she was offering this to him, as she had done so often in the past, as a kind of trophy: "See how smart I am?"

And as he'd done so often in the past, he gave her advice instead of praising her. "She's been done to death, Lin. I must've read half a dozen things about her over the last four or five years. You'd better have a new angle. What's your angle going to be?"

Now, driving his car into the little town of Bowman, she heard his voice again, she remembered how he'd looked, the irritation moving over his face at the news of her coup, the mean way his mouth curved down before he spoke. He'd put a Q on a triple-letter square shortly after that, and she'd tipped the board up to end the game.

She drove slowly, cruising the streets. It was a Friday, and she wasn't due to start with Lily until Monday. She'd given herself the weekend to figure things out, to get used to her surroundings. There was an old town center—five or six buildings clustered around a green, including the requisite church, a clock in its tall bell tower. She'd noted a shopping mall a mile or two back up the road, with a chain supermarket, but here everything was more tasteful. On the first floors of several of the grand old houses there were an ice cream parlor, a gourmet store, an antique store, a bookshop. Linnett stopped in the real estate office just outside of town to get the key to her rental cottage, and directions.

The next day, Saturday, she set up her computer and laid out her books and notes. Then she got into Frank's car and drove again. She found a liquor store and bought a bottle of gin and some beer. She went to the supermarket and did a big shopping, hobbling slowly behind her cart. She sat on a bench on the porch in front of the ice cream parlor and ate a double-dip cone, pistachio and chocolate, while she surveyed the weekend action on the streets in front of her.

It was the kind of town that drove her crazy—mostly retirees, it seemed, the men in green or madras slacks, the wiry, gray-haired women speed-walking in two and threes, wearing expensive warm-up suits. She noticed that a parade of old pickups was steadily passing, some with what she recognized as lobster traps in the back, others with other equipment she took to be nautical. When she'd finished her cone, she headed down the road they'd been driving back and forth on. Harbor Road. It ended at water, at a sheltered harbor, appropriately, with two or three docks reaching into it and some of the trucks she'd seen, or ones like them, parked in a row again a cement half-wall. She sat in her car for a while, listening to a shouted conversation between two men working in solid, beat-up boats pulled against the largest dock—the main one. It was what she thought of as guy talk, work talk: numbers mostly, in this case weights of a catch of some sort, and then money—the price per pound at various places, the cost of fuel, the cost of repairs. The water in the harbor glinted in the sunlight. Bobbing at moorings farther out were what looked like expensive pleasure boats, and on the ocean in the distance, Linnett could see at least a dozen sailboats gliding over the silver water.

That night she found a bar in an old hotel in the next town over that was lively enough—some fishermen here too, she discovered, eavesdropping. Shortly after eight, an entire softball team arrived on a swell of loud voices. They all wore T-shirts that said *Cox Hardware.* Many jokes there, she speculated.

She spent the evening in the bar watching the Red Sox lose on a very large television set mounted in the corner, and the clientele slowly get drunker and louder. Late in the game, they all began to put the moves on each other. Linnett got a little attention, but basically it was a crowd that knew each other, that liked the sense of the familiar. When she wasn't as friendly as she might have been, they left her alone. She went home at about eleven. Almost all the lights in the village were out.

The next day, Sunday, she drove to the supermarket in the mall and bought the *New York Times*. She sat outside on the little deck in front of her house, drinking coffee and making her way though it. When she was done, she went inside and skimmed all the notes she'd made on Lily Maynard. She flipped through the short-story collection, looking at her underlinings and marginalia. She went more slowly through the memoir.

What had drawn Linnett to Lily Maynard in the first place was the memoir. Not just for the reasons that feminists had embraced it, and only initially because she was intrigued by the publicity angle: the old woman and the sensationally successful first book. No, it was as she began to read—even the first few paragraphs—that Linnett had thought she'd like to interview Lily. The world she presented seemed like new territory to Linnett, and also there was something loopy and nearly careless, but compelling stylistically about the way Lily launched herself into the memoir, about the way her prose moved. It began:

W̲e met on Tuesday night for fourteen years. We met to read the Bible, and we did read the Bible, but we also made a world, and with my dying breath I will bear witness, I will testify, that that world worked. We were all women, we were all colors, and when we gathered, all that mattered to us was the love that coursed among us.

"Wherefore seeing we also are compassed about with so great a cloud of witnesses, let us lay aside every weight, and the sin which doth so easily beset us, and let us run with patience the race that is set before us ... For whom the Lord loveth he chasteneth, and scourgeth every son whom he receiveth." So we would read; and by the end of the evening we were speaking of Mattie's son, already a father at seventeen and lost to her, of Shirley's husband, unfaithful again, of the death of my mother or the loss of a baby or the falling away of hope and the belief in the possibility of human kindness. And in that world of middle-aged women gathered in our ordinary living rooms on the south side of Chicago, there was solace, and comfort, and the lifting of even the heaviest of these burdens. And there was laughter and true fellowship.

I never even saw a black person—a *Negro* as we said then—until I was ten or thereabout. I was on a city trolley in St. Paul with my mother when the man got on. My father did not like Negroes, he didn't think they were clean or upstanding. But he held himself to be a Christian and he was an American, and therefore he also believed that if they wanted to, Negroes could live as respectably as we did, that it was possible that they could be our equals. It was, then, a failure of their will and moral fiber that they were not. This man was well-dressed, though his clothes were worn. He sat down on one of the long open benches at one side of the front of the bus, and, unlike the other men riding among us, he took his hat off and held it on his lap. To my astonishment, his hair was a reddish color. I noted too that the brown fingers circling the crown of his hat faded to a pale color on the inside, almost as light as a white person's. I was openly staring at him, something I knew to be rude, but when I glanced over at my mother to see if she'd noticed this, she was staring too.

She felt compelled to comment after we'd gotten off the bus. There was a bit of hemming and hawing. Perhaps I'd noticed, she said, something different about the man who'd gotten on. "Yes, Mother. He was a Negro." Yes, and obviously a very nice man, she thought. She came back to it several times over our afternoon in town. Had I noticed this about him, that? Had I noticed how politely he held his hat on his lap? I had. It just went to show you, she said. Yes. At last she said, "We won't mention this at home," and instantly I understood, though there was no direct hint of this in what she'd just said, that the reason we wouldn't mention it was that my father would then insist we not ride the trolley anymore.

Linnett admired these four paragraphs for their honesty, their quick conveying of a whole way of life. She was intrigued by the way they commented on each other. She liked the sudden turn Lily Maynard made to her father in the third paragraph. She wondered how conscious of her style Lily was, whether an editor might have suggested to her that her father get a paragraph of his own, whether Lily might have resisted that.

The first chapter went on to talk about the church in Chicago that Paul and Lily had come to, about the attempts the preceding pastor and then Paul made to keep it integrated, even as the neighborhood around it turned to ghetto. Lily wrote of her own unpreparedness for this struggle.

I came hearing my parents' voices in my head saying the things they'd never said in so many words to me: that Negroes were different, inferior, and somehow also threatening. That they were tolerable when they behaved with a kind of abject, eyes-averted respect, but not when they were "uppity." But I also believed that all men were equal in the eyes of the Lord. And I believed, with Paul, that to be a Christian meant truly loving our neighbors, no matter who they were. Hadn't our Lord, after all, aligned himself with those lowest in his world, with sinners and thieves, with lepers and Pharisees? Didn't our religion teach that we were fallen too, sinners all, even a man like my father no better than a thief?

Linnett had no experience of religion itself, though she'd attended church occasionally as a girl, mostly at Easter and Christmas with her mother. The idea of Lily's religious principles making demands of her, instructing her in how to conduct her daily life, was fascinating to Linnett. She read through the memoir excited and moved by the opposing forces of belief and loss; interested in Lily's writing; and intrigued by her sense of Lily's character.

Now, in her cramped cottage, she was reading from a passage in the last third of the book, after Lily and her husband began to have difficulties over the direction in which he was leading the church as Paul embraced the politicization of his ministry, as he began to be interested in the teachings of Saul Alinsky, the radical leader then working in the neighborhood to organize the community, to encourage them to press for their rights, to push against the machine and the economics which had virtually imprisoned them. Paul began to feel his role was to encourage black cohesion, black resistance.

One night, long after we'd gone to bed, the telephone rang. I was the lighter sleeper, so I was the one who got up and ran down to Paul's study to answer it, fearing for each of the children quickly and in turn as I went. I recognized the voice at the other end of the line as being that of Larry Sims, in charge of one of Paul's new outreach programs, but he didn't identify himself to me. He just asked if Paul was there and said it was a church emergency.

I waked Paul and lay back down in bed feeling dismissed and shut out of his new world. When he came back to the bedroom and began to dress, I asked him what was wrong.

"Just something involving some of the kids at church."

I couldn't see his face—he was bent over, pulling on clothes by the light from the hall—but I could hear the vibrating excitement in his voice. When he left, he told me he wasn't sure when he'd be back, but that there was nothing to worry about.

He forgot to turn the hall light off, I remember, and I lay for a long time in that half-light, thinking over the course of events that had brought us here, to a point where Paul felt more alive than he ever had, and I felt old and abandoned; and each of us was utterly certain he was in the right.

He didn't return home until almost noon. By then I had regained my equanimity. I made him scrambled eggs and opened some soup. We ate together in the polite silence that marks an experiential gap between people. He was happy, I could tell, and stirred up by whatever the illicit events of the night were—sometimes it was bailing someone out of jail, sometimes it was paying people off so someone wouldn't be thrown in. I was very angry at what I saw as his destructive, cheap pleasure in this new and tawdry world, and then angry at myself too for being so full of judgment, so righteous. When I slid the dishes into the sink to wash them after he'd gone upstairs to take a nap, I did it so fiercely that I broke two of them. It was all I could do not to hurl the shards to the floor. But I didn't. I stepped on the pedal to the trash can and carefully laid the broken pieces in on top of the morning's garbage. Then I put a paper napkin over them so Paul wouldn't see what I'd done. I was afraid he'd think I'd broken them on purpose. And perhaps, in some unconscious way, I had.

In the margin at the end of this passage, Linnett wrote, "Ask about this: unconscious. Anger. Not expressed much in life, no?"

Late on Sunday, Linnett drove down Broom Lane to the mailbox marked *Maynard*, just to be certain how long it would take her to get there the next afternoon. You couldn't see the house from the road—the gravel drive was overarched with trees. Linnett drove on to the next mailbox and turned around.

On Monday, she drove there again, slowly, feeling unexpectedly nervous. The branches hanging over the driveway scraped against Frank's car. Linnett had to pull her elbow in to avoid getting scratched. She came out of the trees to a wide field falling away to the left. Near the top she could see the rows of twiggy apple trees. The driveway circled to the right, where the trees were thicker. Linnett parked under a beech tree next to a big, banged-up station wagon. She opened the door, hauled out her crutches, and leaned them against the car. Awkwardly she pulled the backpack over to herself and struggled to get it on. Then she heaved herself up from the car and slowly made her way on her crutches over the bumpy ground.

The modernity of the house surprised her. She had imagined an old house, a wide porch where she'd sit and talk with Lily Maynard. In concession to the cape architecture of the town, this house was covered in shingles that had just begun to weather, but it was also very much its own thing, a stripe of windows wound horizontally around it, a green-painted pipe railing she leaned against now as she mounted the wide stairs one by one. She rang the bell. Through the sidelight of the door she could see that the space inside was one large room, with a wall of windows on its other side open to the river below the house.

Noreen opened the door, and Linnett watched her eyes round at the sight of her hunched over her crutches. "Hi," Linnett said. "I'm here to see Lily Maynard. Linnett Baird."

"Come in," Noreen said. She stepped back and held the door open for Linnett. "Right over here. She's expecting you." She gestured into the big room.

Linnett surveyed it quickly—a kitchen along the far wall, and in front of the windows to the river, a dining room table ringed with chairs. The furniture in the living area all sleek and modern, except for a grand piano in the corner and the odd Victorian piece. Seated in one of these, tilted awkwardly, as though she were a doll plunked abruptly down, was a skinny old woman, white-haired. She was wearing what looked like pajamas, of a pale green. Linnett lurched slowly across the room, staring at her. Lily Maynard's face was shockingly empty. As her eyes took Linnett in, though, they lighted with amusement at her predicament.

When Linnett was a few feet away, the old woman reached over and touched the two canes leaned against her chair. "Well," she said, in a breathless, rushing voice, "I see we have each come ready to put our best foot forward."

When she got home later that afternoon, home to her rented cottage, Linnett poured herself a gin and tonic. Then she sat down at her computer. *Lily*, she named the file. And she typed:

What you notice first are her eyes, a piercing dark brown, sparkling with a crafty intelligence. Next, her voice, light and girlish, almost unpunctuated in her rush to say things. Then, that she is beautiful, an impossible kind of beauty, composed of all the wrong elements: white hair, the flawless but deeply lined skin, the freckles of age dotting the hands and face. And then, only then, do you really take it in: Lily Maynard is an old woman, more than fourscore years old as a matter of fact. But of course, that's why you're here: to talk to the woman who has made being old—in the literary world in any case—interesting.

chapter 6

Within two days of Lily's arrival in Bowman, Alan shifted most of his working life away from his study in the house to his office in town, an office he had maintained previously mostly as a place to meet clients and as a storage area for his work. Almost every day for the first few weeks of Lily's stay, he's carried something he's pillaged from home—that's how he thinks of it—up the narrow stairs to the door with his name on it. Even now he keeps bumping up against an absence, something he needs that isn't here—slides, a reference book, a catalogue. But he makes do, he stays away from the house. Whatever he needs can always wait until tomorrow. It's a slack period for him anyway.

Though he could be revising the lectures he'll give this fall.

Though he's someone who's always had projects to do in slack periods—cabinetry, competitions to enter. (For several years he'd built harpsichords when he didn't have enough other work, and it was during this time that Thomas's interest in music had been born.)

What does he know of Lily's life at his home? Enough. He knows that there are often visitors. He has seen the shopping lists Lily leaves in her scratchy handwriting for Gaby or Noreen. On this account Noreen has asked for a raise. She hadn't expected, she said, to have to prepare lunch or tea for three or four people several times a week.

He knows that the secretary has started to come this week, and that Lily likes her. Gaby has met her more than once and she says the woman seems nice, but tough. They've laughed about it, actually, that she will have to be tough to work with Lily.

Alan is glad to be able to laugh at something in the situation because he's been surprised by his reactions to his mother, surprised and discomfited. He has never pretended to have an intimate or easy relationship with her, but before this visit, he would have said they had come to a kind of peaceful equilibrium between themselves.

Almost from the moment she moved into his life here, though, he has been angry at her, and then at himself for his anger. He's made excuses to himself, for himself: usually he has visited her, in his old home, her apartment. Never has she stayed more than a night or two in any of his houses. Never has he had to accommodate her life, her patterns. Never has she been so old, so demanding. None of this helps him, or eases his feelings toward her. And he's come to think that at the center of these feelings is his response to what she seems to be using this visit for: the destruction of his past.

For Alan is the one who carries out her trash, and he has seen the carefully torn pages of Lily's history. Of his own history: his father's writing, the words leaping up at him. He allows himself to take just these in, the phrases, the words on the torn sheets that lie on top, before he turns them out into the green plastic bag, dumps garbage on top of them, ties the neck up, and hauls it to the shed. But his indignation at this—is this what he feels?—is something he keeps to himself. He hasn't talked to Lily about it. What could he say, after all? He'd not known that there were such letters, such papers. How could he assert any right to them now, any right to their preservation? What would he do with them anyway? Would he even want to read through them, to know any more than what his mother has already made public of what happened between her and his father? Of his own growing up and what it meant to them?

He would, he realizes. He wants something from this history. It shouldn't matter to him now, but it does. In part because he feels his adult life has been a slow lesson—a lesson for a slow learner—in piecing together the elements in his childhood from which he'd fled then and now wants to understand. To master, perhaps. He has come late, he feels, to some necessary questions about himself. And now he has to watch what he imagines might contain the answers—some of them anyway—disappear forever.

There'd been the memoir, of course. It had brought back a version of Alan's past to him. But it was a version filtered through Lily, through her reading and understanding of events. It did interest him, very much, but he felt a kind of Olympian curiosity reading it. It was too much her story, her take on things, to help him.

There were photographs in the memoir too, a thicket of them between pages 187 and 188, black and white photographs. Of the earlier pictures, most were familiar, he realized, poring over them. He'd seen them in the albums that had sat in the bottom of the sideboard in the hall. Those albums had disappeared when his parents separated and he hadn't thought of them again. In fact, he'd forgotten they existed until that moment.

Some of the pictures were merely curiosities to Alan—those of Lily's antecedents, of her childhood and adolescence, and the later ones of her friends at Blackstone Church, of her in her study, and so forth. Some were merely amusing, or interesting: those of her and Paul together, and of the children as infants, and then in family groupings through the years. Here was Rebecca, for instance, posed perhaps for her graduation photo from high school. Her hair was carefully turned under at the ends, her complexion and intensity were utterly airbrushed away. Her gaze off into her future seemed only foolish and unknowing. A simp. And Clary as a teenager wearing a wide skirt puffed out over white tennis shoes and sweat socks. Here was Alan himself, poised on the pitcher's mound, about to go into his windup, looking, in the baggy uniform of that era, as helplessly skinny as Thomas did now.

But it was the photographs of Paul, of his father, that compelled Alan and confused him. There was one of him as a young man in the pulpit. His arms were resting on either side of it, and his face was earnest and open, the face of a disciple. When Alan as a child had looked up at Paul preaching or praying, his father had frightened him. The pulpit at Blackstone Church stuck out, like the prow of a ship riding slightly over the sea of faces in the congregation, and the view up wasn't flattering. The light glinted meanly off Paul's glasses, and his nostrils seemed to Alan to bristle thickly with dark hairs. As a younger child, Alan was allowed crayons and paper, and he busied himself with them and tried not to look up at this father, the judge. From the age of ten or so on, though, he was expected to listen, to attend without distractions to the sermons, and it was then that he came to understand that there were two quite separate sides to his father. There was the one at home, loving, joking, sometimes a buffoon. And then the one in church, grave, exacting, calling on Alan to be better than he ever could be—he understood this even then. He remembered looking over at Clary and Rebecca in church, at his mother, at the proud love flashing in their uplifted faces. He saw that they were unafraid of this Paul. He was their minister, yes, but also husband and father. And indeed, in the picture, both sides of Paul were present. It made Alan wonder: why hadn't he been able to see him in this way then—whole?

He hadn't, that was all, and from the time his father divided in two for him onward, Alan had understood that the serious side, the grave side—the side that was inaccessible and frightening to him—was the side that was more important to Paul.

When Paul tried in later years to talk to Alan (Alan imagined this as having been arranged nearly always by Lily: "I think you need to have a talk with Alan about . . . " whatever, grades, drugs, girls), it made Alan feel inadequate and hopeless about himself, and angry at Paul for that feeling.

"What is it you're trying to accomplish, son?" Paul had asked once. It was after the separation—Alan was fifteen, and Paul had taken him out for dinner. They were sitting opposite each other in a booth in the Tropical Hut. Paul's face as he asked the question was open and loving in the dimmed, orangy light. He was there, offering all his understanding.

"God! I'm not *trying to accomplish* anything, Dad," Alan had said contemptuously.

But what he'd felt was the sense that he was expected to be more complex and aware of himself than he was. That he *should* have been trying to accomplish something with his behavior, instead of just doing what seemed like the next thing to do, which at that age was smoking a lot of dope and trying to arrange a place and time to be alone with a girl named Mary Ann Singletary.

It had been a relief to Alan when Paul moved to California. He was seventeen at the time, in his junior year of high school. Paul had left the church amid a scandal. As part of his commitment to the community around him, and to what would later be called the black power movement, he'd been letting a gang from the neighborhood use the church for a meeting place. (This was also the last step in the splitting of the church, and the beginning of the flight of the middle-class black members he'd had too. For it was this gang, after all, who'd been extorting lunch money—any money they had—from the congregation's children on their way to school.) A young girl charged that she'd been raped at one of these unsupervised "youth fellowship" meetings. Paul had left at the church's request, and had finally taken a job in Berkeley, a low-paying job doing community organizing. He wrote to Alan regularly, but their relationship was over in any real sense. Paul came East for the appropriate occasions, but his life was somewhere else.

Alan hadn't acknowledged that relief for years. Even when

he was first talking to Gaby about his background, his young life, he spoke of feeling abandoned by Paul then. And of course he was telling the truth when he said this, when he told Gaby he thought it was inexcusable that his father should have left him to the tender mercies of the likes of Lily. But that was just one truth, one among many.

In her memoir, Lily wrote:

A fter Paul's move to California, certainly I, and I think the children too, felt nearly as though he'd moved into another dimension. His letters to them, and his occasional letter to me, spoke of a world which seemed utterly alien, but would become all too familiar in American culture within a few years. In the meantime, though, these missives arrived like time capsules from the world we were all moving forward into, like news of all of our futures: altered states of consciousness, watered-down Buddhism, and always, always, the embrace of the political fury and rhetoric of black power.

Alan could remember only the general tenor of Paul's letters from California to him, the tone of *older friend* he sensed Paul was striving for. And the rage this evoked in him: Paul wasn't even a father, much less a friend! Why should Alan care about the activities of the commune Paul belonged to, about his politics, his causes, his beliefs? He'd abandoned Alan! Why should he care about this side of Paul, this version of him? It was the other side he'd yearned for and now bitterly, angrily, given up on.

Once Lily, having seen a letter from Paul ripped and crumpled in Alan's wastebasket, asked him if he ever wrote back to his father.

"Never," Alan said.

"You should try to," Lily said. "Try to forgive him. It was I, after all, who chose to end things, not he." She stood in the doorway to Alan's room, her dark brows knit in concern. "I mean, if there's anyone you should be angry at, truly, it's me." Her hand rose and rested on her bosom.

I am, Alan wanted to say. But he didn't. He'd shrugged, and turned away, sitting at his desk, waiting for her to leave.

There was one other picture of Paul in the memoir that Alan kept coming back to. He was seated outdoors, under pine branches, wearing an old flannel shirt. He was surrounded by his children. Rebecca had thrown her arms around his neck from behind. Her small, clasping hands made a complicated necklace below his chin, and her laughing face rested against his. Clary was leaned against his side, looking hungrily at him and Rebecca. And Alan, the baby, was seated between his father's legs wearing a knit outfit which left his fat bare legs and tiny, curved feet exposed. Paul's hands encircled Alan's little body, supported him. Alan was tilted back against his father's belly and chest, his head was thrown back to try to see his sisters and his father. He was eager, smiling, sheltered by his father in the center of his own universe. When, Alan wondered, how, had all that, and the wife presumably holding the camera, become so unimportant to Paul, so dispensable, that he could walk away from it to build the new America?

Alan had tried to find the answer to that once. He was twenty-two. It was the summer after he'd graduated from college. Paul had just had surgery and hadn't been able to come to the ceremony. Near the end of the summer, Alan quit his job and headed across the country, to California, on a motorcycle he'd bought with his earnings. In certain cities and towns he had friends from college to stay with. The other nights he slept on the ground, in a sleeping bag. He had talked a good deal about this trip to anyone who would listen in the spring of his senior year. "Hitting the road," he called it. He said he was going to go "get straight with my father." In a hot springs in the Anzo Borrego desert he bought a postcard with a desert scene on it and addressed it to Gaby, in France. (At this point Gaby was more or less just an idea he had, but a compelling one. She was the older sister in a family he'd lived with on an exchange program the spring of his sophomore year.) "Greetings from Nowhere, USA," he wrote. "I've come almost all the way across this endless country at this point on a motor-cycle. It's been a crazy, lonely, exhilarating adventure, with finding my father the goal at the end of it. This brings affection-ate greetings from your admirer in America—Alan."

The truth was that well before then Alan had tired of the trip, of the sameness of the act of driving each long day. And the days had to be long in order for him to get all the way to California and back to Boston before school started. He was tired of the grimy, stained, public showers in the campgrounds he stopped in every third or fourth day. He was tired of crummy food, bad coffee, of the stink of his own sweat, of the ceaseless hot wind on his face.

Paul was dying, Alan could see that the moment his father opened the door, though he'd never seen dying or death before. Paul seemed to have shrunk into himself, and his skin was beyond white, a grayish-yellow. He was wearing a faded denim shirt and khaki trousers that ballooned out from a nar-row belt.

Alan, with his sunburned, windburned face, his Levi's and motorcycle jacket, his bulk and health, felt too large, too loud. Excessive somehow. But Paul's pale, pinched face opened and lightened when he looked at his son. They shook hands.

Alan stayed with his father for two days, and said none of the things he'd meant to say. He tried several times, but his tone as he began was always accusatory and harsh, and Paul seemed determined to keep anything difficult from happening between them. The last time Alan started to say something, they'd just sat down opposite each other in Paul's spartan liv-ing room. Paul was panting slightly from the trip across the floor to his chair. Alan was skirting around the issues, his voice already beginning to harden, and Paul raised his hand as though to ward him off. "No doubt I made mistakes," he said. "For anything like that, I'm sorry. What's important is, you're here. There's no sense dwelling on the past." They were silent a moment.

Christ, Alan thought. Why did I come then?

Then Paul started to cough. Unable to stop, he got up and shuffled slowly to his bedroom. The door shut, and Alan sat alone. He looked around the room, out the window. The bright California sunlight reflected off the naked pastel buildings opposite. There were black kids playing in the street, swearing casually at each other in the language Alan would come to use casually himself in the next few years. For a long time, the sound of the coughing was all he could concentrate on.

Much later, it would occur to him that Paul might have been making him a gift rather than just defending himself. That he might consciously have been keeping Alan from a cruelty to him that wouldn't have time to heal, a cruelty that Alan would have learned to regret. And for that Alan was grateful later. But he felt robbed too, perplexed and sad about the man who was his father. Like Rebecca, he'd taken the answers to all Alan's questions away before Alan knew how to ask them. Who are you? What was I, to you, that you so easily left me behind?

The problem is that Alan can't recall Paul, Paul as he was. And as the pictures make clear. He can't recall that happy, laughing father, that young man gripping the edges of the pulpit in his intensity. Here is what he knows: that Paul had played with them, read to them. That it was he who came in to say their nightly prayers with the children. That he'd taught Alan to ice skate, to throw a ball. He can remember these things distinctly, but without seeing Paul. When he thinks of Paul now, it is the Paul who was dying he sees. He sees him in the naked, harsh light of the empty living room, looking diminished and weak. He sees the pale, sunstruck world of the slum Paul lived in then. He remembers the sound of Paul's coughing, and that across the street, as he listened to his father struggling to breathe, a large, gray-haired black man slowly and tenderly buffed his car until it gleamed in the sunlight.

Now, seeing the letters in his father's handwriting, he is reminded again of his loss, as he was the first time he looked through Lily's memoir and came on the photographs. And he feels angry at Lily for being so deeply unconscious of what she asks of him in assuming he will carry these messages away to be destroyed, in assuming, as she must, that she is the only one to whom they matter, to whom they might bring back that lost world.

He can't speak of this, of any of this, to Lily. He doesn't know how to. What there is between him and her stays entirely superficial. There's the light banter at dinner, often a little barbed, which sometimes suddenly ends in unexplained, unexplored angry silences on Alan's part, silences which drive Gaby wild. And then what Gaby doesn't see, his visit to his mother in the morning, before Noreen has arrived, to bring her coffee, to help her to the bathroom. She is in one of her white nighties then, and often she's pulled on the frayed, stained bed jacket she's so fussy about against the cool of the morning air. The legs she swings out of bed with his help—which Alan has seen too much of, as he has seen too the sparse, iron-gray flag of her pubis—are yellowed and toneless. He stands outside the bathroom in the little hallway off the guest room, his head bent to the door, as she must have stood outside the door when a smaller Alan was inside their bathroom in Chicago, years ago. He listens for her as she might have listened for him, for her most intimate sounds, calling out, "Everything okay?" if she seems to take too long.

What this costs him, he couldn't say. What it costs him to slide the garbage on top of the letters which carry his past away from him forever, he couldn't say. Whether these acts or the anger he comes to feel at her through the course of nearly every dinner is worse, he couldn't say. He cannot speak of any of it to Gaby, except sarcastically, and when he sees the concern for him in her face, he tries to make a joke of it too.

Perhaps it's in flight from all this that within a week of

Lily's arrival, Alan began to leave the office in town too, sometimes fairly early in the morning, often almost as soon as he arrived. At first he pretended this was connected to projects that were ongoing. He checked on the house going up in Bowman until he came to feel that his too-frequent visits were becoming a kind of curiosity to the work crew. He spent one day after that driving all the way to the little town in Vermont where he might get a church to do, just to go over a few measurements that he could have cleared up on the telephone.

Now, increasingly, he's at a loss. A couple of times he's gone down to the docks, to the water's edge, where sometimes at that hour he can sit in the car and watch the fishing boats come in and unload. He feels conspicuously unemployed sitting there. Several times he's driven to the town parking lot and walked the beach, past the husbandless groups of tanned women and little children, the clusters of teenagers with tape decks and Frisbees. He knows these people, he knows they are not from privileged backgrounds; they're townies, with heavy townie accents. But he thinks of how privileged they would seem to most people—the women who don't have to work, who laugh and gossip and complain about their husbands while they turn browner and browner in the sun, while the children run in and out of the seaweedy water and dig and build in the sand and rifle through coolers for snacks.

It had driven Gaby crazy, he remembers, the endlessly long days of supervision and talk with other women when the children were small. What was it that made her uncomfortable? She felt a foreigner. She wasn't used to what seemed to her then the wasteful self-indulgence of the American housewife. She had started the catering business out of their own kitchen when Ettie was not yet two, and that was the end of it for her.

Alan feels wasteful now too, and restless—a man with visibly too little to do. By the end of the third week of Lily's visit, he usually heads farther afield, once the hundred or so miles to Boston, with nothing particular in mind.

He rings Thomas's bell that cool, lovely day, but no one

answers. He finds a parking place in the Back Bay and wanders its busy streets. How it has changed, he thinks, from his student days. He had friends then who lived in rented rooms on Beacon Street or Commonwealth Avenue—jury-rigged rooms, parlors chopped in two by cheap partitions in the grand town houses. You could hear the conversations or the lonely coughing of whoever lived next door.

Now these buildings are divided into condominiums, or in some cases, actually restored to single-family splendor, their windows swagged and shuttered, their entryways gleaming with polished brass.

He walks in front of a building on Newbury Street where he and Gaby lived for the first years of their marriage, in the attic apartment, two rooms and a kitchenette up under the mansard roof. From the front windows they looked out on the Prudential Building and the early plywood days of the Hancock. It was hot under the roof in the summer, and he can remember that they spent most of their time at home naked during those months. The second summer she was pregnant with Thomas. Standing on Newbury Street, looking up at those windows, he feels an unexpected rush of pleasure at the thought of her then, her hips widened, her belly hard and striped, her breasts fattened and silvered with stretch marks.

On another trip north he turns off impulsively at Plimouth Plantation. It's a gray day with a light rain, more like a mist, and he hopes he'll be, if not a solitary visitor, at least a lonely one. But there are six or seven big yellow school buses in the lot. For a moment he considers backing out again and driving away, but something about the huddled forms of the imitation seventeenth-century houses, their dark and cheerless austerity in the weighted wet air, moves him and he stops the engine. The moment he opens the car door, he can hear the children's shrill voices, carrying but cottoned in the thick air. No echo. He pays his entrance fee to a costumed woman and has an abrupt sense of the preposterousness, the strangeness of his being here. How is this connected to Lily? Why should his uprootedness on her account result in his coming to this odd place?

But it's not odd for him, he tells himself. He's an architect. He's interested in these buildings. And he does examine them carefully, the ancient post-and-beam construction, the steep grass roofs, the tiny windows. The windows then, the guide explains, were just this small, to keep the faint warmth in winter from passing out, but they were filled then with oiled paper, oiled to achieve translucence, to increase the dim light within.

God, the misery! he thinks. And all for what? Some ideal of life, some nearly abstract notion of freedom that turned rigid as a prison itself. He tries, standing in the single room that constitutes the entire interior of one of the houses, to imagine a being that could do it, that could live here with his wife, his children, and not go mad. That could live here and then wish to forge even farther in, to push the forest, the Indians, deeper back. His own ancestors on Paul's side of the family had been here then, living in such a village as this, marrying, having children, farming, preaching—sure that God had called them to claim this land, to change forever the way it was used. Sure that God intended them to bring light to the dark-skinned people around them.

It strikes him, suddenly, as nearly apocalyptic that those feelings, that sense of purposeful certitude connected to belief, has lasted in one form or another in the history of this New World until his generation, and then seemingly stopped dead. Rebecca, Clary, himself—none of them has felt *called* in the same way to do anything. Even Rebecca with her radicalism was mostly just expressing rage. Surely some sociologist, some historian, has worked out why this has happened, what has happened. Alan wonders about it now just for himself: what *has* happened, what has changed, to make him, the son of such people as Paul and Lily, what he is?

On another day he heads north and then due west, never even going to the office in the morning. He weaves along the narrow roads in southern Massachusetts, in and out of the old towns from another century, another time, finally arriving at the edge of the Berkshires. He is hungry—he hasn't eaten since he had a quick piece of toast at home this morning, and it's early afternoon by now—but in each town something keeps him from stopping. Here there doesn't seem to be a coffee shop. Here there is, but it's a Dunkin Donuts. And with each town, he's barely into its center before he's out again anyway, back on the twisting wooded roads that break open, suddenly, onto rolling fields with long vistas, the mountains riding low and blue in the distance.

And then he comes to a town, Emmett, whose name seems instantly familiar. He slows below the speed limit, trying to think why. And sees the faded, bedraggled pink ribbons tied here on a tree, there on a mailbox, decorating the newel posts on the front steps of the Emmett Inn. Yes: there's a little girl missing in this town. Missing, he thinks now, for a month or so—he hasn't read about it for at least that long, but he remembers when it happened. Before Lily came: the photographs in the paper of the grieving parents, of the police with dogs straining at their leashes, of the dozens of neighbors who fanned out into the woods that rose steeply behind the town. And of course, the picture of the little girl herself, a school photo, he remembers thinking—the smiling, dark-haired child in front of an artificial sky, wearing glasses that were too big for her. He had been compelled to read each article about her, and there was a flurry of them for the first four or five days.

He's parked now in front of the Emmett Inn, and he sits in the car for a moment. He remembers the description of the girl, and how struck he was that the parents knew exactly what clothes she was wearing, mentioned that she had on new sneakers. It had made him think of his sons at a younger age and the intense awareness he had had then of them physically. Yes, the very clothing they picked to wear each day—a hat one insisted on, a jacket the other wouldn't give up even as it got too small, the new shoes that had magical importance for them. He could imagine himself, like these parents, saying, "He had on black high-tops, with striped laces." The kind of thing you knew about your child, the kind of thing that would tear at you. He could imagine their panic. He could imagine too several nightmare versions of what had happened to the little girl, though he tried to call himself back from that each time. But there was a seductive power to such evil, to imagining it.

He goes into the Emmett Inn. It's a shabby, worn place with linoleum in the front hall. He finds this, oddly, a relief—that it's not furbelowed and spiffy. He steps into the dining room to the left of the wide hallway. The ten or so empty tables are covered with red-checked cloths, and they are all set for dinner with silverware, with paper napkins and glasses. The coffee cups are turned upside down in their saucers. "Hello?" he calls.

There's no answer. In the hall again, he sees the bell on the desk and hits it. From somewhere deep in the building, he hears a responsive noise, a thump. After a moment, a woman about his age, plump, in a plaid shirt and blue jeans, comes sprinting down the wide, curving stairs. She's breathless, and her lank, straight hair is drooping loose from a ponytail. Her sleeves are rolled up and her arms are solid and strong-looking, tanned. Lunch is over, she tells him. "I can give you some coffee and dessert, if you like. We've got pie. But that's it until dinner. There's no one in the kitchen right now."

"That's fine. Pie is fine," Alan says. "What kinds do you have."

"Exactly one kind." She grins. She has a pale, delicate moustache, but she's pretty in some surprising way. "Blueberry. It *is* homemade." It's her voice, he realizes. Its pitch, its softness. It belongs with another woman, and it's strangely arresting on her.

"Blueberry it is," he says. "And coffee. Great."

"Okay." She gestures him into the dining room. "Sit anywhere," she calls out musically as she heads toward the back of the hallway.

Alan takes a seat near the front windows, looking across the wide porch to his car parked outside and the main street beyond it. There are rockers painted white and set in a row on the porch. They stir slightly in the breeze as though invisible old ladies were sitting in them. Lilys. In a moment, the woman emerges through the swinging doors at the back of the dining room, carrying a tray. She sets the blueberry pie in front of Alan, turns his cup over, and fills it with coffee from a steaming glass pot.

She puts his check down next to his place. "If you could pay me now, I'll just leave the coffeepot with you and you can help yourself to more if you want it." She smells lemony, bleachy.

Alan stands, fishes four ones from his wallet. "That's fine," he tells her.

"Thanks," she says. "I've still got some chores to do upstairs." She leaves through the wide doorway to the hall. He hears her heavy tread going up the worn staircase.

Alan sits there for half an hour or so, slowly eating the pie and drinking two cups of the coffee. He feels, oddly, at home and comfortable. The pie tastes wonderful to him, and he realizes, abruptly, how famished he was. Gaby, he knows, would find it too sweet, the crust too chewy. He eats all of it, pushing his fork onto the plate to gather the last crumbs in its tines. Above him from time to time, he can hear the noise of the woman moving around, once her voice in distant, brief song.

Outside the window, the tall trees—horse chestnuts, with their beautifully shaped leaves—flutter suddenly in a breeze. The houses he can see are all painted white, white with black shutters, just as they are in Bowman, in hundreds of New England towns. This could be a life, he thinks, a different life from his own. A solitary man, a man on the road. A man with no mother, no wife and children. Is this what he's been trying to create for himself with these long drives? An illusion of just this freedom, this emptiness? Is this somehow what he would like, to move across this landscape unattached?

And would it have been such a man who would have taken the little girl, taken her in his car someplace and done whatever it was he did to her? A man with no ties, no connections?

Or maybe, he thinks, it was someone here, in the town. Someone like him. Someone everyone trusts, someone living among them now. Someone who tied his own pink ribbons around the trees in his front yard. Someone who joined the search party, who commiserated with the parents. Someone, perhaps, with children of his own. After all, isn't that what history had taught us—that men could be deeply evil, while also being, in a domestic sense, ordinary, or even good?

A woman walks past on the sidewalk, pushing a baby in a carriage. The baby wears only diapers and sits up, sucking on a bottle one-handedly, the other hand twirling a strand of blond hair. The mother is young. She wears blue jeans and she is smoking a cigarette. Her bare midriff shows below a short stretch top. She looks tough, mean. And then she's gone, and the street is back to the nineteenth century again. The illusion of the nineteenth century.

We are what wrecks it, he thinks: this landscape, the stillness and beauty of these towns. The escape they might represent from all that's wrong with contemporary life, with urban America. You can't get far enough away.

The horse chestnuts stir, the ribbons dance on the newel post.

And then he remembers that, in the end, what he is fleeing from is only Lily.

chapter 7

It is probably fair to ask to what extent Lily Maynard is conscious of the effect she makes, but it's not a question you'll easily find the answer to. There are moments, yes, when it all seems deliberated, when there's a pause and what seems a long, sly glance before something provocative or beguiling is said. About her marriage: "Of course, neither my husband nor I really knew anything about each other before we were married—nothing. But then, it was impossible at that period for men and women to know each other at all." Of her success: "I enjoy it absolutely, as I never could have earlier in life. It's taken me this long to understand that what I wanted all along was revenge."

But there are moments too when the dark eyes swim abruptly with tears, when she falls silent in the middle of a sentence and cannot—or will not?—finish it.

"Where is this going?" Linnett had typed. And tried again.

It was, of course, the peculiarity of her becoming famous when and how she did that initially drew me to Lily Maynard as a subject. But it was the mystery of who and what she is now that kept me asking questions. How is it, for instance, that a woman whose background fitted her for nothing so well as presiding at a church social should come to write a book that repudiates the influence of the church itself on the integration movement in America? How is it that a woman brought up to believe in the inherent inferiority of African-Americans should come to believe so ardently in integration in the first place? How is it that a woman taught to believe in her role as helpmeet, keeper of the homefires, spouse, mother, chief cook and bottlewasher—every cliché of the postwar era—should seek a divorce and the isolated life of the writer?

"*Merde,*" Linnett says aloud now.
Another beginning:

At the time of our meeting, Lily Maynard's life is, appropriately enough, again in upheaval. She's about to move from the apartment in Chicago where she's thought and written about her life, in fiction and in the famous memoir, for thirty years, into a retirement community nearby. And, for the moment in transition between the two, she's staying in a little New England town in the sleek, modern home of her son, an architect. If she seems perfectly comfortable in this uprooted state, it may be because Lily Maynard has had nearly as many lives as a cat, and like a cat, has landed on her feet in all of them.

Linnett is in her rental cottage, drinking tea and reading through her various starts on the article about Lily as they come up in the amber glow of the computer screen. It's raining outside, a light, misty rain off the ocean that leaves the windows blurry with the salty air. She's spent the afternoon, the whole week, with Lily, a Lily who seems not at all to have landed on her feet, not at all a mystery or a sly, self-contained woman. Instead she's been faltering, vague, and then finally today, firm, even noble, Linnett would say, in her renunciation of the life Linnett had intended—no, *contracted*—to write about: her life as a writer.

Over. Like that.

After two weeks of interviewing Lily, of taping their conversations, of helping her with her correspondence, Linnett finally suggested the Friday of the week before that it was time for her to repay her debt to Lily, time to help her write the story she'd talked about on and off since Linnett arrived. She'd been looking forward to this, she realized. Partly because she'd come to like and admire Lily and truly wanted to help her; and partly out of curiosity about her writing processes. And then, of course, there was the possibility that it would generate material for her article.

But three times this week they've tried. And three times they've failed.

Lily was fine summarizing it—Linnett has that on last Friday's tape, when they first discussed doing it. "It's an idea I've had as I've been reading through Paul's letters from California," she says. "I'm working my way through them, as you know, all those old letters, one last time."

Linnett asks something that's inaudible on the tape.

Lily laughs, gaily. "Yes, if it's the last thing I do on earth." There's a clinking—they were drinking iced tea, Linnett remembers—and then Lily says, more slowly than usual, "You know, the older you get, the closer to death, the more all those old clichés seem expressive of truth."

Linnett says clearly, "Oh poo, Lily. You'll live forever."

Lily, firmly: "Not if I have anything to say about it. And I will. I do." Her voice grows a little more distant here, and Linnett remembers that she looked away at this moment, out the window.

After a pause, Linnett's voice—flat, slightly Southern—calls her back. "But the story, Lily."

"Ah! the story," she says. "Well, it involves, naturally, a woman not unlike myself."

"Naturally," Linnett says.

"A semi-famous woman, elderly, who's on tour, you know, publicity. Traveling around, doing readings and signings and

the like. Interviews. We'll follow her as she arrives at the airport in San Francisco, and is met, and driven to her hotel. She's
tired, of course. She has a nap. And a little forgetful. Wakes,
can't think for a minute where she is. And then does, and gets
ready, goes to her reading at some bookstore." Lily clears her
throat.

"And I want her to . . . you know, she puts on her reading
glasses, so she can't really see the audience. Just a blur of faces,
really. And then when she removes them, at the end of the
reading, to answer questions—she's very vain, poor thing,
nothing like me in that regard of course."

Noreen calls something over from the kitchen, and they all
laugh. (Noreen's kitchen noises are a remote and intermittent
punctuation to this whole conversation. She's cleaning up for
the day, getting ready to go home.)

After a moment: "Anyway, she looks up and sees this old
man who looks familiar. And then she realizes it, it's her ex-
husband.

"And the whatchamacallit, the woman, you know, running
the reading is announcing that she'll take questions, and she
sees her husband's hand go up, along with some others, and
she deliberately doesn't respond to him first. Or second. She
decides she'll take six or seven questions before she gets
around to him—we'll have some as dialogue, and some will be
summarized. She'll be saving him for last, in some sense, and
aware . . . I want to be very clever about this if I can: she's
aware, don't you know, of preening a bit in front of him, of
really saying to him in a sense, 'Now my dear, it's your turn.
Now you must sit and listen to *me*.' And she's going along,
ignoring him, when the woman, the bookstore woman, gets up
and thanks everyone, says they really have to stop, and begins
to read announcements and so forth. And she has to sit there
and watch this old man get up and leave with the rest of them,
and that's it. And I want her thinking, that night, as she goes to
bed alone in this lovely hotel—oh, it will have a splendid view,
the Golden Gate Bridge, no doubt—thinking of him, calling up

certain images. Wondering, don't you know, what it was he would have asked her. What it was, after all these years, he would have wanted to know. And then almost chanting to herself as she gets sleepier, 'I was coming to you, I was coming to you,' the way a child does to comfort itself, chanting as though she could stop him from leaving as he did."

Lily's voice had gotten weaker over the course of this near-monologue, and she nearly whispered this last, in a way that made Linnett's throat ache even as she listened to it for the third or fourth time on the tape. She remembered Lily's face too, a faraway look on it, as though she'd moved into the story herself and was recounting a memory—though Linnett was fairly sure, given the relative timing of Lily's success and Paul's death, that these events couldn't have happened to her.

There's a long silence on the tape, and then Linnett's murmuring voice, "Oh, that's wonderful Lily. Oh!" She claps her hands once here, a strange, flat sound on the tape. "I can hardly wait to begin. To have my humble little part in it."

"Well, we'll see," Lily says, sounding exhausted, suddenly dismissive.

Linnett asked her how she wanted to work it out, and they talked about possibilities. They decided that they'd try just straight dictation the next Monday and see how that went.

It had gone very badly.

Linnett had sat down in her usual chair next to Lily's, pen and pad in hand. Noreen had put tea and cups down for them, and a plate of cookies Gaby had brought home the day before. Then, at Lily's request, she'd withdrawn to the deck.

As Lily talked, Linnett could see Noreen slowly flip through the pages of her magazine and finally put it aside and stretch out. Lily had been speaking for ten minutes or so by then, and Linnett hadn't written anything down. The old woman was again speaking indirectly of the story, of *how it would be,* as written. Linnett decided to let her go through the whole thing once more before she spoke. Maybe Lily needed this, to launch herself.

"It sounds as wonderful as ever, Lily," she said when Lily was through. "Just great."

Lily murmured a thanks.

"Now," Linnett said, poising her pen over the paper. "What's her name?"

"Her name?" Lily looked confused.

"Yes. The character's name."

"Oh. I hadn't considered . . . " Her hand rose, in front of her face, then slowly dropped again. "Well. I'd like. Let's say . . . Eugenia. Eugenia . . . Weld."

"Ah, good," Linnett said. "So. 'Eugenia Weld was on her way to San Francisco'? Or something like that?"

"No. Oh no." She nearly recoiled. "Something more . . . in medias res, I should think."

"Mmm," Linnett said.

Lily appeared distracted. A stricken, blank look washed her face clean.

Linnett waited.

Finally, weakly, Lily said, "The flight to San Francisco had grown . . . bumpy, over the Rockies, and Euphemia Weld had ordered a manhattan. Isn't that what you call it?"

Writing, Linnett nodded.

"With the cherry?"

"Yes," she said.

"I always liked them," Lily said. "When we used to have cocktails," she said, after a moment.

Linnett waited again. Finally she said, "Excuse me, Lily."

"Yes," Lily said, eagerly.

"Is it *Euphemia* you want, or *Eugenia*?"

"What did I *say*?" Lily asked, irritably.

"Both. At different times," Linnett said. And then, because Lily looked frightened somehow, she said again, "It's really a terrific story." When Lily didn't answer, she read back the first sentence to her, using *Eugenia* without hesitating.

Lily pondered a moment, and then took a deep breath. "She had drunk two . . . no, almost three manhattans by the time the plane landed, and she'd forgotten the name of the woman who was supposed to meet her."

Linnett wrote, rapidly.

Lily's hand moved dismissively. "But the way these things work, you know, they hold up your book, so it's not ever really a problem."

Linnett stopped writing. After a moment, she said, "'Almost three manhattans'? Is that how you want it?"

"I just want you to write it down as I say it. That seems straightforward enough, surely."

"Yes. It is. I'm sorry."

Irritated herself, Linnett determined to wait through the next silence. *Let her do it herself if she thinks she can.* After nearly a minute, she took a cookie and began to eat it, slowly. She tried not to consider Lily, who sat stalled, her mouth dropped slightly open, her hands wildly vibrating on the armrests of the chair. The cookie was buttery and rich, studded with coconut, with chocolate and nuts. When she had finished, Linnett wanted another, but she resisted. She picked up her teacup and sipped at the cold dregs. On the deck, Noreen shifted in the lounge, raised a knee and scratched it.

Linnett began to feel ridiculous. She spoke. "Lily?"

"Yes," Lily whispered eagerly.

"Shall I read you what we've got?"

"Yes."

Linnett read the first two sentences back, using "almost three manhattans."

"And then I said something about the woman meeting her. You don't have that."

"Yeah. I didn't write it down, because you weren't using fictional language."

"What do you mean?"

"You weren't speaking as the narrator then. You'd, more or less, lapsed into conversational prose. With me."

There was a long silence. Then Lily said, "I haven't the least idea what you're talking about."

Linnett took a deep breath. "Okay. I'm sorry. Can you just . . . say it again? Say that sentence again? I'm ready."

"It was about . . . " Lily hesitated. "Here, read me back what you have."

Linnett read it again.

Lily seemed lost in thought. Two sharp vertical lines of fierce concentration formed between her dark eyebrows. She spoke slowly: "But, as it happened, as these things happen, the woman was holding up a copy of Eugenia's book, so it didn't matter. Together . . . they walked, through the airport and out to the parking lot. The woman . . . " Lily paused for a long moment. "Whose name was Laura, or Laurie. Was a talker, and . . . Eugenia Weld, who had the beginnings of a headache . . . " And here Lily's hand rose slowly, as if being levitated, as if being pulled by a wildly trembling marionette string, to her own forehead. ". . . was . . . relieved. Not to . . . have to . . . " The hand dropped slowly. Lily seemed to slump back. "She didn't want to talk anymore," she whispered. "Not about this."

Something's happening, Linnett thought. She can't do this. She let a silence encircle them. Then she said, "Maybe we've done enough for today, Lily."

"Have we?" Lily asked, pathetically eager.

"It's hard work."

"Yes," Lily said. "It is."

"I'll type this up tonight, and we can try again tomorrow."

"Yes." And then she brightened a little. "Tomorrow is another day."

"Ah, well put," Linnett said, smiling. And when Lily didn't answer, she said, "Have you tried these cookies? God, they're unbelievably good."

Lily looked blankly at the plate. "Gaby . . . made them."

"Mmm. I know."

"Say what you will about Gaby," Lily said, drawing herself up. "She is a splendid cook."

"That *is* what I'll say," Linnett answered.

Lily took a cookie and bit it, began the long slow process of chewing and swallowing. When she was done, her hand at her throat as though to help push the food along, she looked brightly at Linnett and said, "Have I told you that we Fletcherized in my household when I was a girl?"

"No," Linnett lied.

"We did. Busy, busy. Too busy chewing to talk, virtually. How glad my father would be to see that Parkinson's has restored me to the habit." She smiled faintly.

"Just a sec," said Linnett, fishing in her backpack. "I'll get out the tape recorder."

And she set the little box on the table next to the cookies and the teapot. "Tell me about your father," she said, and watched Lily relax back in her chair. Her expressionless face somehow relaxed again too. (Later, she thought, she would try to find a way to describe how emotion could be revealed on the blank slate of a Parkinson's face.)

"A mean man," Lily said, almost sensually. "A narrow, narrow man. A man of his time, absolutely. He should have worn mutton chops, and it wouldn't have been out of place. Or out of character."

Linnett poured herself another cup of tea as Lily talked—unlocked, chattery, as if released from a spell. Her voice actually gained in strength as she went on, about the airless world she grew up in, the release into the freedom of her first illness. Linnett reached for the milk pitcher. She tilted it and watched the liquid purl white into the clear, reddish tea.

The next day, they tried again, with the same result, even though Lily took great pleasure, Linnett could tell, in the few typed sentences Linnett gave to her to get them started. Embarrassed and pained for the old woman, Linnett had turned them even more quickly back to conversation, and Lily, in her relief, was more garrulous, even more open than the day before, while her voice lasted. She talked contemptuously and at length on Linnett's tape about the appeal that community organizing "à la Alinsky," as she called it, had for a man like Paul, so used to what she called "the feminized world of the church." "And good works generally," she said. "After all, it was people like Jane Addams with settlement houses, you know *women*"—she let her voice nearly curl with disgust—"who'd by and large been engaged in this kind of good works before. Social workers. Social workers, and the church. Fuddy-duddies. All made fun of behind their backs, as well as to their faces. Poor Paul. And if you think of the civil rights movement at the start, even there there were certainly as many women as men. As many female martyrs. Rosa Parks. And think of those poor little girls.

"Alinsky didn't much like women, I think. As participants. And I can't help believing that some of the appeal his approach had was in restoring a sense . . . well, let's just say, juicing the whole thing up with some testosterone. You know, you could be good, doing good, but you could be manly too, at last. Tough. You could *swear*. It was the same thing black power did in *that* movement.

"Actually, as I think about it, it's probably why all of the movements on the left took this unpleasant turn. Unpleasant to the likes of me, of course. A woman. Silly me." Lily's hand rose to her unwomanly, flat bosom here; she sounded abruptly bitter. "Suddenly women were there just to provide sexual comfort, or to raise warriors for the race, to offer secretarial services. But the movements themselves, everyone at the center, was much more aggressively male. Bad guys. Tough guys. And that had tremendous appeal, I think, to these poor old church fellows."

Linnett asks an inaudible question here.

"Yes!" Lily says. "Silly. Ridiculous. And certainly not Christian. I was furious at Paul." She had stopped here, and shaken her shaking head. "That this long slow labor of love—and of course it *was* long, and slow and often tedious. That it should suddenly seem third-rate and false to him. When it was crystal-clear to anyone, or should have been, I thought, that they were just going for cheap thrills. Posturing. A mess of pottage indeed." She snorted. "It still makes me mad to think of it.

Even the OEO programs that came along later finally got sucked into that macho ... *baloney*, and ended up being discredited. These two-bit hoodlums with their federal salaries!" She paused, and her voice was calmer when she spoke again. "And it did, of course, absolutely nothing for the neighborhood, all that effort and all that money. I can't even bear to go over there anymore."

On Wednesday they'd taken the day off, at Linnett's suggestion. Noreen had helped Lily into the car, and Linnett sat in back with her crutches, and they went to Gaby's shop for a treat. Afterward they drove down to the docks. Noreen got out of the car and talked with several men she knew. Linnett and Lily, "the gimps" as Lily called them, sat and chatted desultorily. Linnett was fairly sure Lily fell asleep for a little while, her eyes shut against the bright glinting sunlight, surrounded by the voices and the noises of the men working, muted over water.

Today, Thursday, Linnett had arrived at Lily's with another idea, one that had occurred to her in the night. She suggested Lily just try speaking the story into the tape recorder by herself. "Maybe it's me, Lily. Maybe that's what's bothering you. You know, it's solitary, writing. It's a solitary process. It's a big adjustment to share it with someone else. I'd have a lot of trouble doing it, I'm sure of that."

Lily agreed to try, and Linnett showed her how the recorder worked and left her alone in her room, with the door shut. After a little more than an hour, she heard the bell ring. She was in the living room. Noreen had the contents of the refrigerator strewn across the kitchen counters. She was washing the refrigerator out. She had the radio on a talk station. Linnett called over to her. "It's Lily, Noreen. She's ringing for you."

Noreen stepped back from the refrigerator and looked at Linnett. "She rang? God, I didn't hear a thing."

"I can tell," Linnett said.

Noreen peeled off her yellow rubber gloves and went to

Lily's room. She was barefoot, and her feet thudded heavily across the floor. In a moment, she came back. "She wants you," she said to Linnett.

Linnett got up and went into Lily's room. Lily was sitting in her chair, erect and pale. The gray light from the windows fell sideways across her face, cruelly deepening every line.

"Got problems?" Linnett asked.

"It isn't going to work," Lily said.

"Is it the machine?" Linnett asked. "You want me to help you with it?"

"No," Lily said. Her voice was unusually strong. "It's *my* machine. My brain," she said. "It's something Parkinsonian that's happened in there." She tapped her forehead.

"What do you mean?"

"I mean, I can't do it, plain and simple. That ... " She paused, mouth open. "Well, you know, I'd thought it was just the physical act, writing ... that had gotten too difficult for me. But, in fact, I *can* write a letter. A weird-looking letter to be sure, but a letter. If I have to. It's too much work and I'd rather not if I don't have to, but I can. But I can't do this again. This kind of writing. It's over."

"You couldn't dictate it?"

"No. It was much the same as when you and I tried it together. I just can't make my mind ... stay on it. I want—or my *mind* wants. To go its own way. I just stop. It's ... it's Parkinson's. I feel it. It's the same way it is with moving. Or talking to you. Or walking with Noreen. If I'm asked to respond, if it's give and take, or if I'm moving beside her, it's fine. But it's too hard, alone. I just stop." She shrugged and faintly smiled.

Linnett sat down on the edge of Lily's bed, thinking. She rested her chin on her crutches. "Maybe there's a way. Something we could do we haven't thought of. Maybe some *way*, of talking it back and forth, and then I could, more or less, extract it. Extract the story, from our conversation."

"My dear. No." Lily's lips pressed firmly together. "That

would be uncomfortable, and humiliating, and nothing I even wish to try. There has to be some pleasure in it, after all, or why bother? And what I have discovered, with your help—and I'm honestly grateful to have discovered it—is that there is no pleasure in this effort. It's an effort to trick my mind into working in a way it no longer seems to want to work, and I find the trick tiresome."

"I'm so sorry," Linnett said.

"You needn't be."

"I am, though. I am, because you did have a story you wanted to write, and *I* did want to help you write it." Linnett felt suddenly swamped by pity for Lily.

Lily clearly heard it. "Now, now," she said. "The story is writing itself anyway. *On me*, don't you see?" She smiled faintly, as though trying to get Linnett to see a joke. "It was a story about an old woman, fooling herself, and then having to see that, and that is what I have seen. And you *have* helped me. There is always something truly . . . restorative, really, finally comforting, in learning what is true. In coming to the end of an illusion, a false hope. I trust I'm not beyond feeling such a thing honestly. That would be the proverbial fate worse than death."

"Oh Lily," Linnett said. Tears had sprung to her eyes. She had never liked her so well as at this moment.

"It's perfectly all right, my dear," Lily said. "And now, I think I'm going to have my rest very early today, and let you have the afternoon off, if you'd be so kind as to send Noreen back in."

"Of course," Linnett said. She picked up the tape recorder and rode her crutches to the doorway. There she stopped and turned back. She was going to say something—she wanted to say something—that might comfort Lily, something about how much she admired her.

But Lily had leaned her head against the back of her chair and closed her eyes. She looked very much the way she had the first day Linnett had seen her, collapsed in on herself, an abandoned puppet. Linnett went to fetch Noreen.

When she played the tape back at her house that afternoon, the tape of Lily alone with her story in her room, it was completely empty. Oh, occasionally Linnett could hear on it a clink or rustle, the stir of the gentle rain outside Lily's windows, or Lily herself shifting helplessly in her chair or clearing her throat. But of the tale she wanted to tell, not a word, not a whisper.

This is the article, of course, the article Linnett should write. The old woman who winds down. Who comes to a halt. It has everything she'd have to struggle to inject into a more ordinary story. Surprise. Pathos. A narrative shape.

She sighs and turns her monitor off. The rushing white noise of the computer itself continues. She pulls her crutches to her and rises onto them, moves to the front door. She opens it and stands, hunched down with the crutches in her armpits. The rain is steady and sibilant. It has plashed up from the deck and silver-dotted the mesh in the lower third of the screen door.

She could make it utterly sympathetic. That wouldn't be a betrayal, surely. She could give Lily all the dignity in the world. Make her a true heroine. As she is, Linnett thinks. As she truly is. For a moment, she considers calling Frank. He'd encourage her. He'd tell her there was no question. No problem. What was the big deal?

What *is* the big deal? After all, Lily had wanted Linnett to write about her, she had wanted the story, she had wanted the attention or the fame or whatever would result. So what if she hadn't known this about herself, that her writing days were over?

And hadn't she herself used other people's miseries in her memoir? Doesn't Lily's own history as a writer give Linnett a kind of permission?

Linnett has thought of asking Lily. But what would she say? "Do you mind if I write up this terrible moment and use it to make my article more sensational?"

Linnett snorts aloud. Come on. That's hardly the only way to look at it. It could be presented in any number of ways. She could say that it would be helpful to other Parkinson's sufferers to have Lily be so open about the disease. She could tell Lily that her audience, knowing so much of her personal life already, had some sort of sympathetic right or claim to this information too.

Linnett shivers and shuts the door. She moves slowly back to the empty chair facing the fireplace. There's a powerful, nostalgic odor of damp ashes rising from it. The room is cold, and Linnett would like a fire, but it's too much work, too much trouble.

Linnett doesn't want to ask Lily for permission. She doesn't want to ask because she's afraid Lily will say no. As long as she doesn't ask and Lily doesn't say no, she can do what she likes, write the story however she damned well pleases. And it will be a good story. A great story.

If she writes it.

chapter 8

The builder was still there, his red pickup truck angled against the back of the house. Alan hadn't expected it, and he was annoyed. He'd been coming to the site in the late afternoons recently, when he was sure to be alone. He'd gotten used to having it to himself. He liked poking around, slowly making notes, things to bring up. And he liked the moments of solitude just before he returned to his own house. Only the day before, a drizzly afternoon, he'd stopped by at about five. He'd stood in the empty shell of the house, the rain pelting outside, and looked down to the river. On the steely black water, a jewel glided, the iridescent striped sail of a lone windsurfer. Alan had stood and watched until the glowing colors rounded the bend in the river and disappeared.

Now Dave hailed him from the front deck. His voice was excited, and suddenly Alan saw why. The windows must have come today, they'd filled in half the wall facing the water.

This house, like Alan and Gaby's, was set on the riverbank, but unlike theirs, was entirely in an old sloping field, part of what had been one of the last dairy farms around here. It commanded a wide view down the river and over its other bank, out to the open sea in the distance. The land alone had cost the Admundsens, Alan's clients, more than three hundred thousand dollars. The budget for the house was four hundred thousand.

Even so these windows were an extravagance—a wall of them at double height facing the view, the panes all three by three. Alan stood in the open space where the living room would be and grinned with Dave at the way the first four panels looked.

Dave spoke now in a countrified way. "Yep, she'll do, I guess. In a pinch. Kinda cute really." He was a short, stocky man with a full black beard.

Dave and Alan had worked together often, and Alan was familiar with the nuances of Dave's vocabulary. It was only when he was deeply pleased that he was this inarticulate. Disapproval sharpened his use of language. He'd once called a detail Alan had worked out "hermaphroditic," because it used elements of two quite different styles.

But you could live with *hermaphroditic*. It was when something was "bogus," "incredibly bogus," or "quite extraordinarily bogus" that you had trouble with Dave. He'd grouse about it regularly. He'd delay doing it. Occasionally he'd complain to the clients, trying to form an aesthetic alliance with them. He'd once said to Alan that he found something he'd designed so extraordinarily bogus that he wouldn't be held responsible for building it. "Unless you give me a direct fucking order, I'm not going to do it."

"Fine," Alan said. "This is a direct fucking order then."

Dave hadn't spoken to him for several days after that, but he'd done what Alan told him to do, and in the end had to agree it wasn't as bad as he'd thought it would be.

They stood together now in the shell of the house. The meadow had been mowed recently. The air smelled of it, and of the raw wood around them. Alan nodded over and over, nearly giddy with pleasure. "You've made me a happy man, Dave," he said finally, and then realized, with some surprise, that this was true.

"Hell, this might even make the Admundsens happy, and that's going some," Dave said.

"They'll be out this weekend they think." Alan gestured to the windows. "Too bad you couldn't get them all in."

"You can see how it's going to look, though. Not a bad design. Not bad at all."

"Well, we'll see how he takes it. You can never be sure with him." Peter Admundsen had stood in the open platform of the house some weekends earlier, looked around slowly, and made his only comment: "This all feels much smaller than I thought it would."

Alan had reported this to Dave, and it had become the punch line in a series of dirty jokes the builders tossed back and forth as they worked.

Now Dave's dog arrived, a clot of wet black fur with a dopey grin, zigzagging through the framing, and it became clear that that's what Dave had been hanging around for. "Hey, *here* he is," he said. "Been fishing, you useless sack of bones." He looked up at Alan. "He spends all day down there and nothing to show for it. Why don't you get a paying job, you mutt?" He swiped at the dog affectionately.

"Anything he caught down there would have so much *E. coli* all you could use it for would be fertilizer anyway."

"Well goddammit Alan, you know, you're right. That's what he must do when he catches 'em, throws 'em back on account of excess *E. coli*."

They both laughed.

"He's not so dumb," Alan said.

Dave bent over the dog and hooked his finger under its collar. "See you next week, then," he said, pulling the dog toward the open doorway and then releasing him. "Good weather, Monday."

Alan watched him let the dog into the cab of the truck, then swing his tool kit into the back. After Dave had pulled away, Alan moved slowly around inside the building, and then hiked down the field to the river's edge and looked back up at it. The new windows glinted in the afternoon light.

It was too big. Sorry, Peter, he thought.

Alan had wanted something smaller or more horizontal on this land, and that was what he'd originally designed. He'd

done an elaborate, careful rendering of the plan to try to persuade the Admundsens. It hadn't worked. They had been clear
about their desires. They wanted a second floor, with a long
view. They wanted to lie in bed and watch the light change out
over the ocean.

It was going to be beautiful, Alan knew that, but if he lived
in the little shingle house across the river, he'd be pissed—he
knew that too—about having to stare across the water at the
glass palace opposite him.

Back inside again on this way to the car, he forgave himself,
he forgave the Admundsens. And it could be a lot worse for the
people across the water, he thought. It could be some garrison
colonial monstrosity. The Admundsens could be wanting to
make a lawn of the meadow. Alan had talked them out of that,
and into the ease of keeping it wild, mowing it a couple of
times a summer.

He climbed the ladder to the second floor—the staircase
wasn't built yet—and stood looking out through the top of the
new windows. Beyond the riverbank opposite, the ocean darkened in the blue distance. There were several tiny sailboats
moving nearly imperceptibly north into the harbor hidden
behind the riverbank. The Admundsens would have what they
wanted up here.

In fact, Alan had enjoyed their decisiveness, and even the
argument itself. He especially liked Peter Admundsen, a large,
unflinchingly direct man. He'd used the word *spine* with Peter
once in talking about the house. A mistake. They were sitting in
Alan's office in town, with the drawings spread out in front of
them, and Peter had asked a question about the flooring, about
which way it would run. Alan had indicated the direction he
thought it should go in, he'd said it wanted to run in that direction, because of the spine of the house.

"Oh, come on, Alan!" Peter had said. "The *spine*. It *wants to
go*. That's bullshit."

"Petie . . . " his wife began. She was big too, stout really, and
she treated Peter like a naughty, overgrown child.

"No, I mean it," Peter said to her. He turned back to Alan. "*You* want it to go in that direction. Why don't you just say that? I want it to go this way." He stabbed at the drawing. "And you want it to go that way. All this talk about *spines* and *wanting*—what are you trying to make yourself believe? That it's alive? That you're some sort of surgeon?" He snorted. "It's a matter of what you want and what I want. Period."

Alan had laughed. He had appreciated Peter's bluntness, and he tried after that to be more conscious of the jargon he sometimes used, he tried to be simpler in his explanations of why he believed certain things made sense for the house. And in the end, he thought, Peter had come to understand the house he would own better than most clients did. He felt he'd really taught him something about the building's integrity, about siting, as well as some simple facts about what could work and what couldn't.

And now the house they'd argued over was taking shape. Alan loved this stage of the building process, the first sense you had of the reality of the house, of the way this thing you'd thought so hard about would have its life in three dimensions. He felt an ease, a peace he hadn't felt in weeks as he moved around in the space.

He carried it home with him. And when he pulled out from under the overhanging trees at the foot of the drive to his own house, he was suddenly freshly pleased with it too, with its modesty, with the way it hugged the land.

Then he noticed: there was an extra car, a third besides Noreen's and Gaby's, parked in the drive. He pulled far over to the right to give it room to get out. Lily's friend, he thought. The amanuensis. He tried to remember what Gaby had said her name was, but couldn't.

When he opened the door, he could hear Lily's watery, onrushing voice, almost a whisper now. She was usually resting it for dinner at this hour of the day. Alan tried to time it this way: Lily in bed, Noreen gone or about to leave, Gaby still asleep.

But there was Noreen, doing something in the kitchen. The woman sitting with Lily looked over as he started across the room to the hallway for the bedroom. He tried to signal a greeting with his uplifted hand and keep walking, but Lily's looping sentence stopped and she called in an urgent whisper: "Alan!"

He turned and came back. Lily introduced him. The woman, the secretary, grinned up from her chair, her legs stretched out in front of her on a hassock, the toes of one foot sticking out from a dirty white cast. Her toenails were polished a dark red, Alan noted, narrow crescents of white grown in at the base. "Linnett?" he asked.

She nodded. "Baird," she said. Lily's whisper had been exhausted.

Alan reached out his hand to her, taking her in quickly. She was thirty-fivish, maybe a little older. She was slender, but big-boned, with long, wild hair turning gray in a frizzy tent around her head and shoulders. She had pale skin, touched with pink at the nostrils, the eyelids. She wasn't really pretty, but she had a kind of palpable sexual confidence that he'd always found attractive.

She stretched her hand up, and they shook. She withdrew her hand first. "I'd get up, but . . . " She shrugged.

"What happened?" Alan asked dutifully, withdrawing his hand. Her grip had been strong, firm.

"I was jogging. Now I jog no more." She seized her thigh above the cast with both hands and made a face. "Flab." The flesh dropped away from her fingers, marked with red from their pressure.

"It would be . . . confining," he said, feeling an odd embarrassment.

"Oh I can do anything I want to," she said glumly. "As long as I keep my damned *leg* straight out in front of me." And then she flashed a broad smile.

Alan laughed, and turned to meet Lily's sharp, appraising gaze in her otherwise blank face.

"*You're* running late today," he said. "I thought you'd be napping by now."

"Oh, I know," she whispered. Linnett looked quickly at her wristwatch. "But I was going on and on about myself and finding it so fascinating. As one does."

"Well, I'm getting Gaby up now, so you better quit soon if you want a rest before dinner."

"And I need to leave in about ten minutes," Noreen called over.

"Oh God, it's my fault," Linnett said. "I was a little late getting here, and we were having fun today, and we just went on much longer than usual."

"Oh you mustn't let *Alan* bully you dear," Lily said. "But I suppose Noreen does need to go home sometime. Noreen!" She tried to call it out, but the extra effort failed in her throat, the word was a croak.

"Noreen," Alan said. "I think Lily's ready to go."

Lily bowed her head to Alan. "My gallant interpreter," she whispered.

Alan grinned at her. She wouldn't bother him today. He felt too celebratory, he wouldn't let her. He leaned forward and helped her up. Her weight, pulling on his arm, was negligible.

Noreen was right there, easing Lily away from Alan. "Want your canes?" she asked Lily, a little too loudly.

"Oh, it's too much bother," Lily said. "Let's just do the Parkinson's shuffle together, shall we?"

"Fine with me," Noreen said. She smiled at Alan and Linnett Baird.

Together Alan and Linnett watched the two women move slowly back to Lily's room. Noreen's head was bent to Lily, and the old woman must have spoken, because Noreen laughed loudly, and said, "You're not kidding." The door shut behind them.

"I've been admiring your house," Linnett said, after a beat. Alan turned to her. She had her arm lifted to gesture around the room. She was wearing a sleeveless red blouse, and the flesh of her arm was white, the veins a faint blue map within. "Lily tells me it's yours in every sense—I mean, you designed it, too."

"Yes," he said. "Thank you. We're happy in it. Though there are always things you'd change." He made a vague gesture.

"Oh yeah, unlike the rest of life," she said.

Alan laughed. He sat down—just for a moment he told himself—on the edge of the chair Lily had been in. "And what do you do when you're not taking dictation from my distinguished mother?"

"More of same, I'm afraid."

"A sort of traveling secretary?"

"Oh. No, I'm not really a secretary." She made an odd face. She was a little put off, he thought. "This is just a deal I've struck with Lily."

"Oh?"

"Yeah, I'm a writer. A journalist. I'm writing about Lily actually. An article." She watched him for a moment. "Didn't you know that?" she asked. Then she smiled, the broad, easy grin. "No, you didn't. See, I just offered to help her with her mail and writing and stuff as a way to . . . well, I suppose, justify hanging around as much as I thought I'd want to."

"I see," he said. He was startled that he hadn't known this, and suddenly uncomfortable. "I see," he said again, and nodded.

"You don't like that, I think," she said. "Am I right?"

He shrugged. "It's not my business, is it? To like it or not to like it."

"Yeah, but you *don't*. Like it." She was smiling at him, but there was a note of irritation in her voice too. "C'mon. 'Fess up."

"What do you want me to say? No. I don't."

"Oh, I'm not hurt. I'm used to it. People either really, really like you, if you're a journalist, or they kind of really, really don't."

"It's just I don't want to be a part of it," he said coolly. "I don't want to be quoted, for instance. Or even make an appearance. 'The son of the famous . . . ' Whatever. You know. What Lily does is her business. Whatever . . . use she wants to make of her life. That's her business. But I . . . I've never been a part of any of it, and I don't want to start now."

"I understand." She was watching him intensely, with light eyes, her face utterly sobered.

"And I so much don't, that I don't even want to be quoted, directly or indirectly, as saying that in your article."

"I understand." She bobbed her head. "And believe me, Lily *is* my only interest here. This piece I'm doing?" Her eyebrows went up. "I think it's going to be pretty much standard fare. I mean, I hope it'll be better. Deeper. But the stuff that draws me to her is the same stuff"—her hand made a circle—"that everyone else has written about."

"Which is?"

"Well, it sure isn't you."

"But it is . . . ?"

"Uh, you know."

"No, I don't. I don't read about Lily when I can avoid it."

"Well, you know. The feminist angle. The woman at fifty, sixty, seventy, striking out on her own. And the racial stuff. Whether integration is a passé ideal. And the religious stuff too: the patriarchal nature of the church and all that."

"Patriarchal." He smiled. "A word I'm sure Lily has never used."

"Patriarchal?" Linnett tilted her head and smiled back at him. "Nope. You're right. And I actually don't either, except *as above*, to describe, to encapsulate, as it were, a way of talking. Or of thinking really. But you get my drift. What I mean, really, is that you have nothing to fear from me." She folded her hands neatly in her lap and rounded her eyes, a parody of innocence. "Honest."

Noreen came out of the guest suite.

"All set with her?" Alan asked, getting up quickly. He felt, somehow, caught at something.

"Yep. And I'm on my way, once I get my purse." She crossed the room to the kitchen island, hauled her enormous bag to her shoulder, and started back to the door.

"So long, Noreen," Linnett said. "I'll see you Monday."

Noreen stopped. "Oh, you're not coming in tomorrow?"

"No. I thought I'd give it a rest. Give Lily the weekend off."

"Well. Monday then."

Alan walked to the door, more or less behind Noreen, and stood there momentarily after she'd left in a kind of farewell. Outside, her big station wagon roared to life, unmuffled.

"Noreen doesn't like me," Linnett said, behind him.

"You think not?" He turned. "Why?"

"I *interfere*." She made a stern face. "She'd never say it, but I know it. They have their oh-so-peaceful mornings together. Monastically peaceful, really—Noreen out here, doing what, I'm not sure, and Lily alone in her room with her *things*, as she likes to call them. And then I hobble in and wind Lily up. In Noreen's space, at that." She gestured around her. "No place to hide, the way you designed it." She was smiling at him, as though she were teasing him. "But at any rate, she gets an earful." She sighed. "You can't ask for more than that in life. Can you?"

Alan came back and sat down again, again just on the edge of the chair. "I suppose the odd earful is the cornerstone of your business."

"I suppose it is. Whereas *your* cornerstone is more like your honest-to-god basic cornerstone."

"I suppose it is."

They were smiling at each other. My, my, thought Linnett, at the sense of the possibility in the air. Or was she imagining it? "How *is* business?" she asked.

"What do you mean?"

"Oh, just I know it's a slow time for construction. I know this 'cause I *read* the papers."

How odd her inflections were, Alan thought. Almost as odd as Gaby's, which came from another language. Linnett's, though, were her own, a quirk, apparently. "Well, so far I've been lucky," he said. "It's slow, certainly. But this is a wealthy community. Well, partially wealthy anyway. And with land prices generally lower now—still absurdly high by any rational standard, of course—anyway, there's the occasional house to build. Or addition." He shrugged. "But I've had a couple of mighty slow years."

"Oh God, haven't we all."

Alan had just started to speak again, to ask her how that went in her business, what "slowness" was, when there was a little mechanical noise, a clicking, and she started abruptly forward, picked up a small black box he hadn't noticed from the corner table.

"Oops. Tape's over," she said. "I forgot about it."

"This was all taped," he said.

"Yeah, I'd been taping Lily, earlier."

He leaned back, grinning. "Jesus," he said. "*Trust* me, she says."

Linnett was smiling too. "I forgot all about it."

"Yes and no, I suspect."

"Well, yes and no," she said. "Hey!" She pointed at him. "You didn't give me anything anyway."

"I don't know anything to give you."

"Oh, I suspect you do. You're Lily's child, after all."

He snorted. "Motherhood was not Lily's strong suit."

"Ah?" she said.

He looked steadily at her, and then shook his head.

She laughed. "I should say 'Ah!' I mean, *there's* a gift, if I wanted to use it. 'Motherhood was not Lily Maynard's strong suit,' and you take off from there." She shrugged, watching him.

"Do it, and I'll break your other leg," Alan said, smiling back at her.

And now, suddenly, Gaby was there in the open doorway to the back hall, puffy-eyed, looking from one of them to the other, Alan and Linnett, slouched in their chairs. Their voices had finally waked her, a full twenty minutes past the time Alan usually got her up, past the time he usually sat and talked with her. She was befuddled, still remembering a dream she'd waked with, a dream that her brain, moving toward consciousness, told her she should save to tell Alan, who wasn't there. Who was here.

"Hello," she said. And cleared her throat. "Hello," she said again.

Linnett started, then turned to reach for her crutches.

Alan stood quickly. "You're awake," he said, taking two steps toward her, then stopping almost in the middle of the room to watch Linnett, who was struggling with the crutches, trying to get up.

"Yes," she said. "I'm late to the shop."

"I'm sorry," he said. "I got talking."

"*I'm* terribly sorry," Linnett said. "It's all my fault, Gaby. I stayed on later with Lily than I was supposed to, and then I waylaid Alan too. I've been *bad*." She was balanced on one foot now, and she began to shove things into her backpack.

Gaby watched her stupidly for a moment before saying, "Oh, it hardly matters."

Alan stepped back toward Linnett. "Can I help you with that?"

"Yes," said Gaby, suddenly seeming awake, moving toward Linnett too. "Let us help."

"Oh, thanks, no," Linnett said, "I've learned to manage it." She looked at Gaby again. "Really, I'm so sorry to have stayed this long. The time just kind of flew by with Lily, and I didn't notice how tired she was getting, how late it was."

"It's all very nourishing to Lily, I'm certain of that," Gaby said.

Linnett swung her backpack up over one shoulder and propped herself on her crutches.

"Do you have far to go?" Alan asked her in a new, polite voice.

She looked at him, amused, he thought. "Oh no. I'm just down the road a couple of miles."

"Where are you staying?" Gaby asked.

"I've rented a little house. A little cottage kind of thing. At the Thayers'? Do you know them? On their sort of enormous property. It's charming, really." They'd begun to follow behind her as she clumped to the door.

"So you're all alone?" Gaby made it sound tragic.

Linnett turned around and laughed quickly. "Yes," she said. "Completely solitary."

"Well, but this isn't right," Gaby said. She looked over at Alan, who was already by the door, waiting to hold it open for Linnett. Linnett could sense a kind of signal pass between them. "I didn't realize you were ... At any rate, why don't you stay? Stay for dinner. You can wait here, if you don't mind." She gestured back toward the open room. "And have some wine or something, while we go to the store. We have to close it up, but we won't be much more than forty-five minutes or so, really."

Linnett turned to Alan, behind her at the door. His face was as blank as a child's. As Lily's. He didn't want her to stay then.

"It's no trouble, I promise you," Gaby was saying. "I work with food, you know, and often I bring dinner home, which is what I planned for tonight. It will be simple, but good. If I say so myself."

"Well," Linnett said, looking back at Gaby. "That's a tempting offer, all right."

"Then it's settled," Gaby said. She looked at Alan again, and then quickly back to Linnett.

"Well," Linnett said. "Thank you. That's lovely." She turned and smiled brilliantly, warmly, at Alan. "That's so kind of you all." Her voice became a little Southern, suddenly. "Ah will."

chapter 9

After Alan and Gaby had left, Linnett got up again and hobbled slowly around the big room. Though she'd been coming to Lily for three weeks, she hadn't yet been left alone in the house. Now she hunkered on her crutches in the kitchen area. She pulled open the handsome drawers, noted the array and arrangement of gleaming utensils—the matching knives, the whisks, graduated in size, the measuring things. There were two fancy ovens, she saw. More amazingly, two dishwashers. The refrigerator was one of those huge, stainless steel things with the freezer on the bottom. When she slid open the packed freezer drawer, the first thing that caught her eye was a package of frozen duck breasts, round and white as snowballs. Duck breasts! She snorted and shut the drawer.

She came out from behind the island. At the other end of the long living room was the piano. Linnett worked slowly over to it and sat down. She leaned her crutches against the bench. She struck a few chords. Who played? she wondered. The son—Alan—seemed somehow an unlikely candidate, but you never knew. Linnett had had a lover once who'd never mentioned such a talent in the months they'd slept together, but at a party at someone else's house sat down and improvised the blues expertly for more than an hour. Linnett had felt betrayed, somehow, that she hadn't known he could do this.

Betrayed, and aroused, she recollected now.

Linnett herself played a little, but the only things she knew by heart were leftovers from long ago: "Für Elise." The opening bars of the "Moonlight Sonata." The piano's tone was marvelous though. It made even her primitive fumbling sound musical and rich. Quite a little toy indeed.

Then she remembered Lily and stopped abruptly. No need to wake her. An affectionate and unlikely picture rose quickly in her mind of the old woman, curled like a baby on her side in sleep. She'd worn her out today.

After yesterday's final defeat at writing and Lily's brave acceptance of it, Linnett had arrived this afternoon determined to make the time easy for Lily, easy and lighthearted. She'd concocted a series of harmless questions that would lead Lily into those corners of her life she seemed most relaxed in.

And it had worked. Lily had talked at length and animatedly about her mother, about her college years and Paul's courtship of her, about the first inkling she had that she might have a gift as a writer. Linnett had kept her going with one open-ended question after another, and hadn't really even noticed as Lily's voice lost strength.

Nor had Lily. She'd been taking something, Linnett felt, from the memories, from the sense of herself they brought to her, and Linnett was unwilling to stop her, she wanted so much to help. She'd been amazed when she looked at her watch after Alan arrived, to see how late it was, how long she'd kept Lily at it.

She got up now and made her way down the hallway to the room Gaby had emerged from. The bedroom. The door was open. The bed was unmade, a tangle of white sheets with a faded, frayed quilt sliding off to the floor. The view out these windows—they were French doors, really, left flung open to the winds—was over the deck toward the river too, but it was a little more overgrown at this end than in front of the living room windows.

What was she looking for? She didn't know, but she couldn't not have looked.

There was a group of family pictures sitting in tilted frames on the bureau top. Linnett crossed to them and picked them up one by one. Children and parents in various combinations over the years, the kids gradually becoming young men. There was a picture too of Alan and Gaby, very young, in what looked like a French restaurant.

Of course, they must have met in France. This American life, this house on a river in a town of comfort and bourgeois safety, was just the way it had all turned out. In the picture, Alan's hair was longer than Gaby's: it must have been the sixties or early seventies. They were bent toward each other, each resting elbows on the table, and the person taking the photo seemed to have startled them.

Gaby was ready to be startled. Her quick glance toward the camera was sly, flirtatious: oh, me? Alan had had to turn a little over his shoulder to see the person taking his picture. Maybe he'd been saying something intimate to Gaby. I adore you. I must have you. At any rate, he was frowning at the intrusion, he seemed almost alarmed.

He was incredibly handsome, Linnett thought. She felt a pang of resentment for Alan and Gaby, for the romance implicit in this picture. For the luck of the way it had all turned out.

Linnett set the picture down and pushed the door next to the bureau open: the bathroom. It was all tiled in here, a pale greenish-blue. There was no tub, per se, but a tiled box you stepped down into. Room for two, Linnett saw. Cozy. Next to it, on the floor, a stack of sumptuous big towels in a matching color. There was a bidet, a pedestal sink. Who had this sybaritic taste? The pretty, slightly plump French wife, formerly of the gamine charm? Or Alan, so skinny and seemingly sober?

Until he laughed, Linnett thought. Then he was a very attractive man. And he'd been attracted to her too, she could tell.

Linnett went back into the bedroom, stood at the foot of the bed. Each of them had a nightstand. The one she took to be Alan's was neat, books stacked just so, the clock squared against them. On the other side of the bed, closer to the French doors, the books and magazines were splayed out on the table and even on the floor around it. Down there too, a pair of flowered underpants. A sock. Some cooking magazines, Linnett saw. She started to move toward the heap, when a door banged in the house.

A voice, male: "Anybody home?"

Linnett teetered, then decided quickly: the deck. She will have been out on the deck. Yes, looking at the view. She moved herself carefully toward the screen doors. She pushed them gently open with her body and eased herself out. She was breathing deliberately, slowly and evenly.

Once she made it safely outside, she exhaled. Ah. No rush now. The question occurred to her only after a moment, her heart calming in the light hiss of the breeze through the pine trees at this end of the deck: who was this? Some friend, meandering in for a drink, maybe. Someone connected with Alan's work. Or Gaby's. Mighty familiar, in any case. Linnett moved down the deck toward the glass wall to the living room.

And then a wash of rich sound, of music—the piano!—poured over her and she stilled. It was some adagio, Linnett didn't know it, but the yearning chords slowly pulsed out the opened doors at the living room end of the deck. Linnett, suddenly cradled in the lush sound, was caught unawares. Tears sprang to her eyes. She closed them and stood frozen for several minutes, letting herself be held in the sound, in the light air, in the sense of deep desire and loss the music carried.

Then there was a hitch. The music stopped abruptly. "Ah, *fuck!*" the voice said, and there was a deedley jazz riff, a little ragtimey dance. Linnett felt as though someone had slapped her. She opened her eyes and moved down the deck to where she could see through the reflection of herself to the figure inside on the piano bench. A big kid: dark, curly hair, gangly body, all elbows from the back.

After a minute of that fooling around, the music, the real music, started again. Linnett, more cautious now, hobbled to one of the wooden chairs on the deck and lowered herself slowly. The music swelled around her once more, and she closed her eyes again and leaned back in the chair, greedy for it. The audience.

The Gaby in the picture Linnett had looked at with envy was about to step from one world into another. Alan had been in Paris for only a few weeks this time. It was early September, and he had to go back to architecture school in only a few days. And Gaby had decided to go with him, to go to America.

In the photograph they're sitting in a little restaurant near St. Sulpice. They're celebrating. Alan is spending nearly all the money he has left on their meal. It is a moment of unalloyed happiness for him, a moment he always remembers for that, for the purest joy he's ever known. Looking at this photograph now sometimes has the power to call him back to a sense of that possibility.

Gaby, happy as she was then, was also more practical. She saw Alan more simply as the answer to the dilemma that was then her life.

She had met him three years before, when she was in love with someone else. Alan was in France for a semester with an American exchange program, and he was placed for six weeks in her house because she had a brother two years younger—Alan's age—and her parents thought it would be a wonderful opportunity for him to perfect his English. What she remembered of Alan then was how handsome he was, and how shy, how silent around her. She was home only a few times a week for family meals, to do her laundry and the like, so she couldn't have been said to have come to know him, but she understood he had a crush on her. Everyone in the family understood that. They joked about it sometimes in French too rapid, too idiomatic for him to catch, and he sat among them and smiled sweetly, waiting for their laughter to be explained. She thought of him at that time as the beautiful American. She spoke of him that way to her lover, Gerard. "Be careful," she would say, "or I'll run off with the beautiful American."

Alan, actually, knew a great deal more about her. The brother his age—there were three other, younger children as well—was a font of willing, scandalous information. And of course, there were family photographs around, stories he pumped from her mother about her childhood. When he went back to the States, he wrote her occasionally, very short, friendly notes. His intention was simply to keep himself alive in her memory. The first one thanked her for her kindness to him while he was in France. He said he would never forget her. It was signed, "Your American brother, Alan." Later notes would report that he thought of her, would tell her about whatever was changing in his life—he had decided to become an architect, he was accepted at graduate school, he finished college.

Meanwhile, Gaby's life was unraveling. In the explosions of the late sixties, she was trapped and divided by her loyalties. She wasn't bold enough for Gerard, and she was far too radical for her parents. While all of Paris, all of France—all of the world, it seemed—convulsed, she stood and watched. When it was over, she followed Gerard to the country near Dijon where he and five or six friends of his had rented a house they were all going to live in together, communally. But sex was part of what was being shared, and this was impossible for Gaby, as she discovered. She came back to her parents, where she lived for a few weeks surrounded by chilly silence; and then she found an attic apartment off the Rue Monge, and a job tutoring foreign businessmen in French.

She had sent a postcard or two to Alan in response to his notes the first year after he'd left. Nothing after that. But her brother had kept him informed in a general way of Gaby's path in life. (Not of her misery, because her brother couldn't see that.) When Alan came back to France in 1970, he had a tiny grant from architecture school to research the shape and func-tioning of town squares in various medieval villages in Europe, but his aim, his goal, was to present himself as an adult to Gaby and to win permission to woo her.

In mid-June, he checked into a youth hostel near the Marais, and walked the distance to Gaby's apartment, wishing, actually, that it were even farther, that the approach would take even longer. He wanted to be walking toward her forever. He saw himself from time to time in a storefront window, and was startled that he looked so much himself, striding along, tall and skinny in blue jeans and an old jacket, his long pale hair lifting in the light breeze that stirred too in the fresh green of the trees. He felt so transformed by his mission, his desire, that it seemed he should also, somehow, look different.

She wasn't home. He left a note for her. To his surprise, he had a message waiting by the time he returned to the hostel at the end of the day. It stated a place and a time she would meet him the next day. He almost didn't recognize her in the cafe. She'd cut nearly all her hair off, and gotten very thin.

But she didn't disappoint him. She'd ordered a drink, a clear liquid in a small glass, and she was smoking a strong-smelling, unfiltered French cigarette. She talked, excitedly, in her rhythmic, lilting French, slowed down for his benefit, about her tutoring job. She mocked the businessmen she worked with—their accents, their clothing. She asked him about himself and expressed interest in his project, her eyes steady on him, her mouth slightly opened, a faint smile sometimes playing on it. She was as nervously animated, as brittle and charming, as Alan remembered her.

What Alan couldn't tell was that this was an effect he was having on Gaby. She had thought her life was over. She had unfitted herself, as she saw it, for every universe she might have occupied. She had made a mistake too, in taking an apartment near the Sorbonne. It pained her to be surrounded by students. Though many of them were the same age as she, or only slightly younger, Gaby felt used up, damaged, as she moved among them. She was twenty-five.

Now here came Alan, offering her a version of herself she

had thought no one—not even herself—believed in anymore. And Gaby became for him the person she'd once been. What she thought about it was that this was fun, this was good for her. She would flirt with him and repair herself.

But Alan wasn't willing just to be flirted with, just to adore her, though it wasn't actually until a few days before he left for the summer's project, having idled much longer than he meant to or was supposed to in Paris, that he talked to her openly about it. He insisted, actually, on taking her to dinner, which she knew was a great expense for him. They went to the tiny, very good neighborhood place near St. Sulpice (the same place the picture would be taken later, in September), and before the meal even started—they had eaten only the appetizer—he blurted out that he wanted her to think about coming back to America with him.

"What!" She laughed, excitedly. "You mean, to live with you?"

"Yes. Exactly. No, to marry me, actually." His hands nervously played with the heavy silverware at his place.

"Alan." Her head tilted. Did he mean it? "But this is mad."

"It is not mad. It's what I want. I'm sure of it."

Gaby's face was flushed with pleasure. She was flattered and thrilled, though she didn't take him seriously.

She persisted in her amused resistance. They argued first in the abstract—was this mad or not? Could this be a way people began a marriage or not? How well did you need to know someone to be in love?

Finally Gaby leaned forward, her elbows on the table, and said in a lowered voice, "But Alan. My dear. We haven't even slept together."

He smiled at her. "Well, that's easily remedied."

"No, no. What I mean to say is, you don't even know really, if we're compatible in that way."

"Yes, I do. We are," he said.

"Pffft," Gaby made a dismissive noise, and a gesture with her hand. "Perhaps. Perhaps not. And then what? If not?"

"Gaby." His voice was intense. "I've watched you move. I've watched you ... set a table. Light a cigarette. Walk away from me down the street. I know. I'd be only too happy to demonstrate this, how right I am. How *correct* I am, about this. Any time you'd like a demonstration. But I don't want to get distracted here. I want you to think about this while I'm gone. And what I want, when I come back in September, is for you to say you'll come home with me."

Gaby sat across the table and looked at him with her mouth open. There was a candle on the table. Its light glittered in the tears that suddenly sat on the lower rims of her eyes. He felt that she was truly seeing him for the first time, that she was feeling the stirrings of what would be a deep and abiding love for him.

She was thinking of the last argument she'd had with Gerard, which had begun when she told him she'd slept with both of the other men they were living with. He had said carelessly, "As you wish, Gaby. I don't own you," and she had slapped him.

She looked away, now. Down at her hands, back at Alan. Here he was, this beautiful child, really, from another universe, saying the things she'd wished to hear from someone else.

"I think we'd better have the demonstration," she said.

At this moment, the waiter came with their dinner plates. They both looked up, startled, as if they'd been under a spell he'd just broken.

"Oh, waiter!" Alan said. "Look, we'll just have the check please."

"But you've ordered the prix fixe, sir."

Gaby grinned.

"Yes, that's fine. We'll pay for the prix fixe. We'll have coffee." Somehow Alan felt this was a compromise. "And then the check. Please."

In the dark of the little hallway that opened into Gaby's two attic rooms, he held her. He whispered, "You'll tell me what to do to please you. Whatever you want, I want to do.

You be the French woman, I'll be the American boy."

Gaby knew this was a kind of joke, and she laughed, hoarsely, but it thrilled her too, the idea of the power she had over him, a power she'd never had before, with anyone. She was panting a little from the long climb up the stairs, from excitement. She could feel his heart pounding in his chest. "Kneel down," she said.

He did. She placed her hands on his head for balance and stepped out of her shoes. She kept her hands in his hair—this thick hair, longer than hers! His face was tilted up to her in the dark, she could see its whiteness, the black hole of his mouth. He was panting too. She touched his lips.

"Lift my skirt," she whispered, and when he did, she moved her own hands to push down the black tights she wore.

How could Alan have been so sure? How could he have loved Gaby so convincingly when, in fact, he did hardly know her? Perhaps it was the idea of Gaby he loved, and the idea of someone loving her that she loved.

He knew very precisely, of course, where she came from: the old suburban house with its ordered garden, the lush vines hugging the trellises, the windows curtained in lace. He knew the concern for grace that marked the way she'd lived in that house, the particular way coffee was always made in the morning, the careful presentation of food, the long ritual meals. He knew very precisely her relations to those people who lived there, he knew the formal solicitudes that marked these relations.

And these were the very things Alan had never had. Even before his parents' divorce, there had been nothing encircling, nothing comforting or sensual in his home. Lily was a terrible cook and an indifferent server of meals. The things they did together, as a family, usually involved going out to something uplifting—to hear music, a preacher; to see paintings. Though Paul Maynard could often be a warm and loving man—it was he who read to the children, who played games with them,

Parcheesi and Monopoly, and later chess, until they got the TV—both he and Lily felt that the raising of the children was her job, as the church was his. But Lily's capacity for affection unfortunately seemed exhausted by the single-minded and intense focus she had on him, her husband. There was always a sense among her children of feeling shut out from that love. It seemed to make everything Lily and Paul shared—their religion, their joint intellectual pursuits, certainly anything sexual—very much a secret between them. (Later Clary and Alan had talked about this, actually, about how Lily and Paul seemed to assume that the children would understand and partake of their lives' deepest meaning without anything ever having been made explicit about that, without any effort having been made to include them. They would be offered the things that Lily and Paul had had, a fine education, a religious upbringing—in the sense of Sunday school and confirmation and prayers at home on a regular basis. They would have sexual information from excellent books written specifically for this purpose. But there would be a great silence about what all this was to mean or what it had meant to Lily and Paul. And the divorce then held all of it up for questioning anyway.)

When daylight slowly filtered into Gaby's tiny apartment, Alan hungrily watched the objects in the room emerge from darkness. There was a little bamboo chair in the corner, spindly and knuckled, and hooked over its back, a furled umbrella slowly revealed as red. There was a striped cloth draped over the tall, narrow chest of drawers, and a vase of flowers resting on that. The walls were a deep, intense blue. Even the laundry strung neatly on a line across the opened casement window, a bra, black tights, two pairs of white underpants—glowing flags in the dawn—seemed arranged to give pleasure.

The tiny table he could see through the doorway to the other room had a white cloth on it. And when Gaby had gotten up between their bouts of lovemaking in the night—they were both ravenous since they'd eaten so little dinner—there were bread and cheese in the next room she could fetch. There was wine. They sat cross-legged on the bed and Gaby served them, spreading the cheese on the ovals of bread she lifted one by one from a little basket she'd carried in. In all of this Alan felt a sense of order, of sacrament, as strong as anything he'd ever felt in church.

And so it was that Alan lay in Gaby's bed for the next two and a half days—except for those hours she was at work—and used all his powers of persuasion, his body, his words, to try to win her. And when he came back from his travels at the end of the summer and she said yes, they went to the same restaurant they'd gone to in July to finish the meal they'd begun then, and an American friend of Alan's happened by as they sat there and took a picture of this extraordinary moment in their lives.

It wasn't until they were living in the United States, in his apartment just over the Somerville line from Cambridge, that Alan thought to ask Gaby much of anything about her life, that he found out that she'd needed him as much as he'd needed her, that she'd taken the life he'd been imagining her in for the three years he waited to woo her and smashed it up with a deliberate and reckless abandon equal to that of all the students who had hurled paving stones at the police. Perhaps most wounding was to learn that Gaby's engagement to Gerard had ended not because she left him, as her brother had reported in a letter to Alan—it was, after all what Gaby told the family—but because of his indifference to her.

They married anyway, but Alan couldn't help believing at that time that something had changed in him forever, some capacity for deep feeling. Gaby had been like a bright flame burning within him for more than three years. Everything he knew about her was holy to him, and something hardened in him when she explained those years of her life. He felt like a child. He felt humiliated. He felt he'd needlessly, uselessly given Gaby some power over him that he wished to seize back.

And after a fashion, he did. It was the early seventies, after all. There was the sense abroad that all vows, all institutions were worth reexamining or reinterpreting, even a marriage vow newly made. Alan began sleeping with others.

This was something Gaby could understand, though it hurt her. She felt by acceding to it she was helping Alan do something necessary for himself. And she didn't feel it was important to tell him the one time she too took a lover—though it also felt like something necessary for her.

By the time Thomas was born in 1972, they felt settled enough, sure enough of themselves and each other to put all that behind them, to turn eagerly, tempered by fire, they felt, and truly adult, to the life they could make together.

Now Thomas sat on the deck his father had designed to woo his wife a second time and talked to Linnett about his parents. By coincidence, he was almost exactly the same age Alan was when he went to France to win Gaby the first time. "Their *lives* I mean, are just so . . . ordinary," he said. He had gotten them each a beer from the refrigerator. The sun was still high in the far western sky, but the sky itself was beginning to be touched with pink above the trees on the opposite bank of the river. Linnett was facing him. Her long frizzy hair was lighted from behind in a wild corona around her head.

She made a face that pinched her features. "Come *on*! Everyone says that about their parents. More originality please."

He grinned. He was taken with Linnett, delighted to have found her here on what he'd thought would be the standard night at home. (She'd applauded from the deck when he'd finished playing. He'd spun around on the bench to stare at her, hunched over the crutches, standing in the open screen doorway to the deck. "Who *are* you?" she'd said.

"More important," he'd answered, "who are you?")

"Okay, here's the thing," he said. "You know about my grandparents, right?" She nodded. She'd told him she was writing an article on Lily. "Well, their marriage was like, this intense thing."

"Intense, schmintense. As it happens, your parents' marriage is the one that lasted."

"*Lasted!*" he said contemptuously.

She smiled. "Someday you won't think of it as such an easy achievement."

A thought occurred to him. He drank his beer, watching her. He set the bottle down on the arm of his wooden chair. He hadn't brought out glasses for them, and Linnett hadn't objected. "Are you married?" he asked.

"No longer."

"Oh, you're divorced."

"Yes. Like half the rest of the world. And I wouldn't ever look down my nose at someone who'd made it work."

"Hey. I wasn't looking down my nose. It's just not what I want for myself, is all. You know, the house in the little town." He gestured vaguely around him. "The kids, the routine."

"Well, if you get your wish, you probably won't be able to have those anyway." He'd told her he was studying piano, that he hoped, maybe, for a career playing.

After a moment, looking at her, he asked, "When you were married, what kind of life did you have?"

"On balance"—she nodded judiciously—"I'd have to say shitty."

He laughed and she smiled back at him. Then she said, "But only because it took so long, so very long, to fall apart. We had a lovely beginning. Lots of fun." She shook her head, remembering Frank then. Herself.

"Was he a writer too?"

"Yeah. And a teacher. *My* teacher, as a matter of fact. Of journalism. Therein lies the et cetera, et cetera. Once I began to be as successful as he was, the shit hit the fan, as we used to so charmingly say." She took a deep swig of the beer. "It reminded me, actually—my marriage—of your grandmother's marriage. Or rather, Lily's book reminded me of my marriage. I think that's partly why I wanted to write about her. Because of that pattern, you know, of catching up with the person who's taught you something? Maybe even passing them, or surpassing them—this is as I *saw* it of course. And of course how Lily saw hers too. Anyway, how that all plays out. I really identified with their conflicts, Paul's and Lily's. With her disillusionment. You know, I saw why that made it end."

"But it was so fucking high-minded in the meantime, that's what interests me about it. God, even the way it ended was high-minded." His legs and feet, as he spoke, were in constant, jiggling motion.

"Well, yes and no."

"Yes! I mean, you've read it, right?"

"Yeah, and so I know how Lily saw it anyway. But maybe she was just tired of him." Linnett was peeling the damp label off her beer bottle with her fingernail. "Let's say she started to think he was kind of a . . . jerk, really. And used that high-minded stuff as a way of . . . being high-minded about that. Instead of just saying, 'Gee, you know, I actually find you kind of dorky now.' I've heard of worse strategies."

"God, you're cynical."

She shrugged and smiled at him. "I need to be cynical in my job. Or at least very, very careful whenever anybody uses the word—hmm: the words?—high-minded around me."

"I would hate that. Being that way."

Thomas spoke fiercely, and in the conviction, Linnett could hear it, that he would escape this. *Oh my dear,* she thought, but she said to him, "Sometimes I do." And gripping the edge of the label, tore a jagged strip straight down through its middle.

chapter 10

In the shop, Gaby and Alan worked with a practiced ease, silently. They hadn't really spoken on the way over, either. Alan was annoyed with her, Gaby knew, for having invited Linnett to dinner. Well then, he shouldn't have flirted with her. Gaby could tell the moment she entered the room that that's what had been going on. It was an unconscious gift of Alan's, flirtation—Gaby saw Ettie as having inherited it from him—and she never even thought about it when he used it with their friends, or with clients. But every now and then it startled her, as it had this afternoon, and before she'd really even taken it in, she'd asserted her claim on Alan by transforming Linnett into a guest of both of theirs.

Though she might have asked her to stay anyway, even without the sparks in the air. It was always Gaby's impulse to enlarge the table, and now, with Lily here, she welcomed almost any addition, to keep Alan from getting angry or upset with his mother over the meal.

She looked at him now. He was wiping the shop counters, bending, putting all of himself into it. Ah Alan. He was so dear to her, and she'd been feeling so far apart from him. She moved to him, encircled his waist from behind, and when he stopped, rested her head on his back. Her head came just between his shoulder blades, and she could feel the broad, flat muscles of his back under her cheek.

"Don't be angry," she said, after a moment.

He turned around in her arms and cupped her cheeks in his hands, tilting her head back. "I thought we'd be alone after we got old Lil to bed."

"Ah." She nodded. "Well, we wouldn't have anyway in all likelihood. Thomas phoned this afternoon, and he's probably coming down for the night."

"You mean, if nothing better turns up."

She smiled. "That wasn't precisely what he said. He needs to borrow a car to get down here, and he wasn't entirely sure he'd be able to."

"Nonetheless."

She swayed against him. "You were having a nice time flirting with Miss Whatyoumacallit." Gaby pronounced this very exactly, as no American would, and Alan was charmed, suddenly, and intensely aware of the pressure of her compact body against him.

He smiled at her. "I was thinking of you. Every moment."

"Hmm. I shall try to believe you. Still, she seems a nice woman."

"Nice enough, I guess."

They rocked slightly in each other's arms for a moment.

"What is it Lily is telling her, do you suppose?" Gaby asked dreamily. "I mean, it's all there in the books, wouldn't you say?"

He lifted his shoulders. "Dark secrets."

"But there are precisely no secrets anymore."

Alan sighed. "One would think. But there's always more to come, with Lily."

"Hmm." Gaby leaned her head back and looked at him. "What would you like for dinner? Out of all you survey." It was her habit to bring home parts of dinner from the shop. Soups and vegetable dishes in winter. Salad, cold pastas in summer. Cheeses. Breads, desserts.

He bent down and bit her earlobe. "A little of this," he said. "A little of that."

She moved her body against him and felt, slowly, the stirring of his erection. Her hand reached down and rested on it. "Hmph. Perhaps you could make yourself a little *more* useful, dear."

Alan smiled. This was a joke between him and Gaby, a joke on Lily. She'd said it to Gaby the first time they'd met. They'd been trying to converse—Gaby's English was still fairly rudimentary at this stage—and Lily, visibly impatient, had finally left the room to prepare dinner. Gaby, not knowing what else to do, trailed her to the kitchen. After a moment of watching Gaby stand there awkwardly, Lily had taken pity on her. She'd thrust some onions and a knife over the table toward her. "Here, perhaps you could make yourself useful, dear," she said.

The knife was unspeakably dull, had probably never been sharpened, and was flimsy to boot, not intended for this task. The onions were being cut up for kidney stew, one of Lily's morally edifying meals. On the table in front of Gaby, there was an opened can labeled *gravy*, with a horrible, brownish pudding in it. Gaby realized abruptly that this was a two-way street, that if she was failing Lily on the basis of some standards she couldn't have named or guessed at, Lily was likewise a failure in a world she understood and Lily knew nothing of. Lily had used paper napkins that evening too, and as she unfolded hers and laid it across her lap, Gaby had the sense that she would not have to be afraid of her mother-in-law again.

Now she and Alan separated and went back to their chores. Gaby disappeared into the kitchen, carrying a tray of cheeses. Alan finished wiping off the counters, and then began to bag the day-old bread. He was lost in thought: the Admundsen house. Peter. Gaby's hand, warm on him. Linnett Baird.

The door rattled. He looked up. It was one of the kids who seemed to hang around the center of town all day, Alan recognized him. He wore the uniform they'd taken to—the baseball cap turned backward, the voluminous shorts that hung below the knees. Alan pointed to the sign in the door. "Closed," he shouted.

"C'mon man," he heard the kid whine.

Alan shook his head and went back to work.

There was the sharp slam of the kid's fist on the door, the rattling vibration of the glass. "Asshole!" the kid shouted.

Alan felt the adrenaline of rage so powerfully he didn't even want to look at the kid again. He quickly turned and went into the kitchen, his breathing slightly accelerated.

Gaby was moving around back here, from the counters to the big walk-in refrigerator. Watching her, he tried to calm himself, but abruptly he saw the kid's face again, the sullen, stupid look under the half-moon of the baseball cap's opening. He wanted to hit him, to cause damage.

He remembered Linnett Baird then, the cast on her leg, her fingers gripping the white flesh above it, leaving their red print on it as it fell back. He had been coming on to her a little, but he meant nothing by it. It was Gaby he wanted. They hadn't made love for several weeks, and he knew it had to do with Lily. Or not so much Lily maybe, as his response to Lily. Today, though, she seemed to be signaling an interest.

His eyes followed her now. She'd taken her shoes off—she liked to go barefoot in the summer—and her small, wide feet made a light noise as she padded back and forth. She was talking to him, but it was more a conversation with herself: she was speaking about food, what would work with what. He tried to relax into her voice, its familiar off-rhythms. Slowly he felt it work on him. He thought of her body. There was nothing about it he didn't know, intimately—its quiet colors, its rich smell. He felt as encircled, as surely embraced, he realized, by the familiarity of Gaby's body, as he did by their house, or their bed, or the sound of the river in their room at night. It was where he lived, he thought. Where he'd made himself at home. In her.

She squatted to put something onto the lowest shelf of the

refrigerator, and he watched the flexion of her strong thighs, imagining his fingers pushing at the flesh, imprinting it.

"Just bread and cheese afterward, I think, no dessert," she was saying now, and he was breathless suddenly with the strength of his desire.

When Linnett began to talk about herself, what she'd wanted for herself in life, everyone else fell silent. They watched her attentively. She was their outsider, after all, their news from another world. Besides, they had all talked too much about themselves—Linnett had somehow made this happen—and there was some sense of a balance being restored with her revelations.

"It was an absolute wall," she said. She pressed her pale lips together. "I could not surmount it. I mean *bang*!" She clapped her hand on the table, and the silverware and dishes jumped. "That was it. It was devastating to me. See, here all along the whole reason I was writing at all was 'cause I was going to write this novel, and finally, to find out, with the time and money, that I just *didn't* have it, well ... " She shook her head, and looked around the table at them. "It was devastating."

The table was covered with crumbs—Gaby had brought out the promised crusty French bread and several soft cheeses after the meal—and all their empty coffee cups sat tilted at oddly different angles on their saucers. The short, fat candles on the table were flickering low in their little glass dishes. Here and there on the brightly printed tablecloth were wine stains or dollops of food from their earlier courses. Lily's voice was long gone and she'd hardly eaten a thing. Every now and then through the meal she whispered something to Thomas, seated next to her, and he announced to the table what she was saying, but she'd been silent for a long while. Now she was almost nodding off in her fatigue, but she wouldn't be put to bed. She'd refused twice.

Linnett focused on Thomas. "It'd be like if you ended up playing cocktail piano for the rest of your life. Or"—she turned to Alan—"if you never did anything else but kitchen renovations. You know, like you'd never have an important building."

"I wouldn't mind playing cocktail piano for the rest of my life." Thomas was grinning at Linnett.

In the dimmed light, he looked older, she thought. You could see how handsome he'd be in a few years. "Oh you would too," she said.

"No, I like cocktail piano. There's some great music."

"But for the rest of your life?"

"Sure."

"What absolute horseshit."

He shrugged, a carefree, stupid expression on his face.

She shook her head, and her tent of hair swayed as a mass. "You know you're fully as unpleasantly ambitious as I am. As I *was*," she corrected to the table at large.

Thomas shook his head. "Not so," he said. "I'm innocent of all charges."

Linnett had a moment, looking at him, of seeing him as innocent. As pure. She looked quickly at Alan, then Gaby, what she saw as their open, good faces. How had she come to inhabit a world so different from theirs?

"I think in France we don't suffer so much from this idea," Gaby said conversationally. "From this kind of ambition. We are much more realists. It makes for an easier life."

"It's not realism, Mom. C'mon," Thomas said.

She stared at him, focusing. "What is it then? What would you call it?"

"It's . . . like, *fatalism*. It's that everything is . . . ordered. You don't have the choice."

"That is changing all the time."

"It's changing maybe in Paris or a few other big cities. But most places it's not. Most places, I bet, you do what your father did. If your father was the butcher, then you become the butcher."

"If that were true, why has the number of farms dropped so since the war?"

Thomas squinted in thought. There was a moment of silence.

"What's your argument, Gaby?" Alan asked then. "That the French *are* ridden by ambition? I thought you were on the other side."

Gaby looked puzzled. She'd drunk too much, in her pleasure at not being alone for another meal with Alan and Lily. Abruptly she laughed. "Well, I seem to have painted myself a little into a corner." She shook her head. "Perhaps I was just arguing. Enjoying the argument."

"But I know what you mean," Linnett said. "It would be nice not to feel responsible for *inventing* yourself all the time."

Gaby was grateful. She smiled warmly at Linnett. "Yes! That is what I mean. Americans take this responsibility so seriously. If they are not absolutely . . . great, or something, they feel to blame."

"It's all or nothing," Linnett said.

"Yes, that's it," Gaby agreed.

"No way!" Thomas said. "Americans *forgive* themselves for everything. That's why we're the inventors of the dysfunctional family. True!" he proclaimed. " 'Nothing's *my* fault. My mother drank too much and my dad was an asshole.' Oops!" he said to Lily. " 'Scuse me." She seemed not to have noticed.

"It's both, I think," Alan said.

"Both what?" Gaby was confused.

"It's both that we feel uniquely responsible for our fate, for what we are, and that, on account of that, we try to put the blame everywhere else. Anywhere else."

"So when I do become a cocktail pianist, I can blame you guys." Thomas was grinning.

"Please do," Alan said. "I'd like to feel I influenced you somehow."

"Well, you'd hear it from this group if you really settled for that, I bet." Linnett tried to smile at Gaby and Alan, and met their serious frowning gazes. "I mean, really, you have a kind of *investment*, I would guess, emotional and otherwise, in Thomas's career. Don't you?"

There was a few seconds' silence. Then Gaby said, "Of course, we hope both our children"—she pronounced it *shildrun* in a way that moved Alan—"can achieve what they've set their hearts on. Whatever it would be."

"Oh yes! you've another child." Linnett suddenly remembered the photographs she'd lifted and looked at in the bedroom, and she blushed, though in the dim yellow light no one could see this.

"Yeah. Ettie," Thomas offered.

"A girl, how nice. A woman, I mean," Linnett said, and rolled her eyes at her own correction.

"*Not*," Thomas said. "Etienne. A boy." He grinned. "A man."

Alan cleared his throat. "He's interested in business. In finance, actually—there's a difference, as we've learned."

"Yeah, he's out there in some bank wearing a suit and tie every day. God."

"We know it's not what you would choose, my dear," his mother said. "But every profession has its liabilities, Thomas. Even yours."

"But see, Mom, the thing is, I don't see mine."

"No," Alan said. "Everyone has blinders at the start, or we wouldn't be able to start. Later there are the things you regret."

"What is it you regret, Dad?" Thomas was serious suddenly, the mask dropped.

Alan looked over, startled. He hadn't thought it through. "Well. I suppose . . . I don't know. I think, though, at the time I was a student, I thought that architecture could *do* more. We all thought that. That it could change the world." He shrugged. "Maybe it was self-important, but we thought, at the time, that it would be a great force for social change. We thought, I guess, of architecture as revolution. We talked about it that way. We were radical young men. And the odd woman."

Thomas and Alan, frowning seriously at each other across the table, suddenly seemed like mirroring images to Linnett, their family resemblance was so strong—Thomas the negative, though, the dark one.

"But everything was politicized then," Alan said, more lightly. "You know, journalism." He nodded to Linnett. "Education. Since we believed we could change the world, that we *would* change the world—that even *we* would all be changed eventually—well, we thought of every profession, every . . . activity nearly, as radical. Or potentially radical. It was the same in music, in the arts."

"Not, I think, cooking," Gaby said.

"Oh, I don't know. What about that whole discovery of ethnic food, peasant food from every corner of the world. Remember, suddenly everyone had a wok?"

"Were woks then?" Gaby asked. "Were they before or after everyone slept around?" She looked deliberately puzzled.

"Gaby! C'mon!" Alan laughed for a second, like the sound of a quick clearing of his throat. "Children are present."

Gaby turned to her son. "We were observers, of course, Thomas dear," she said. "Amazed observers." She smiled at Alan.

"So, Dad, you don't feel that way anymore?" Thomas hadn't made the shift to the lighter mood. He had leaned forward now in his earnestness, elbows on the table.

"What way?"

"That, you know, that your work is important in that way."

Alan shook his head. "No. I think not. As I've practiced architecture—as most people practice it, I think—it's been often of interest, aesthetically, or intellectually. Or both. But more a personal consolation than anything else." He looked around the table. The faces—all except Lily's, which seemed utterly remote—had opened in sympathy to him.

"That's a great deal to get from work, my dear," Gaby said gently. "Work that also interests you."

"Yes." Alan shifted back in his chair and smiled. "But it is a bit like playing cocktail piano for the rest of your life."

Thomas was serious a moment, his head nodding. Then he

jumped up, and in two leggy strides was at the piano. He sat down and turned on the lamp which arced over the keyboard and started to play a tune Linnett recognized after a moment as "Tea for Two."

Gaby leaned forward and smiled in the candlelight. Alan began to tap the table in rhythm with his spoon. The music bounced along regularly, Thomas's left hand striding over the bass keys in octaves, the right teasingly dancing around the melody.

Suddenly Linnett felt Lily's hand trembling on her arm. She leaned across Thomas's empty seat to the old woman, but couldn't hear the whisper over the music. She raised her hand, and Gaby, reading the signal, called out, "Thomas, wait a moment. Gran has something to say."

The music stopped. "What?" His face was shadowy in the light from the piano lamp when he turned.

"Gran has something to say," Gaby repeated.

They all watched Linnett and Lily. Linnett nodded as Lily whispered breathlessly. Then the old woman sat back. Linnett looked at her, at the smoothed false guilelessness of her face. She turned to the table.

The room was silent, waiting. Linnett made her voice brisk and, she hoped, inconsequential. "Lily says there's no surer or shorter route to heartbreak than having high expectations for your children."

There was a moment of silence. All of them except Lily would have thought it lasted longer than it actually did. Time enough for Alan to feel a quick shock of anger, and the impulse to respond by hurting his mother. Time for Gaby to check him with a cautioning frown. Time for Linnett to feel oddly ashamed of herself, and furious at Lily for making her repeat such a hurtful remark, surely a deliberately hurtful remark.

And Thomas. Whatever it was he felt, he did the only useful thing, a beautiful thing. He began to play again. Not "Tea for Two," but the third movement from the Schumann Fantasy he'd mastered for his performing tryout at the conservatory. It began with somber broken chords in the bass, and then a light singing voice in the right hand.

They were all silent. Thomas's face had changed at the piano, the careless, affably goofy expression he wore to meet the world had vanished, and a look of fiercest concentration took its place. One foot danced on and off the pedal, the other moved freely in the air several inches off the floor, in connection with the music somehow.

He looked, Gaby thought, like a man. To Linnett, he looked compellingly attractive.

Alan wasn't looking at his son. He had bent his head, resting his forehead in his hand, listening.

The music moved forward, the voices in it somehow gradually merging into a triumphant, yet grave, song, which burst forth once and then retreated; and then came forward again, insisting on the possibility of a joy made deeper by sorrow, offering, somehow, a vision, musically, of a boundlessly wide and painful beauty.

Thomas's playing had always been marked by a singing quality, a grace and clarity, and Alan could hear now what it gave to this music. He felt, listening to Thomas play, that his son was answering Lily, was telling her that what she had said and done was not so much wrong as irrelevant.

Alan was moved, grateful beyond measure to his son. Thomas's *gift*: he understood the word newly. It had been given to Thomas to give to others, and he was doing that now, at this unexpected and necessary moment, in a way perhaps no one at the table could have set in words, but which each of them, in some way or another, understood.

Linnett drove slowly home, preoccupied. As a result, she missed her driveway and was in the village before she realized it. She went all the way down to the docks and made her turn in the lot there. Even now there were a couple of pickup trucks parked against the concrete abutment, the men in them drinking beer and shouting their conversation from vehicle to vehicle under the single, glaring light high overhead. Linnett drove even more slowly back up the dark road. There was one couple walking on the sidewalk in the village, startled and squinting in her headlights. Otherwise the occasional lighted house was the only sign of life.

She spotted her driveway this time—*Thayer* on the mailbox—and turned into the woods. In a hundred yards or so, the drive opened out to the meadow and the vast shingled house, every window hot with light tonight it seemed, and the driveway still studded with cars. A party. Linnett kept on the gravel, past the house, and headed down the hill to where her cottage was.

In the dark she used her crutches as probes, sweeping them over the ground ahead of her, surveying it for rocks or knolls before she put her weight down. Her head was tilted up to the sky, the way a blind person's sometimes is. She could hear the noise from the Thayers', the music, the raucous voices raised above it carrying through the still night air. When she reached the safety of the little deck at her cottage front, she heaved a sigh of relief and relaxed for a moment, slumped on her crutches.

In the light of the small wall lamp she flicked on, the cottage interior looked tiny and messy. It consisted of one room, with a double bed in the corner, a large table taking up most of the space. There was a fireplace with two chairs facing it (one covered with Linnett's clothing), and a kitchenette on the opposite wall—no stove, but built-in burners, a sink, and a half-refrigerator. Linnett thumped over to the one available chair, swung her backpack down to the floor, and sat.

Her mind whirled for a moment with the evening's events. She shut her eyes and saw again the table in candlelight, felt the warmth of the conversation; the shock, then, of Lily's remark.

A burst of laughter from the Thayers' floated down, and she looked around herself again at the cheerless little room, the nicked furniture, cast off from the big house, no doubt.

Linnett didn't like the Thayers. Their vegetable garden was near her cottage, and occasionally they came down with friends carrying drinks to survey it, to pick blueberries or the earliest tomatoes. Usually this occurred at the cocktail hour, when Linnett was just back from being with Lily, when she was trying to make rapid notes on things she'd noticed—gestures, the minimal shift in Lily's facial expression—things she couldn't get on tape. It was for this reason that the Thayers irritated her.

And others too. She had heard them explaining once to a guest with a kind of pride of possession that she was a writer. "We've got a writer living there now." Just before she heard this, she had been thinking that she might make the effort to heave herself out to the tiny front deck and stare at them to let them know they were bothering her; but it occurred after they spoke that if she did this, she would become part of the tour—the appearance of the frazzled writer: the greetings, then the comments and speculation afterward.

A writer. She smiled, grimly. Well, she'd certainly blown her cover tonight.

But maybe Lily had seen through her all along, had known that Linnett must have failed at whatever it was she truly wanted to do to be trailing around in borrowed cars, in rented housing, on spec, on spec, on spec, sucking up to people like her.

She reminded herself that she liked Lily, that she'd been enchanted with her in a sense.

And now? Well, now she saw that Lily could be a bit of a bitch. More than a bit.

But she'd known that all along, hadn't she? And been charmed by that too? The elderly woman who was *not* sweet and kind, who did not think it was a perfectly lovely day.

Tonight, though, she had seen how damaging that quality could be. She'd felt for the first time a genuine dislike for Lily. And to be unkind to Alan, who seemed so defenseless.

Linnett laughed aloud, recognizing her first symptom of being attracted to someone. A very married someone, she told herself. She pushed herself painfully up. She'd better get ready for bed before she dropped off right here.

Once she'd slid into the rumple of sheets, her hair yanked fiercely back into a ponytail, she reached out for Lily's book, her memoir, which was lying on the floor by the bed. A woman's voice was audible in a long monologue from the Thayers', angry and *on a roll*—Linnett recognized the spiteful, percussive quality. Remembering again Lily's innocent, bright commentary on children, her blank face after its delivery and the sudden shift in mood at the table, she flipped through to the section of the book which dealt with the end of Lily's marriage.

We fought daily. Yes, this was what she'd been remembering. This high-minded ending, as Thomas had characterized it. She adjusted the pillows behind her, and propped the book on her knees.

This is to say nothing, of course, as every couple's style of fighting is different. The question is, then, what was it we were doing when we fought?

Talking, mostly. Talking and then weeping, both of us. It seemed to me that for weeks, months, we were always closing doors—the door to Paul's study, to the kitchen, to the bedroom. We'd begin to talk, once more, and from somewhere else in the house we'd hear one or several of the children. One of us would get up and shut the door, and suddenly we would be enclosed with our differences. By the end of that time, I think we both felt that they were all there was anymore.

We tried again and again to bridge the gap between us. And then turned away from each other again and again in silent defeat. And slowly, slowly, over those weeks and months, those long silences of defeat were victorious. The talking simply dried up, the turning away became the state of things between us.

In the beginning of the talking, I suppose it must be said, I dominated, probably in decibels as well as in minutes logged. It struck me as amazing that I could not make Paul see that I was right, just as, I'm sure, he was amazed and confused that I could not—perhaps he might have said *would* not—see his point of view. Plainly put, he thought the black people around us had chosen their path, their leaders, and it was not up to us to wish for paths or leaders more palatable to us. If we wanted to help, if we felt their cause was just and Christian and right—and we both agreed on that—then we needed to make ourselves of use, of service to them in the path and with the leaders they had chosen.

I argued that they had chosen their leader when they joined the church, that Christ was their leader,

and that Christ commanded love, not anger and
hatred. He said Christ was a white man. I said Saul
Alinsky was a white man too. I pointed out that
Martin Luther King, who happened to agree with
Christ, was a black man. He said the community had
not chosen Martin Luther King as their leader. I said
that was chance, and even partly perhaps the result
of the encouragement of people like him to go in
another direction. He said it was not chance, it was
the necessary result of this being a northern movement for equality and power. And so it went, endlessly back and forth, each of us utterly convinced of
the rightness, the greater integrity, of his side.

From somewhere up the hill, Linnett heard a glass break,
the woman's rising voice break too. She tilted the book down
opened on her chest.

Could it have been this way for Lily and Paul, this civilized?
This *high-minded*? When she had read this earlier, she had
believed it completely. Why not? But tonight, with the memory
of Lily's quick eyes as they waited behind her mask of illness
for the effect of her remark, Linnett thought otherwise. She
thought things might have been phrased just so in these arguments, calculated to wound, to draw blood, to provoke anger
and rage.

She thought of her own fights with Frank before their
divorce. Near the end, spent by a struggle that had lasted for
years, there was an exhausted, bemused, but true discussion of
what had gone wrong that an observer might have read as
high-minded. At least they were kind to each other at that
point. But before then there had been the requisite broken
glasses, the names.

The names. She smiled. In desperation once, fumbling for
the deepest insult, the darkest profanity she could attach to
Frank and his hateful face, his whole odious physical presence,

Linnett had called him a "sneed." It just slipped out. "You! You fucking . . . *sneed*!" There'd been a little beat of silence.

"*Sneed*, Linnett?" he asked.

She nodded, a choking laughter rising. And in a moment, they were both laughing, shrieking this epithet intermittently.

Now Linnett shook her head. A moth lightly tapped the inside of her lampshade, bringing her back. She picked up the book again, flipped through slowly, and stopped at a spot several pages later.

What was slowly dawning on me too, was that in giving up Paul, I would also be giving up Blackstone Church, that it was his church to lead, and I could no longer be a part of its life. This may seem a small thing to some readers—there were of course many other churches to choose from, and I might have looked forward to the pleasures of searching for the one which challenged and comforted me in equal measure, as Blackstone had for all these years.

But Blackstone was my home in a profound sense by now. I had, in fact, grown up there, and every vault, every golden star painted on its ceiling, the slatted racks for the hymnals, even the worn velvet cushions in the pews—each was as dear to me as someone else's memories of the curtains or the furniture or the chipped china in his parents' house might have been.

I had come to Blackstone as a young woman, a child really, though I was myself the mother of two children by then, and soon to be pregnant with Alan. But there was no sense in me at that time of understanding that my beliefs would have consequences for others which I would have to take responsibility for. I was held safe and youthful in my marriage, embraced and protected by my love for Paul, and his for me, and the deep and—it seemed to me then—enduring connection all those feelings had to my faith. My life was seamless to me, a fabric, all of a piece.

I did not yet know that it is by rending, tearing, and then slow painstaking repair that we become adult, that we become truly whole. And if you had told me then that the efforts to make Blackstone an integrated church would divide me from Paul, would lead me to examine my faith and end my marriage, I would have said no, take this from me, I do not wish it.

And even in the midst of that division and examination and separation, once it had begun, I often wished I could go back to what I had begun to think of as my *girlhood*, when I felt safe. And indeed I felt that Paul wished it too: that what he was asking from me when he asked me to accept his version of truth, of the events we were living through, was that I return to that blinkered, girlish life which saw only the spiritual and marital path he had set out in front of me. I saw that he regarded my dependence on him, my childishness in our early marriage, as the finest part of who I was. I saw that my own anguish and questing and growth were not steps and changes he wished to comfort me through or nurture, but were threats, problems, inconveniences, willful and perverse defiance.

During this period, I would sometimes relax my eyes in church, and let the confusion of faces, of men and women and children, swirl into color and mass alone. I would see us, brown and black and white and yellow, as one, together raising our voices and our faces in singing and praise. Was this not as it was supposed to be? Had I not helped to make this happen? Could I not stay, even if Paul and I were no longer together?

But then he would begin to preach in the hard, new language he had learned, the language of power and of anger, language in which he insisted that all of us who had loved and struggled together could be in no true relation to each other without acknowledging the falseness of our positions in society, without coming to terms with the anger and rage he insisted we felt, without turning that anger and rage into an instrument of political action.

And I would look around at the faces of the people I'd known so well, lifted, listening, intent. I'd search particularly for the women in my group, and seek reassurance in their presence. Iva, with her six boys arrayed in Sunday splendor down the pew, Anne-Marie, who'd married a white man and thought she would pay for it forever, until she came to Blackstone—all the women I'd told my most secret sorrows to, women who'd held me and comforted me when I felt most alone in the world; and in my mind I'd say to Paul, what do you know about our love?

But then gradually I noticed what seemed to me the closing up of those faces, the tightening in rage and anger, the change that was coming, that Paul was invoking and making happen. And so I began to understand that I had to prepare myself to leave the church, as well as Paul, in order to take that final step on my own, into what I believed. I had to force myself to look carefully at this dear world, and accept that it was no longer mine.

Each Sunday toward the end was an agony of leave-taking. Of noticing something I'd never noticed or even seen before, of noticing it and feeling I could not be happy or whole without looking on it every Sunday of my life. How could I?

But how could I stay? I could not.

Linnett remembered how intrigued she'd been to read this the first, and then the second and third times. The sense of Lily's honor-driven, conscience-bound choice between two intense attachments, between two different lives, really. For herself, nothing ever seemed so clear. She was always full of skepticism about her own motivations. Especially in any impulse toward renunciation, she sought to discover what was self-serving. And usually found it.

Once she'd turned down a teaching gig at the university because she hoped Frank—who'd had a run of bad luck and was depressed—would be next in line. When he got the job and took it, she allowed herself too often to remember her "kindness," to remember that she'd been the first choice. She'd used both to feel superior to him.

Lily she had imagined as an exception to this kind of behavior, but now she didn't know.

She thought abruptly of her various stabs at writing the article. All pathetically adulatory, she saw now,

She thought of her joke with Alan this afternoon, about starting, "Motherhood was not Lily Maynard's strong suit." Maybe so. At any rate, something more like that.

She sighed, and bent over the side of the bed to set the book back on the floor. She turned out the light. The woman's voice had stopped long since at the Thayers'. There was just the tinny, distant music, the rumble of voices. Occasionally the sound of a car starting and driving away over the crunching gravel. The way it was in childhood, Linnett thought. In bed in the dark, listening to the grown-ups. She slept.

Alan and Gaby had started to make love and then stopped, as though by mutual agreement. They lay now, side by side, listening to the sounds from outside. Over the rush of the water below, the night air carried only faraway birdsong and the occasional sudden flutter of wind in the trees. The room was bright with reflected moonlight.

Why hadn't they finished, once they'd begun? They were

too full, Alan might have said. They'd drunk too much wine. They were tired.

As for Gaby, she knew differently. It was her choice, she felt. She didn't want him. Why?

Lily's face rose in her mind's eye. Lily, who made Alan different. And it was through Lily's eyes that Gaby sometimes saw Alan now—as a boy. A beautiful American boy. She smiled slightly, remembering him then, and shifted in bed to look at the black trees beyond the deck.

Of course, what Lily had said tonight was unforgivable. Cruel. Gaby understood that, and it made her angry at the old woman. How hard, how awful for Alan to have his mother announce—openly, if obliquely—such disappointment in him. And, Gaby felt, by extension, in her. For she knew that Lily blamed her, in part, for the course Alan's life had taken. She saw Alan as having become, perhaps, *Frenchified* by Gaby, as having refused—what? what would Lily call it? America, of course. The good fight, maybe. Political involvement.

And it was true that it had been Gaby's wish not to live in the city anymore, if that was any part of it. She had fallen in love with New England, with the countryside, the open hilly farms, the amazing palette of the woods in fall. And this had turned Alan's life in a certain direction. He'd left the firm he'd started with in Cambridge, he'd set up a private practice in Bowman. That meant houses, vacation homes, kitchens, additions.

But it was he who had wooed her with the countryside. That first fall when she'd followed him over, he'd borrowed or rented cars nearly every weekend, and they'd driven—up the coast of Maine, in the Green Mountains in Vermont, through the Berkshires. Gaby had been dazzled and amazed at the piercing bright colors, the clear hard air, the vast reaches of green pine and red and purple forest, dense and promising and mysterious in a way completely unfamiliar to her—in France there would have been fields under cultivation, or another village just over the hill. The country here invited Gaby, made her feel a sense of possibility. When Alan finished architecture school, she began to try to persuade him to make the move out of the city.

But he'd been tired of Boston too. He'd agreed when the children got close to school age that it was too expensive. Besides, he'd never had much success, anyway, in that world of competition for public buildings or public spaces—that other, more glorious life of the architect.

Still, she'd never heard him say before what he'd said tonight, that he regretted some part of it. And this house, which she'd always thought of as connected, somehow, to her affair— his wish to bring her home after it—must also have been a kind of concession of the possibility of that public life, a sign that he saw that it wasn't going to happen that way for him. It was, then, a kind of giving up. A giving up that was part of his love for her.

Gaby thought of her brothers, her father. Her father still worked in the pharmacy he owned, her brothers were both bankers. They were all private men, like Alan. They went to work, they worked hard—or perhaps not so hard, it occurred to her—they came home and were family men.

But French family men. Different. In fact, this was precisely what Gaby couldn't stand anymore when she visited—their self-importance, their ponderousness, their endless delivering themselves of opinions on this and that, while the women did everything at home. She knew she had not made her choice accidentally, finally. She had chosen America, and Alan. Escape.

Alan had chosen her and her Frenchness. In part, then, for escape too. And they were stuck somewhere in between.

No, not stuck. She would never say stuck. But each had given up a great deal, apparently. There were disappointments. Things you couldn't know you had wanted, or even things you were quite certain you hadn't wanted, but still, as you discovered, missed some aspect of.

Had her mother ever, ever, thought of her father as a boy?

Yet wasn't this part of what had drawn Gaby to Alan? His boyishness. His openness. And certainly it was part of the adventure she hoped for when she said she would go with him to America, that she was moving into something with no familiar form, no predictable shape. Just what she chose.

And what he chose too, of course.

She thought again of Lily's empty face at the table tonight, of Linnett's shamed face as she spoke Lily's words. Of Thomas, playing in answer to that. That was enough, surely, that she and Alan had raised a child capable of this? This beauty, as well as this generosity?

Gaby was beginning to drowse in the silver light.

Suddenly there was a piercing shriek from outside. She started violently and turned to touch Alan's arm. "My God!" she said. Another cry of high-pitched pain and terror followed quickly. "My God! What is it?"

Alan stroked her arm. "An animal." His voice was hoarse. He'd been asleep. "Maybe a squirrel. Something's killing it."

"My God," she said again, as the long, bright, rending screams filled the night air. "Oh! Can we do nothing?"

"No. We can't," he said.

They listened together. It stopped, then started again, over and over, the shrilling, agonized cries.

Gaby cried out and turned into Alan's chest. He held her until finally it ended, until the screams died into a throaty last whimper and stopped.

Until they both turned on their backs and lay still and exhausted, but now wide awake.

As for Lily, she slept the dreamless, deep sleep of a played-out child.

chapter 12

Alan's office was on the second floor of a house in the village, above an antique shop. The stairs up were steep. They were made of uncovered, scarred wood, and they twisted sharply into darkness at the top. Was it worth it? Linnett wondered. She didn't even know that he was there—she hadn't called ahead for fear he'd tell her not to come. She stood for a long moment weighing it; and then spun, suddenly, and lowered herself into sitting position on the third step. She was surprisingly quick going up this way, hoisting her bottom from step to step and pulling her crutches along with her. At the top, though, she had to struggle to get up. She stood resting on her crutches, almost panting for a moment with the effort of accomplishing this. The hall light was out up here, but one of the four doors had a frosted glass pane through which a pale light filtered. Alan's name was stenciled on this pane, though she could hear nothing when she bent her head toward it. She knocked. She heard footsteps and then he opened the door.

"Hey," he said, sounding not entirely pleased. He was wearing half-glasses. They made him look spinstery.

"Hey, yourself," she said. "I was in the neighborhood, so I thought I'd just painfully *throw* myself up your very steep staircase, drag my *body* through your pitch-black hallway, and drop in." She tried a warm smile. She hoped it was warm.

"Well, hi." He hadn't moved.

"May I come in?"

He stepped back. "Sure. Sorry. Come on in." He shut the door behind her as she moved forward, and then he strode past her and pulled a modern, rolling desk chair from under the table by the window. Linnett looked around. The walls and woodwork were all painted white. The room was flooded with light from a large bay window in the front. The tables—there were three of them—were white Formica, the lamps white too. There were four of the desk chairs, in blue and green wool, and against the wall, a blue wool loveseat. Everywhere on the walls were hung architectural drawings and photographs of buildings.

Linnett took off her pack and swung it, and then her crutches, to the floor. She sat in the blue chair Alan had pulled out for her, and leaned back, looking around. Alan had sat at one of the tables, facing her. It was as though she were a client. "I'll be straight," she said after a moment's silence. "I wanted to ask you a little about Lily."

"I suspected as much." He took off his glasses and rubbed the bridge of his nose. "But I told you, I don't want to talk about Lily."

"Well, I know that, and I wouldn't, I *won't* quote you or anything. It's just that I'm feeling, a little, at sea, at the moment. I can't seem to get . . ." She frowned and looked out the bay window in the direction of the voices rising past: all she could see from here were the trees across the street, the spire of the church. "Umm. A footing, journalistically speaking. So to speak." She looked at him. "As it happens. As it were."

He looked back, a long steady gaze. Blue eyes, thought Linnett. Nice.

He lifted his hands. "No," he said. He smiled, as though to soften the blow.

"Oh, pretty please," she said.

He shook his head, looking slightly embarrassed—for her? for himself?

"Okay," she said. "Look. Let me apologize anyway. For my

part in Friday night's little . . . insult, whatever. Somehow, I guess, I got Lily going. Or I felt she used me. Anyway." Linnett shrugged. "I thought she was unpleasant. And I was surprised that she was unpleasant. In that particular way. And, tired as I was Friday night, I went home and reread some stuff of hers and saw in it, this time, I guess, some new possibilities."

He had begun tapping his pencil. "Such as?"

"Such as. Such as. Well, for instance, she talks about being angry with your father over the church stuff. At Blackstone. Obviously. But she kind of points, herself, to a wish for you— for *me*, I mean: 'the reader' "—Linnett made quote marks with her fingers—"to understand how their anger worked, to, like, picture their fights. And she draws them as these very lofty discussions, really. Tearful, but lofty as hell. But while I was reading it, I was thinking of her tone to you on Friday night. And I wondered if maybe there wasn't a more . . . *explosive* quality there. If it ever got down and dirty, maybe."

He smiled, a small, grim lifting of the corners of his mouth, and shook his head. "Nope. It never did."

"Do you remember them? The fights?"

"There were no fights. That's what I'm saying."

"The discussions, then. That whole breaking up thing with the church at the time."

He shook his head. "I don't really. I was only twelve, thirteen then. I didn't really care about it, frankly."

"Well, didn't they talk to you about it?" she pushed. "Explain it to you?"

"Nope." His face was closed. "Not until the end, until they were splitting up. And even then it was very . . . summarial. 'This has happened, we have disagreed, Dad is moving out,' that sort of thing."

"Well, when did you understand it then?" Linnett leaned forward on the edge of his table and rested her face in her hand.

He sat back. He raised his light eyebrows. He grinned at her, teasing. "Did I say I understood it?"

"Don't you?"

"I have my theories. I didn't, though, at the time. At the time, I recall, I was concerned exclusively about me. About whether I'd be considered weird or be dropped socially somehow, because my parents were divorced."

"And?"

"No. It didn't really work that way. I was actually able to parlay it into sympathy, in fact, in some quarters. But that was my fear. There were only a few kids I knew whose parents were divorced—or the father had died or something. And—of course we never thought of this, that their lives were economically fragile. To us, to me, they just seemed strange. Unattractive. And that's what I cared about. That's all I cared about. That somehow I would become similarly, I don't know, marked."

A warm wind from the open window passed into the room, ruffled the papers on the desk and the corners of a few of the drawings tacked to the walls. Both of them looked over at the leafy noise for a moment.

"But that didn't happen," Linnett said after a few seconds.

"No. I was entrenched enough socially, I guess. And Lily had the family money which she tapped into then, so there were no big changes. We did move, but the new apartment was closer, actually, to school and my friends than our house had been. So that seemed even a benefit."

"Wow, lucky you."

Alan shrugged. "As I said, I was really mostly concerned with myself at that age. You were no doubt a selfless humanitarian at thirteen or fourteen."

Linnett raised her hands, palms up, as though to deny she'd been accusing anyone of anything. "Hey," she said. And after a moment, "Well, so what are your theories? Now?"

"Theories of . . . ?"

"You said you had some theories about your parents' divorce. About why they broke up."

"Oh. Well." He began to slide his glasses around on the table's surface. "You're not using this."

"Not directly, no."

"How, indirectly, then?"

"Just . . . to help me define my own stance toward Lily. I just feel *enclosed* with her at this point. With her version of things." She looked out the window for a moment. "I need help. " She slipped into a Southern accent. "I'd be mighty grateful, suh. While just downright reverential, if you wish, about your privacy."

"No quotes? None?"

She crossed her heart.

"Okay. It's pretty harmless anyway, I think. But here it is. My theory. It has to do with their whole earlier relationship too." He looked at her. "I assume you remember all that—her upbringing, hermetically sealed off, nearly, and then the experience of meeting my father, true love, deep faith, da *duh*, da *duh*."

Linnett smiled at him. "Sure, that's about how I remember it."

"Well, my idea is . . . Actually it's not just mine, my sister's too. We both think that Lily's conversion experience, as it were, centered really on my father. That he was her God, her Christ, whatever. He sort of embodied that for Lily. He had a kind of virtually papal infallibility. And when he began to fall into error, as Lily saw it, it wasn't as though it was just a human being making a mistake, it wasn't like the disappointments the rest of us have in our marriages, you know?"

Linnett nodded, thinking she'd ponder this revelation later.

"That teach us how to love another human being. Because Lily, frankly, isn't interested in loving another human being." He heard how his voice had hardened and he stopped. After a moment, he smiled. "This is my *theory*, understand."

"Oh, *I* do," she said, with one of her odd inflections.

He smiled again, hearing in this way of emphasizing it— would she have intended this? he couldn't tell—her opinion that others wouldn't. "Anyway, my father, as I see it, didn't have a chance. I mean, yes, the issue was incredibly important to Lily, and yes, she did feel he was wrong, that the whole black power thing was a dead end. And she felt in her heart, I think—wherever that vestigial organ may be in old Lil—that her friendships with some of the people in church, some of the black women in particular, were true. Were real, you know. So she *did* feel that he was, what? 'Invalidating her experience,' I guess. She did have those kinds of"—he changed his voice, became a pompous announcer—"prefeminist intimations of feminist anger." Changed back. "I'll grant all that. But I think the basic truth and the reason the marriage ended was that she saw he was human, that he could make mistakes. What she thought were mistakes. Remember, she'd turned her life completely around for him, because she believed in him. And now he was betraying that belief. And I think she found that, literally, unforgivable."

Linnett had been watching his face carefully while he spoke. After a moment, she said. "And you think that's pretty unforgivable of her."

"Don't you? Wouldn't you like to imagine that your husband, if you're married . . . ?" She shook her head. "If you got married, or even your . . . boyfriend, your beloved, would find a way to love you even after he discovered you weren't perfect?"

Linnett sat up. "Hey, you think I'm not perfect?"

He laughed. "Only because you're wearing a cast, of course." He gestured at her leg. "I took that as a kind of . . . hint. A metaphor."

"There are some times, my friend, when a cast is just a cast. Don't forget it."

They smiled at each other.

She angled her head to see what was on the table in front of him. "What's this?" She tapped the edge of the sheet, and rolled her chair closer to the table. To him.

"Ah. Just doodling. It's a maybe, could-be church. In Vermont."

"Mmm." She bent over it, frowning. "Interesting."

"Can you read it?" he asked.

She sat back. "No. Not a bit. I just said that, actually. I was being officially interested."

He put his glasses back on and traced it through for her, floor plans and elevations, porch, nave, choir, sanctuary. He showed her where the windows would be, the doors, the skylights, and described the way light would enter the space, the sight lines the congregation would have out the windows. Bent close to her over the table, he could smell her perfume, the faint animal odor of her hair. If he leaned a little toward her, wisps of it tickled his cheek.

She looked up. "It's lovely. I hope it gets to be."

"Well, thank you."

She tilted back again, rocking in the chair a bit, and looked out the window, saw the finger of the church spire, the belling clouds above it. She looked back at him, squinting her eyes a little. "It's curious, isn't it, that you're working on a church?"

"Well, no, honestly. I see the connection you're trying to make, but lots of people with not a trace of religion in their backgrounds do churches. Anyone offered one would. Would be happy to." He gestured. "A church, a mosque, a temple, a shrine. We don't discriminate. Or I wouldn't. So it isn't connected. And I'm not even a believer, after all that."

"But you were brought up that way. You went to church each Sunday to hear your father."

"Oh Lord, yes. Sunday school, church, church choir, church sports, the works."

"So. Um." She leaned forward over the table again, resting her chin in her hands. "You were sort of part of that, then, that attempt to integrate Blackstone too. I mean, what were your experiences? Were yours anything like Lily's? I mean, I guess I'm asking how you'd vote, in terms of what the reality of the situation was."

He shrugged. "I don't know. I really don't. As I said, I didn't think about it the way they did."

"But how *did* you? That's what I'd like to know."

"I don't know. I was confused, that's probably about the sum of it. About race."

"Because your parents disagreed."

"No, no. God no. I mean, as I said, I really didn't understand the nature of their disagreement at all. Until later. No, it was just ... Well, Lily and my father came to the question of race as adults, having had virtually no experience of it in their lives growing up. You remember that passage about Lily's first seeing a black person, about how amazed she was?"

Linnett nodded.

"Anyway, they came to Chicago, and the church was in flux. And they made their decisions about what the right way to feel was, and they felt it. That is the kind of people they were. They were good people. They saw life—Lily still does to some extent I think—in terms of right and wrong. Good and evil. It makes things kind of thrilling in a way, I imagine."

Was there something wistful in his voice? Linnett couldn't tell.

"And the black people who came into our church—which had been after all, a white church at one time—were ... Well, they rewarded those feelings. They were, you know, aspiring to the middle class, or they were middle class. And they were interested in being among white people, or they wouldn't have joined that church. And that was my experience in the church too.

"But I was also going to public school, where from kindergarten on, the number of black kids slowly increased with that whole migration north. And these kids were different from the kids I knew in church."

"How?"

Linnett saw Lily in the way the line of concentration deepened between his eyebrows. "Poorer. Fresh up from the South. Not particularly interested, or even aware, at first, of integration, of what was happening around us all. God, *with* us all. Older than we were, because they'd been so badly educated they couldn't perform at grade level. Also sexually sophisticated. If not active. Rough. Profane. Scary. To me." He lifted his hands. "I was scared. That was it, basically. I was scared all the time around them. They embodied all the things I'd been taught to be scared of. Ashamed of. Never to mention or show understanding of. But on the other hand, being scared of black kids was utterly taboo. The biggest taboo of all. That was not a thing I was allowed to feel in my house. With my parents." His lips firmed against each other in a tight smile. "And if I so much as hinted at it, they'd point out how well I got along with kids at church, at Sunday school. But the fact was, I didn't. Those kids seemed, somehow, *too* good to me. Maybe because they *were* conscious that we were being integrated. Anyway, I felt that they were sort of pious, holier than thou. Than I anyway. I suppose, in my confusion, I thought they were all secretly like the kids at school, that they were somehow *pretending* to be this other way." He paused and frowned. "No, that's wrong. Nothing was that clear to me. Here's what I felt actually. That there was a kind of authenticity—though I would never have used the word—about the kids at school that there wasn't about the black kids at church." He shook his head, slowly. "And as for myself, I felt inauthentic everywhere. Completely false."

"So that's it?"

"That's it. That's the nature of my confusion. That *was*."

"And you couldn't talk about it with Lily and Paul."

"No, I couldn't. I felt it ... depressed them, or shocked them, somehow, when I began even to get close to talking about it. The closest I came was with Lily a couple of years later, after the divorce, when I got beat up. By some black kids."

"Jesus." She rocked back in her chair. "Badly?"

"No, not too. Cracked ribs, some loose teeth. I went down fast—there were four or five of them and it seemed like the wisest course. They kicked me a little before they left, in the ribs, in the head."

"God, you must have been terrified."

"No. No, I don't think I was, once I was hit once or twice.

It's hard to explain." Here's what Alan was remembering: his panic in the long teasing moments as they caught up with him, surrounded him, pretending to be talking casually. "Hey man, hey faggot, where you going? Why you in such a rush?" Their smiling faces, the tension in their forced relaxation. And the relief, the relief, with the first blow. And the second. "You know, there weren't so many guns then, so I didn't really think of that. And they hadn't pulled a knife, no one had cut me. It hurt like hell, later, but then . . . I don't know. Maybe I was in some kind of shock." He had lain there after they left, tasting the blood in his mouth, the odd metal flavor of it, listening to their footsteps, their voices, moving farther off, and feeling a deep peace settle on him. "But the point was, Lily was just undone. Not because I was hurt, but because I might be angry at blacks. She almost literally wouldn't let me speak."

"But how did she stop you?"

"Just . . . by talking for me. 'Now I know you must be feeling this, but I think what you'll come to see is that.' And so on."

"And what did she expect you to 'come to see'?"

"That they were the victims, of course. Not I."

"Ah." Linnett nodded. "And did you?"

"Well." He grinned. "I did and I didn't. I mean, I wanted my anger. Not at blacks, but certainly at those particular guys. And I tried to talk about it to Lily, to make her see that for once, I'd earned a feeling. I really tried to talk. About all the feelings, the foggier ones earlier, and now this one, this clear one. And she was terrified, I could see it in her face. I mean, I was a person . . . By now I had black *friends*. I mean, I was going to the university high school, which was a little bit integrated anyhow and they were, you know, really middle-class kids, kids whose lives I finally did understand—and still she couldn't allow me . . . anything. To lift the curtain one little bit was like tearing it down for Lily. She just couldn't allow it. She gave me the party line, and she tried to shut me up. And I'd bought the general argument long since, so I did shut up. I don't know." He shrugged. "And that was how she talked about it to other people too. I heard her. You know, 'Yes he was hurt, but not too badly, and he understands why these things happen and he doesn't blame anyone.' "

"How very politically correct."

"Lily was the queen of political correctness. In that way. And my father too. Paul." He shrugged. "So you see, I didn't have a side in either one of their arguments, because for me the truth . . . No, not the truth. The *issue*, anything worth arguing about, lay elsewhere. And wasn't allowed."

"But later on . . . " She smiled, suddenly, sheepish. "This is coming back to Lily, I'm sorry. Later on . . . Or no, actually." Her finger touched her mouth. "*Earlier* than that, it was earlier. Her stand, her position, being sort of against this kind of community organization and that whole black power thing, that wasn't politically correct, was it?"

"No, no. Though she had a few friends who supported her. But no, she swam against the tide on that one. And it cost her a lot. A whole lot. 'Cause that's the way liberal politics were going then. And certainly the church was, our church was going that way. You know, Alinsky and all that. I mean, in effect, it cost her her whole community at church. Certainly the marriage, in some ways. And she got called a lot of names, implicitly or explicitly, for standing up to all that. Even when she wrote the memoir. I give her credit."

"Reluctantly."

He grinned. "It's hard for me to feel exuberant about Lily."

"You don't much like her, do you?"

"Ah. *Like* her." He frowned, smiling slightly. "I don't think of it in those terms, I guess." Then he sat forward and was suddenly serious, looking down unseeing at his drawings on the table below him. "Lily is . . . she's phenomenal, really. I admire her, what she's done with her life, the *use* she's made of it, I guess." He shrugged and met Linnett's eyes. "I may even be envious of some of that. What I know is that I don't think of my own life the same way. At all. I don't wish to *make use* of it. Or to have *Lily* make use of it, for that matter. But in some—I don't know—not very intimate way, I would say I even love Lily. There's a deep, serious connection, based on how I understand her." He smiled again. "If I do."

Now he shook his head, relaxing back in his chair again. "But there are so many things about her I dislike. And some of them I can't forgive her for. As I said."

After a moment, Linnett said, "It must be tough living with her now."

"It's pretty bad. I hadn't thought it was going to be, honestly. I thought I'd made my peace, now that I'm a grown-up." He smiled sardonically.

"So why are you doing it? Why didn't you ask your sister to?"

"Clary?" He shook his head. "No way would she do it. She said that loud and clear. And she'd gone to Chicago and done all the work, you know, getting Mother ready to move into the center, which then had to be postponed. So I owed her. But believe me, Clary has maybe even more trouble with Lily than I do."

"And did your other sister? Did Rebecca?"

"I'm not sure. You know, she was older than Clary. She was out in the world even earlier, and much less interested in me, so I knew much less about her, even then." He laughed quickly. "I think she pretty much had contempt for all of us, the whole bourgeois troop. Except she was interested in the radical stuff my father was doing, so she probably did have ... Well, she probably joined the argument against my mother. If she cared that much. I suspect Christianity was pretty irrelevant to her."

"Do you ever hear from her?"

"Rebecca? No. Clary does, every couple of years, and there are sometimes messages—greetings, really—for me. They were pretty close." He looked at her. "None of this is what you wanted to know."

"Oh it helps. It all goes into the hopper."

"But it doesn't get at what went on between my parents. Which is where you started."

"But you *did* offer me your theory."

He bowed, a little inclination of his head. "Correct. Which, of course, you will not use."

"No. I swear."

His eyes met hers and lighted warmly. "Where's the tape recorder?"

She smiled. "Come on. Don't you find me an eminently trustworthy person?"

"Eminently? No."

She looked at her watch.

"Are you due there?" he asked.

"In a little bit. I don't need to rush, if you have anything else you want to tell me."

"I didn't want to tell you this."

"It's my charm, I guess. It gets them every time."

"Your persistence anyway."

"Hey, c'mon. Give me charm. Make me feel good."

"Charming persistence. How's that?"

"I'll take it," she said.

"Do *you* like Lily?" he asked, abruptly.

"Oh, I love her. But she's a great subject. And she's not my mother, praise the Lord."

"And what constitutes a great subject?"

"Well, it can be different things. But with Lily, it's partly her egocentrism, certainly. She's damned well interested in herself, so she's ready, you know. She does *half* the work for me. She knows what she wants me to write. Sometimes a modest genius, let's say, is the worst. Then you really have to work. Lily lays it out: 'Here it is, my life, ain't it grand?' and that makes my life easy. But ... " She shrugged. "It's also the stuff she's laid out before, for everyone else. So I'd like to try for more. I'd like to know some deep, dark secrets."

"Well. I haven't got any."

"Oh no, you do. You've told me some. In a way I can't quite articulate yet. And I won't, I *really* do promise, use them directly."

"Why is it that every time you say that, I get more nervous?"

Linnett was pulling herself up now, onto her crutches. She looked over at him. "You're cute when you're nervous," she said.

He turned away quickly, and she could feel herself blush. A mistake.

The hall was newly dark to her light-struck eyes when Alan opened the door and let her out. She touched her shoulder to the wall and moved slowly. "Please don't watch me do this," she said. The light shone from behind him in his pale, curly hair. She couldn't read his shadowed face. "It's *about* as graceless as you can get."

"I'll try to have a working bulb in next time you come," he said.

She turned to look at him again. "Great. I'll see you, then." She lifted her hand, and he stepped back in and shut the door.

She inched to the top of the stairs, feeling her way with her crutches, listening for Alan's retreating footsteps in his office.

Next time, she was thinking, as she lowered herself to the top step.

chapter 13

—

When Lily was in her early forties, her father, Henry, had taken several years to die, from something no one then would have known to call Alzheimer's disease. Violet spoke of it as his being "addled." "Your father seems more and more a little bit addled," she'd written to Lily. "I think he has too much leisure and not enough to fill it with." Lily had gone up to Minnesota four or five times during those years and stayed for a week or two at a stretch, usually taking Alan, or Alan and Clary, with her. Her function was more to provide her mother with companionship than to help. There was, after all, ample paid help.

The last summer of her father's life, she went up in June, taking all three children, and stayed until just after his death, in mid-August. At this time Henry didn't even recognize Violet anymore. He had forgotten what food was, and had to be forced, occasionally, to eat a bite or two. (It was this that he would die of actually, that old Fletcherizer. When he stopped breathing, he'd taken no food for three weeks, no water for four days.)

Henry's bedroom had been moved downstairs long since. He was allowed to wander the first floor, but the outside doors were all kept locked. The nurse, an enormous, meaty woman named Mrs. Engel, dressed him tidily every morning. By nine-thirty or ten, though, he was usually already a shambles, draped in dirty towels or tablecloths he found in the laundry room, or having torn his shirt, or simply taken off pieces of his clothing. For the most part, his activities were harmless and self-contained, but occasionally he had what Violet called a "wild day," when he struggled to escape, when he struck out, when he rained obscenities on her or Mrs. Engel, or cowered in fear in the back hall, or simply screamed and screamed. Then Mrs. Engel, whose instructions from Violet were to let him alone as long as he was peaceful, would descend on him with her heavy tread and whisk him off to his bedroom. There she would give him what she called "a little something to help him sleep."

Henry, who'd been stout all his adult life, was tiny and wizened now, his skull sharply visible, his face shuttered blank, his mouth an open, empty hole in which his restless tongue danced wildly. The children hated him, and Lily found herself, out of a perverse loyalty—for she had never loved her father, either—trying to explain to them what he'd been like in her youth, who the person had been who was Henry.

To no avail. They shrank from him, as from a sick and therefore disgusting animal. Once, when he was having a bad day and Mrs. Engel had been summoned, Rebecca stood halfway up the front hall stairs—where she'd fled from him—and shrieked, "I can't believe it! I can't believe I'm going to have to spend all summer locked up in this smelly old house with this *cretin*, just because he's your father."

Behind her, Lily could hear Violet's sharp intake of breath. As soon as Mrs. Engel arrived and led Henry away, Violet moved past Lily and slowly climbed the stairs. Lily stood in the front hall and watched her mother's effortful ascent, a painful imitation of Rebecca, who'd turned after she shrilled her hateful words and run upstairs. Now Lily could hear Violet's door shut too. She followed Mrs. Engel and held her father while the sweating, heavy woman prepared the syringe and plunged it into his spindly arm.

Then she came out into the front hall again and stood for a

long time trying to decide what to do. Alan and Clary were in the living room listening to a record of her parents' that Clary played over and over that summer, about the Stellenboschen boys: she was memorizing the lyrics, and Alan was caught up with her in her project, as he so often was. "Stop your mooooaning," they sang with the hearty men's chorus. "Stop your grooooaning, the Stellenboschen boys aaaare here."

Lily mounted the stairs in rhythm with the music and crossed the wide upstairs hall. She knocked on Violet's closed door. After a moment, her mother called softly, "Come in," and Lily entered.

Violet was still a pretty, plump woman at seventy-four. Now she was sitting at her dressing table. Clearly she'd been repairing the damage that her tears had done. Her rouge was too dark, and Lily's heart wrenched at the sight of this fat, elderly clown, trying to behave with so much dignity.

"I'm so sorry about what Rebecca said, Mother," Lily offered. "She was just frightened, really."

Violet looked at her with watery eyes. "But to call him a *cretin*, Lily!"

Lily nodded, thinking she would not even try to explain the context to Violet: the cretin jokes that even Alan knew by heart. *What did the cretin say to the one-armed man? Why did the cretin cross the road?*

"In *front* of him. As though he weren't even a person. As though he were invisible." Violet's eyes swam with tears. "Oh, here I go again." She drew a long breath in and turned to the mirror.

Lily didn't know what to do. She was afraid if she touched her mother, Violet would collapse. She sat down on Violet's bed and waited.

"I want you to promise me something, Lily," Violet said at last.

"Of course," Lily said.

"It's not so easy as that," Violet said. "I want you to help me if I'm dying as your father is. I couldn't bear to . . . " Violet stopped, but after a moment her throat made a little involuntary whimper. She cleared it then, and said firmly. "I want you to help me."

Though Lily wasn't sure she'd ever be able to do what Violet seemed to be asking, her devotion to her mother was deep and absolute. "I will," she said.

"I'll rely on you. You are far braver than I. I've always been . . . too fearful. But I count on you, Lily. On your courage."

"I understand."

"And you will? You will do as I wish?"

"I will."

"Thank you, dear."

Fortunately Lily hadn't had to do anything. Violet's death had been as discreet and unobtrusive as her life. She died in her sleep, at age eighty-one, with her clothes for the next day neatly laid out over the upholstered bench at the foot of her bed.

When the doctor told Lily she had Parkinson's disease and explained the possible sequelae, Lily had remembered Violet's request. She was looking at the doctor, but she was seeing in her mind's eye her mother's face as it had looked then, in the mirror—the curious reversal of her features, the watery eyes, the hectic circles of rouge, the fear.

There was no one in her life with whom Lily had the intimacy Violet had had with her, no one of whom she could exact the promise Violet had exacted of her. But Lily did have more courage than Violet, courage of one sort anyway, and she was certainly more resourceful. All by herself she did the necessary research, she told the necessary lies to her doctor, she made the necessary arrangements.

How could she have decided such a thing, prepared to implement it, with apparently so little doubt, so few second thoughts?

Of course, Violet's veiled request had given her a kind of permission. And then, too, Lily had been alone with her will and her own sense of right and wrong for many years by then. Even her religion was something she experienced in isolation from others. Though she had continued to meet with the Bible group until it finally dissolved, she had never joined another church after Blackstone, preferring for a while to call, as it were, on one church or another, or the University Chapel, on different Sundays. And then increasingly she didn't stir herself on Sundays at all.

Not that she didn't believe, or didn't pray. But prayer had become for Lily a concentrated and other-focused way of thinking, a yearning state she sometimes gave words to in her mind and sometimes didn't. As she said in her memoir about her withdrawal from organized religion, "Sometimes I fear I hear God less well now, I understand less well, perhaps, his intentions for my life. But I also know that I don't hear the false voices speaking for God that would silence my own, inner voice, that would come between me and him."

In any event, God did not seem to offer her an objection to her decision.

Monday was a bad day for Lily. She'd hardly eaten anything through the morning, and the cereal sat now, a little skin congealed on its surface. To move seemed something beyond volition. She'd simply dropped the few letters she'd managed to read into the basket by her chair. She couldn't close her fingers with enough force to tear them. She felt undone by the letters too. Or perhaps it was just that she'd virtually reached the end of them, of this long history she'd decided to put herself through one last time before it disappeared. Before *she* disappeared, she thought.

Outside the window, the sun did its lively dance in the long-skirted, curtsying pine branches. To Lily it was just blurred and shifting light. Irrelevant. Everything seemed irrelevant.

Through the long weekend, Lily had closed in on herself. She had come to understand that she was to live a life in which the words would simply be stopped. The writing, the endless imaginative arguments about life, wouldn't be there anymore.

Her disease seemed for the first time a visceral thing to her, a tree trunk growing inside her, filling her with thickness, woodiness, and now tentacling into her thoughts, her soul itself, hardening them.

The week before, when it had first come to her that Parkinson's was taking this part of her life away, she'd had a surge of energy—the will, as she felt it, to rise to this insult. To surmount it, in fact. Even, perhaps, a sense of this as adventure. The last adventure. The last drama. She had wondered where it might come from, the final thing that would happen to her, and now here it was. Well, then.

She had believed the words she'd spoken to Linnett. She had never feared the truth. She had tried always to meet life without flinching, and she thought she could in this case too. She had felt Linnett's admiration for her as she made those first efforts, and she'd been nourished by it. This is who she would be then, until death. This brave person. *This* Lily. Her afternoon on Friday with Linnett had been almost gay, and it was Lily's sparkling flirtatiousness that had kept Linnett long past the time she usually left.

Almost from the moment Alan had come in to wake her Friday night though, it seemed Lily would be asked to accept something less triumphant about all this.

"Put on your dancing shoes, Lily," he'd said. "We've got company." There was a secret, teasing smile on his face, but he wouldn't tell her who it was. He smelled of liquor too, and Lily, as though she didn't drink herself, felt a sense of indignant repulsion.

He'd had to shake her several times to wake her. She was tired after the long afternoon with Linnett, and, in all likelihood, also from the effort of accepting her new diminished life—though she hadn't yet dwelt on that. Still, as she rearranged her hair and smoothed out her clothes (how fortunate that she'd put on this pale lilac outfit this morning), she felt the familiar anticipatory pleasure in the notion of company, the hungry eagerness to occupy once more her public self.

Imagine then her hurt, to discover Linnett, *her* Linnett still there, sitting at the table, laughing with her grandson Thomas. The conversation had begun without her, and it was quick, too quick for Lily to join it—Linnett to Thomas, Thomas to Alan, back to Gaby, over to Linnett, to Alan, to Thomas again. They were all, Lily thought, *flirting* with each other. Something in this struck her as deeply perverse, disordered. What's more, they barely seemed to notice Lily. In fact, as the evening wore on—and on, and on—Alan asked several times if she didn't want to go to bed. As though she were a child. She could have slapped him. Once or twice she managed to say something, to speak up, but then they all pretended she'd said nothing. The conversation simply continued around her as though she hadn't spoken. She felt canceled out. Erased. And then, at the end, Thomas played that terribly loud and melodramatic music—which she found, somehow, upsetting beyond words—for far too long. Someone should tell him there could be too much of such a thing.

Lily's sleep that night was deep and yet somehow not refreshing, not restful. She woke from it on Saturday with a sense of a thick, woolly fatigue or remorse she couldn't have named the source of. Though her routines through the weekend were unvaried, the days seemed interminable. Was this what life would be now, this vegetable creep of time?

We have many little deaths to prepare us for the final one, and often we have to struggle to find God's loving hand in them. For me my separation from the church was one such death, and my divorce another. I think that what accounts in part for the depression I allowed myself to fall into in the years that followed these two changes in my life was partly the sense they brought me of being cut off from God's love in a way that other events—the deaths of my parents, for example, or the small unnoticed deaths of my children as they became adult—did not. I found it comforting to read Job through this period, not that I thought of my own suffering as in any way comparable to Job's, but that I was similarly shaken and distressed by it. And that the answer God gave to Job seemed the most strangely reassuring one possible.

But I think what finally reconciled me to God's shape for my life was the gift he made me of self-understanding at the time of Paul's dying.

Paul had been ill throughout all of 1968 and 1969. I had written to him oftener in this period than I had before. Neither of us had ever asked the other about our personal lives after our divorce, but I think friends had probably kept him informed of what I was doing as they kept me informed in a general sense about his life. I knew, for example, that Paul had had one long and serious involvement after he moved to California, and I knew also when it was over. Is this a kindness or a disguised cruelty, this passing on of information by friends? I don't know. However, I could tell simply from the tone of his letters to me through the period of his illness that he was alone then. I wouldn't have needed the tender mercies of a friend.

I suppose it might fairly have been said of me that I was alone during this period too, but I did not feel this to be the case. I had begun to write, both the occasional story and this memoir, and I felt my life had never been more crowded—with memory, with the will to understand what memory was telling me, and with fictional explanations, too, of what I understood. In addition, in order to maintain some discipline in this activity, I'd enrolled in not one but two writing classes, and I often felt that my days and

evenings were fuller than they'd been since I was
Paul's wife.

Now Paul was writing me sadly and often about
his failure of faith, and about his inability to make
sense of or to come to peace with the course of his
life—the losses he'd endured, the pain he was experiencing in his final illness. He spoke of our life
together nostalgically, as of a golden time, a time of
sweet innocence.

I came to feel uncomfortable with this tone, and I
discovered it reminded me of the period before we
were married, when he'd written to me from his exile
in Ohio, "You are going to be a marvelous woman one
day, Lily Roberts, and I want to be the man there to
witness that transformation." At the time, I remember, I was nothing but thrilled by this idea, but it later
seemed to me the height of the unconscious conde-
scension that marked the relations of men to women
in that era.

I wrote him back now and called up that remark.
I said the tone he was taking now reminded me of it,
and that I found his easy nostalgia for our believing
youth belittling and sentimental. That I thought he
misjudged my faith if he imagined it had been
untested or unexamined. That while there was almost
nothing I wished more than to be of comfort to him
at this time, I couldn't write to him again if he continued to seem to ask me to accede to this way of
remembering our life together.

He wrote back immediately and apologetically
and said he was shocked at the picture of himself he
encountered in my letter, but also grateful for the
encounter. He felt as though he were seeing himself
"face to face." It made him recognize, he said, the sin
of the pride he'd been taking in his desolation—"I
see I've had a real sense of pleasure in the notion of

myself as so rigorously honest as to have let my questioning lead me to despair. And how strange that while I no longer believe in God, I do, apparently, still believe in sin."

He wrote, "I don't remember writing you that foolish remark, Lily, but I can easily believe I did. The irony, of course, is that you have grown into that marvelous woman, and that I am not there to see it."

I wept when I read his letter. I wept with a combined sense of the most painful loss, and gratitude—blessedness, even,—for that loss. For the first time, I understood how much who I had become was necessarily intertwined with it. "For whom the Lord loveth he chasteneth." How could I not have remembered that, not have understood it? Now, through Paul and our rapprochement as he drew near death, I did.

Over the weekend, Lily had come to the point in Paul's correspondence with her when he'd written the letter she'd quoted from in her memoir, one of her last letters from him. Holding it in her trembling hands this time, she read it in its entirety, she met again the words he'd gone on to write after his apology, the words she hadn't included in her account of things then. These words:

But I think you underestimate even your youthful self. Because always under your seeming devotion and compliance was the warmth—I would even say the heat—of your bracing coldness. (And you know there is heat in coldness, do you not, Lily? At this age I have used cold packs enough on various arthritic joints to welcome the pain of the cold for the soothing fire of blood heat that follows.)

I had the easier version of faith, and of love, for you

Lily. Because you came to faith, and to love, so slowly, so carefully, that it required far more of you in the end. You were always more analytic, and then, once you'd satisfied yourself with your examination of things, more passionate, more radical in your feelings. I sometimes worried that the more instinctive forms of love were not so available to you. That easy maternal devotion, for instance, that seemed so natural in some women and which, as we spoke of from time to time, was something you had to struggle to feel. Or the simple neighborliness of people like Adele Footman, or Polly Mayer. Sometimes, yes, I wished we had that more comfortable life together, the sense of a table at which angels might be entertained, unawares. But never, never would I have substituted those creature comforts for your fine coldness and the exacting passion it brought with it. Even, I think, as that exacting passion drove us apart. It was the bedrock of our life together, while that life lasted, the force in you that compelled me in every way, and that fed my deepest hungers—spiritual, physical, intellectual.

Why hadn't Lily included these comments in her memoir, these remarks by Paul about her coldness? At the time, she remembered vaguely, she had dismissed them quickly as not apropos to the discussion of her recovery from depression, her renewed sense of connection with God. But reading them now made her almost reel, a sick, dizzy feeling.

How dishonest she had been! She had used Paul, used his letter, used everything about their life together, to justify herself. To bear witness to her own virtue. The shame of it! the endless pitiable shame of knowing yourself so badly! For Lily had thought, of course, as she wrote the memoir, that she was peeling off layer after layer of herself, getting closer and closer to some essential core.

Vanity. She wouldn't live long enough to arrive there, she

saw that now. "Now I know in part." She whispered these words to herself. That would be all, until death released her. What arrogance to have presumed she understood the truth! And what dishonesty to have revealed only part of Paul's truth. Particularly when it was a truth—she saw this now, she felt it in rereading the letter—so lovingly offered.

And so coldly received. So calculatedly turned to her own uses. Her spiritual triumph. Over him.

She moaned aloud, and Noreen, who'd been cutting coupons from the newspaper in the living room, set her scissors down to come and ask what was wrong. Lily's appearance shocked her, and when Alan came home that afternoon, she reported that his mother was having a tough weekend, that maybe he should try to get her to rest more on Sunday.

In bed that night, Saturday night, Lily had tried to pray, but these words too seemed stiffened and locked inside her. She was terror-stricken, abruptly, her pulse pounding in her head. What, who would she be if the disease consumed even her belief?

Looking up in the dark, she made herself recite the Lord's Prayer, the General Confession—anything, the Twenty-third Psalm, whispering the words in a rushing, panicked voice. Hearing her, you might have thought she was in a race against time to finish up.

Later, Alan would think of those odd moments during the weekend when Lily seemed to wake from a half-sleep and thrust herself forward with a mislocated will and energy. He would blame himself for not knowing something was wrong. When he spoke of it later, of his failure, Gaby would defend him: "But she had been so horrid to you that Friday, Alan. You were doing quite well to be as kind to her as you were."

At dinner on Saturday night, Lily had suddenly started to speak of Paul, to speak of him as though he needed to be defended against Alan. "Your father," she'd said abruptly, "was a man of his time, a narrow, narrow man, to be sure. But he was a very fine man, nonetheless."

"I would never have said otherwise, Lily," Alan said, after a long moment when he and Gaby held each other's eyes. There was a silence at the table.

"I know he seemed very remote to you, but he could be very generous too. He tithed, you know."

"I didn't know."

"He did."

And then she fell silent. Gradually Alan and Gaby began to talk to each other once more—about the Admundsens' house and the payment schedule, about when the boys would come home for the end-of-the-summer break.

"He broke his foot once, he was so mad at me," Lily whispered urgently. They both looked at her. "I'd driven the car into a streetlight, backed right up into the post, and when I told him, oh, he was mad! He wouldn't say anything, that wasn't his way. He didn't get angry with me. But he went outside and kicked the car." She smiled, the slight demented rictus of the Parkinsonian. "Kicked it hard, I would say. I remember the cast on his foot very well. Like our friend, you know." Her hand fluttered helplessly at her chest.

"*Lin*nett," Gaby said.

"*Lin*nett," Lily corrected. "Yes." Her head bobbed. "But there, you see, he never yelled, never scolded. That wasn't his way."

"No," Alan said. "No, it wasn't."

And then she subsided, as though Alan had conceded some necessary point about Paul, a Paul who seemed oddly unlike anyone Alan had ever known.

And on Sunday, when Alan stayed home reading the paper—Noreen had Sundays off, and it was one of Gaby's busiest days—Lily appeared suddenly, effortfully wobbling on her canes across the living room. She looked, Alan told Gaby later, like the madwoman of Chaillot. She had done her own makeup with an unsteady hand, and her eyebrows trailed off upward toward her hairline. Her hair itself had escaped in drooping strands from the bun she'd tried to make. She wore her absurd frilly bed jacket over her clothes, and its odd, faded, fleshy pink made her own flesh look more bloodless, more ghostly, than ever.

He got up as soon as he saw her, and went quickly to her. He'd never seen her so frail, so crazy-looking, and it frightened him. As he took her arm, she opened her mouth to speak, but nothing came out.

"What is it?" he asked. "What is it, Mother?"

She shook her head, with great effort. Alan was panicked. He thought perhaps she was dying, that she was having a stroke. He got her across the room, into a chair. He fetched her a glass of water, and then, halfway over to her, thought better of that and went back and got a glass of whiskey. She recoiled when he held it to her lips. Her tongue pushed out at it, the way the boys' had as babies when they were offered new foods.

He sat, then, helpless, holding her hand and patting it.

"What is it?" she whispered at last.

"What is what? What?" he asked. And then, because he sounded so impatient, he said, "I'm listening."

She stared at him, as though trying to understand who he was. "I needed . . . your help."

"With what?" he asked. She didn't answer, and after a moment he said, "I'm right here, Lily."

"I needed your help," she said again.

"Okay," he said. And he remembered that he had begun at this point truly to be impatient with her. He looked at her painted face, the puzzled, halted look in her eyes, the strange, doubled eyebrows, her opened mouth, and he'd felt irritated. Finally, when she didn't speak again, he said, "But you did get yourself up, Mother. All by yourself. And you got your makeup on, and your . . . jacket there."

She lifted her arm and looked at the jacket sleeve hanging loosely off it as though she didn't recognize it.

"So you didn't really need me, you did it yourself."

"Yes," she said finally. "Yes. That must have been it."

*   *   *

And now, here it was Monday, and Linnett would arrive soon. Lily needed to gather her energy. Often in the past, the reading through of her papers and letters in the morning had fueled her for her afternoons with Linnett. The younger woman would arrive and find Lily ready, eager to recreate for her the world of Hyde Park and Woodlawn in the forties and fifties, for instance. Or the life of a young minister's wife in a small-town parish.

Today though, Lily wished Linnett wasn't coming, that she could have Noreen help her back to bed and just let go, let go of it all. It seemed to her, looking at the pages lying curled but intact in her wastebasket, that all of life was simply diminution and loss, the paring away by degrees of what had seemed necessary, the learning to do without. She thought of Rebecca the last time she'd seen her, her beautiful, passionate daughter, about to disappear forever. She thought of Paul. She thought of Alan, and Clary, and their lives, so unconnected to hers, so full of *things*. Her hands hung, curled down from the arms of the chair, spotted, trembling the more now in repose. She felt done in, done for, nearly invisible. She wasn't sure she even had a voice. She opened her mouth and made a squawk, small and high-pitched. Over her vacant face as she heard it, something faintly amused passed, and was gone.

Since Lily didn't have much of a voice, Linnett said she wouldn't stay long—just until Noreen got back with the groceries. (The Ph.D. candidate writing her thesis on early efforts at integration was coming for tea the next day, and Noreen had "a bunch of stuff" she wanted to get.) Linnett read Lily's mail aloud to her, and copied Lily's whispered indications of how to respond on the back of each letter. To the request for a signed copy of the memoir to be auctioned off for charity, regrets. All copies were in storage in Chicago. To the request to lecture next spring in San Francisco, regrets too. "No voice," Lily whispered. "By then, probably no body."

Linnett laughed.

To the woman in Chicago doing a collection of memoir excerpts, instructions on whom to contact in Lily's publishing house for permission. There was a long silence. Lily's face looked remote, dead but for the color.

Linnett had arrived today steeled against Lily. She'd decided on the drive over, after this morning's talk with Alan, that she wouldn't be susceptible anymore, either to Lily's charm or to her weakness. But there was something nearly childishly bereft about the way she looked now, and Linnett felt sorry for her in spite of herself. "Why don't I get us each a good stiff drink from Alan's supply, Lily?" she asked now. "Maybe you could use one, and then a long, long nap today."

Lily nodded. "But just wine," she said, as Linnett started to struggle up.

"Righto," Linnett said. It was laborious, her trips back and forth on crutches to get the glasses, then the bottle of wine and the corkscrew, but once she was seated again, she served them quickly.

Lily held her glass with both hands and lowered her head to the rim to sip. Even so a little wine splashed onto her bosom. Linnett pretended not to have seen it.

"Noreen shouldn't be too long, Lily," she said. "As soon as she's back, I'll go." Lily made a little noise of assent. "I wish I could help you up, but . . . " Linnett gestured at her crutches, at her cast.

They sat in silence for a while. Lily had set her glass down now, and her hands, lying in her lap, moved incessantly, a repetitive, curling, jittery motion of the fingers against the pads of her thumbs. Linnett had the impulse, which she resisted, to reach over and put her hand on Lily's two hands, to hold them until they stilled. She cleared her throat. "Why do you suppose, Lily, that we each kept our . . . infirmity, so to speak, from the other?"

For the first time this afternoon, Lily looked at Linnett with a spark of true interest. She shook her head slightly and her mouth made an O. No. Don't know.

Linnett smiled, glad to have roused Lily a little anyway. "If

I were being fancy about it," she said, "I'd diagnose *denial*. You know, that we're both people who deal with difficulty that way. But I don't really believe that, because we don't deny anything *to* ourselves. We *know* our problems."

Lily's eyes were guardedly alive.

Linnett leaned forward and adopted something close to Lily's whisper. "We're liars, Lily. A much, much better thing to be." She grinned and sat back. Lily's eyes were steady on her.

"No, no, no. I should speak for myself, Lily. *I am* a liar." Linnett rested a hand on her bosom and sighed. She took another sip of wine and watched Lily. "But I do think, also, that anyone who writes a memoir has got to be a *little* bit of a liar too."

Lily's hands fluttered, and she directed them to her drink, set on the edge of the table next to her. Linnett watched her, checking the urge to help. When Lily had successfully managed a swallow and set the glass back down, Linnett continued, "You want it to have a shape, after all. A memoir. Just as I, when I write a piece, an article, I need a shape for it. But life is ..." She sighed. "Well, the famous loose, baggy monster itself. Hideously shapeless. Ain't it?" She smiled again. "If I were writing my memoir, for instance, I'd be tempted just to jiggle it over this way a bit here ..." Linnett lifted her shoulder and imitated this motion. "Tug it into shape there. And whatnot. What not? *Why* not?"

Lily had looked away now, maybe out the window at something. Linnett couldn't tell whether the old woman was really listening, but after a minute she went on anyway, a little louder. "I could tell you how much fun it was, for instance, traveling around, staying in the odd hotel or motel, moving into a new world with each article. Why not indeed? It's partly true. Why bother with the other part? It messes up the *story*."

Linnett's voice had grown hard a little earlier, and Lily had looked away because she heard accusation in it. Now she wondered: had she said something to Linnett about Paul's letter? about her own editing of it for her memoir? She was confused, suddenly, about how much Linnett might or might not know about her, about whether she'd just thought things, or also spoken them aloud.

Now Linnett sat back. She stretched her legs out, and lifted the one in the cast onto the coffee table in front of her. "I don't know," she said. "Maybe it's all like dreaming anyway, Lily. Our lives. You know."

Lily's head swung back to look at Linnett. She shook it. No. She didn't know anything.

"Oh, you've read the stuff, I'm sure. About dreams. Our dreaming is just chemicals getting readjusted in our brains, and we give it visuals. Or we find explanations for the visuals that the chemicals create. It's a version of watching clouds drift across the sky. You know—'Hey! here's a camel. Here's St. Nick. Here're the Four Horsemen of the Apocalypse.'"

Lily looked blank.

But Lily always looked blank, Linnett reminded herself. "Maybe life is just like that. Is only that. We're busy *firing* away on these synapses or whatever in response to things, and trying like crazy to make sense of what is senseless, just this *traipse* of chemical life."

She laughed, suddenly, and had another sip of wine. "Nah. Pay no attention to me. I wouldn't even be here, Lily, if I didn't think you could tell me the truth. If you wanted to." She smiled over her glass.

Lily gave her the faintest of smiles back, which Linnett read as the sharing of her joke, but what Lily was thinking was that she hadn't told her, she was certain of that. She remembered abruptly Linnett's betrayal of her the other night, her intimacy, her alliance, with the others. The way she'd ignored Lily. She wouldn't have told her. Not after that.

"I went to see Alan today," Linnett said after a long silence. "At his office."

Lily didn't respond.

"He showed me a project he was working on. I liked it. Just as I like this house. Don't you, Lily? Like this house?"

Slowly and with effort, Lily raised her shoulders. Indifference.

Linnett's lips tightened. She was remembering abruptly Lily's remark to Alan Friday night, her own forced complicity in it. She said, "Course we talked some about *his* memories. About how his memoir would go of that same period you wrote about. It was interesting."

Lily's looked at her sharply, and Linnett went on. "To him it was not as clear-cut as it was to you." She could hear a car coming down the driveway. Looking out, she saw Noreen's crumpled station wagon swing up into the parking area. "Not as simply a matter of who was right and who was wrong. Which is how you seem to have seen things, Lily. Isn't it?"

Linnett waited. Noreen moved around in the dappled sunlight under the tree, slamming various of the car doors.

She thought she saw Lily shake her head, just slightly, and her mouth opened.

Then Noreen was bumbling up the stairs, rushing with too many bags, making a great deal of noise. She kicked at the door and it opened. The wind ruffled Lily's hair, but her face was made of stone.

Noreen's voice was loud and energetic: news of the world out there. "It was ten degrees warmer in town than it is here," she yelled. She hurried across the room to set the bags down on the island. "I thought I'd die!"

"Well," Linnett said. "We've been sitting here in the cool sipping this excellent wine. We've been *comfy*, haven't we Lily?"

Lily slowly turned her head. This word was like a blow to her, for reasons she couldn't have explained. (That comfort was what Alan had chosen for his life over what she might have wished for him? That it was her failure not to have been able to offer it—comfort—to any of the people she loved?)

At any rate, she spoke now.

"Comfy!" she said, with all the energy she could muster, and in it Linnett heard anger, and judgment, and something else a little like despair.

*   *   *

At dinner that night, Lily could hardly eat anything, but her thoughts seemed to have completely cleared. She felt as though a generous hand had brushed her brow as she napped in her room after Linnett left, and settled all the chaos within. Looking at Alan across the table, she remembered, oddly, a game he and his friends had played when they were small. But not too small. Perhaps nine or ten. And what was strangest, she thought, was that she'd never heard the girls play anything like it. "How would you rather die?" one of the little boys would ask. "Would you rather be burned to death, or shot? Would you rather be put in the electric chair, or hung?" The choices were always violent. "Would you rather have your head chopped off, or drown in boiling water?" They would actually discuss the ramifications of these deaths in terms of how much pain you'd have to endure, at what point you'd "pass out," and the like.

She told Paul about this, and they'd laughed together about the high drama implicit in all the choices, laughed that the more likely forms of death, and the less thrilling, were never considered—cancer, heart failure, despair. Being old. Being tired, done in.

They had laughed, Lily remembered. She had stood in the doorway to his study, where she'd come to offer her report of the boys' game. The light from the window behind Paul's desk whited his hair around his face, and he'd leaned his head back to laugh with her. And with their laughter, weren't they too, as surely as the little boys were, pushing away the very possibility they thought they were recognizing? *Denial*, as Linnett would call it.

How beautiful he had been then, Paul! his head thrown back, laughing with her at death.

From across the table, Alan watched the faint play of his mother's smile. "What are you thinking of, Lily?" he asked.

For several seconds, her mouth worked. "I am thinking of your father," she said at last. "Of his laugh."

chapter 14

Twice before Linnett had sat by while Lily entertained visitors. Sat by, sat in—whatever. Once it had been another divorced minister's wife. She'd begun a memoir too, and, it turned out, wanted to read some of it aloud to Lily, wanted to "pick her brains" about how to get a book contract. Lily's disease had suddenly become much worse, she'd actually managed to seem a bit non compos mentis before the afternoon was over, and the woman left, clearly disappointed, but full of a satisfying pity she signaled to Linnett with long, pointed glances when Lily began to circumnavigate a subject peculiarly.

The other had been a pair of feminist scholars working on a book they were going to title *Redefining Heroism: The Female Mode*. With them, Lily was prickly, a bit Red Queenish. Which Linnett had pointed out to her afterward. Lily had laughed.

This was different. It was different because Linnett felt differently about Lily at this point. Certainly not so allied with her. Much more critical. She'd decided to delay her own arrival to avoid the prolonged settling in, with Noreen offering things per Lily's instructions and Lily playing hostess, pouring things interminably, unsteadily passing the agitated plate of cheese and crackers, or cookies, with what seemed a deliberated mischief. (Linnett was reminded of a friend she'd had with a wandering eye. He'd toy with people sometimes, trying to confuse them as to which eye they should be trying to meet.)

She called Noreen to let her know she'd be late, and then fixed herself a tuna sandwich for lunch. She carried it and a bottle of beer to the metal table on her small, square deck and settled herself down in the matching chair. Both were enameled a sharp citrusy green, gone to rust at the bolts that held them together. The chair rested on a single bent tube of metal that traveled under the seat and across its back, and Linnett bounced lightly in it as she ate and drank, looking out unseeingly over the Thayers' garden.

She'd been working all morning outlining the piece on Lily, filling in a paragraph here or there. She thought she might finally have the distance, the correct distance, to do the work. She'd gone through what she recognized now as familiar stages with her—enchantment, then disenchantment or antipathy, and finally, magically—it usually happened this way—a bit of elevation, as she thought of it, that let her see all of these emotions and where they applied, that let her see her subject whole.

She would use the illness, she'd decided. Or it had been decided for her, as she saw it, by Lily herself, by what she'd said to Alan last Friday. She'd write too of Lily's apparent bravery in facing the illness and what it had done to her. Linnett had convinced herself this was the right way, the fairest way, to use what she knew.

She'd begun:

What happens to the writer when the writing is done? Lily Maynard's life offers one answer to this, and those who have taken heart from her appearance on the literary scene at age seventy-two, from the fine work she's done in her memoir and her fiction since then, may also take a kind of courage from her example at this juncture in her career, when that chapter seems to be closing. Lily Maynard has Parkinson's disease, and its slow progress seems finally to have brought an end to her life as a writer.

But not to her life. Because Lily's Maynard's story is nothing if not the account of a woman triumphing repeatedly over defeat, and it's with that same indomitable force and energy that she has confronted this painful fact.

She didn't know quite where she'd go from there, but this was the start, the hook she'd been waiting for, she was certain of that.

The sun heated Linnett's skin. A wasp settled on her sandwich, but was amenable to hovering when Linnett had her turn, so she didn't even try to shoo it away. She closed her eyes and slowly bobbed the chair. She could hear the buzz of a distant mower, the sound, faintly, of cars rushing by on the road. She dozed.

The shift in the air woke her. A thin veil of cloud had drawn itself across the sky, and there was a steady breeze. Linnett rolled her head from side to side, horizon to horizon. Dark clouds were moving in slowly from the south. Goose bumps had formed on her bare arms and legs. She picked up her beer and sipped it. Tepid.

She went inside. It was three-thirty. Good. The visitor was to have arrived at three. They would be, as Lily put it, in medias res, and Linnett could come in and be an observer, rather than a co-hostess, as she felt she'd been perceived before. She changed to a skirt, brushed out her wild hair. At the last minute, she grabbed a sweater—it was really getting chilly—and kathunked slowly out to Frank's car.

Lily's visitor today was the Ph.D. from Brown, with the thesis on early integration movements. As she'd explained in her letter, someone had recommended Lily's book to her, and she thought she might be able to use the women's group. Her approach, she'd said, was to try to talk to everyone she could find who'd participated at the time in a particular effort at integration, and to get their collective memory of the nature of the experience and the quality, retrospectively, of the interactions between black and whites. Lily had been very tired the day Linnett had read the letter aloud to her and she dictated her answer. They hadn't talked about the student, but Linnett had assumed she was black.

She was. She stood to be introduced to Linnett and held her hand out, waiting patiently for Linnett to lodge her crutches in her armpits so she could extend her hand back. She was tall, quite a bit taller than Linnett, which meant almost six feet, and she had mahogany skin. Her hair, like Lily's, was smoothed back into a bun. Her gaze was sober, measuring, and Linnett found herself wondering what she'd been making of Lily, how the exchange had been going.

Lily was sipping tea, Linnett noted, and her visitor—Marcea it was pronounced (had it been spelled Marcia? Linnett couldn't remember) McKendrick—also had a cup of tea by her place. There was an opened bottle of wine set out too, with three empty glasses by it, and an extra empty cup by the teapot, presumably for Linnett if that's what she chose. Lily, via Noreen.

"We've been discussing Blackstone Church," Lily announced, as Linnett began to unload her backpack.

"Well, go right on. I'm just a fly on the wall," she offered to Marcea. "I'm here to eavesdrop. I'm—did Lily already tell you this?—I'm doing an article on her. For *The New Yorker*. So ignore me if you can."

"*The New Yorker* magazine?"

"Is there a something-else *New Yorker*?" She was holding the little tape recorder in her hand. She grinned at Marcea.

"I guess not." Marcea's gaze was level and unamused.

Uh-oh, Linnett thought. But she said, "Do you mind if I record?" She sat down. "It's just to get Lily, really. Really Lily."

"No, it's fine," Marcea said.

"And of course, I love it," Lily said. "More *me* for posterity."

She was in high spirits today, Linnett thought. "Oh, come on Lily," she said. "You're hardly ready to accede to posterity."

"One never knows," Lily said.

Linnett clicked the box on and set it down.

"Lily's been telling me about the church," Marcea explained to Linnett. "The women's group."

Lily's hand went trembling up and they both turned to her. "Bible group," she said. "It was a Bible group. Not . . . not, not a women's group as we understand that now. A reading group, for discussing the Bible. The other part of it . . . well, as I was telling you, it evolved."

"But it *was* consciously integrated. A consciously integrated group." Marcea was asking, but it was a statement.

Lily frowned slightly. "Not as such. I mean, it was the church that was consciously integrated. It *had* been white, and then, as the neighborhood changed, the pastor that preceded Paul, and then Paul—Paul and I, in my role as helpmeet—felt our mission was to prevent, in this one community anyway, the sin of prejudice, of white flight. To make everyone think about what it meant to *be* a Christian church in such a neighborhood. About what being a 'neighbor' meant, as Christ used the word. The group became an expression of that, necessarily. And that was certainly one of the things we talked about."

"So, at any rate, you were conscious of *being* integrated," Marcea asked.

Lily smiled the frigid Parkinson's grimace. "Yes. That."

Suddenly rain lightly tapped the window. Lily seemed oblivious to it, but Linnett and Marcea turned and watched it for a moment. The trees rocked in the wind.

"I heard on the radio that there's some big storm passing out to sea tonight," Linnett said. "This must be the beginning of the rump end of it."

Lily barked—a laugh, a startling noise—and Marcea's head jerked toward her. Then, to recover herself, she looked down again at her notes. Linnett could see a list of questions in a girl's handwriting, the letters rounded and prettified. The kind of handwriting in which you'd find a happy face in the dots of the *i*'s, or heart shapes.

Marcea lifted her head, asked away, and Lily was set in motion again. How many times had she told this story? Linnett wondered. She'd heard a couple of taped interviews with Lily—NPR, and a talk before an arts council in Chicago—and she must have read at least a dozen, anyway, in various newspapers and magazines. Lily had the patter down. She repeated some phrases verbatim. Linnett found herself barely listening to the history of the church, a history she knew by heart anyway. She reached over and poured herself a glass of wine.

As Lily talked and Marcea kept her going, the rain slowly intensified, the sky grew darker. At some point, Noreen came out from somewhere in the back of the house, and, seeing them sitting in the dim light, crossed the room and turned the lamp on. Linnett lifted her hand to signal a greeting, and Noreen raised her eyebrows back.

Now Marcea was asking something specifically about integration and Alinsky. Lily's mouth prissed a little. "Well, he may have thought integration was the right thing, but he never publicly argued that. That was the point. That he took no stand on that publicly."

"But what's the problem with that if he believed in it?"

"Because he never tried to call up that behavior in people. He missed a great opportunity, I think. Because *there* was the civil rights movement in the South demonstrating that calling on a sense of shame, of justice, of morality, could work. Did work. Really, they had the courage to insist on what was best in the white community."

Marcea had listened to this with a little half-smile playing around her mouth. She sat for a moment, and then she said, "But see, I don't think the black community is responsible for the spiritual health of the white community."

"No, no that's true." Lily frowned. "But finally, it has a strategic interest in it, à la Alinsky, Mister Strategy himself. Because unless the white community is called on somehow, to behave morally, the black community suffers. And it really can't—I'd argue—give up on the moral health of the white community without losing something morally itself."

Marcea waited a moment, and then said firmly, "I think the black community had every right to give up on the white community."

Lily leaned her body forward, a tremulous tilt. "My dear, I thought you were here to interview me, not to argue with me."

Linnett looked at her tape recorder. Still going. Good, she'd have this. She poured herself another glass of wine.

Marcea had seemed a bit startled by Lily's comeback. But she recovered herself. She smiled. She said, "Let me rephrase that then: Don't you think the black community had the right to give up on the white community?"

"Yes. Yes, of course they did. But I'm saying that they achieved so much more where they did not. And I'd argue that it has been a disaster that they did. That they let the white community off the hook. A perfectly useful hook. Because it's too easy to say, *mea culpa*, I'm a racist, of course I am, and then not do anything more. And I'd also argue, I do believe, actually, that sometimes that moral impulse needs to be called up from outside."

Marcea seemed to start to speak, but Lily's whisper rode on.

"But that's neither here nor there. What the black community didn't have the right to do was to cast aspersions on the other part of black community that wanted to continue the struggle for integration, that thought friendship with whites was possible, was a kind of ideal, actually."

"And those were the black women in your group."

"Yes. Later known as *Toms*, as *oreos*, and the like. Those were my friends."

Marcea was writing something down now. After a minute, she looked up. In a genial tone, she asked, "I wondered about language."

"What do you mean?"

"Well, this is part of what I'm interested in—how members of groups back then, integrated groups, behaved together. And one of the measures I'm using is language. I wondered about the nature of the language used in the group. Whether the speech was . . . comfortable."

"Of course it was," Lily said quickly. Then she paused. "Well. Within certain limits. We were speaking of our most intimate feelings. That was sometimes hard. And we may have struggled for words occasionally, as one does . . . "

"But I meant specifically whether black English was used." Marcea's voice was crisp.

"Well. There's black English and there's black English." Lily seemed to have pulled herself up a little in her chair.

A quiver of amusement—or irritation? Linnett couldn't tell—passed over Marcea McKendrick's face. "And what kind of black English would you say was spoken, in your group?"

She thinks Lily is a fraud, Linnett thought.

"My dear, first of all, we were middle-class ladies. That is what we were. The black women in our group spoke middle-class black English."

"They spoke white English, then." Marcea's voice was gentle, but firm. A kind, strict teacher.

"I would say not."

"And I would suggest that it's possible you may not be aware of the distinction I'm making."

"My dear. I don't think you are aware of the distinction I am making."

"Perhaps you can explain it to me." Marcea never wavered in her politeness. Linnett was impressed. She must have been all of twenty-five, twenty-six or so.

"I think I am speaking of a different world from the one you understand so well, from the one you're used to operating in. This was, you'll remember, the fifties, then the late fifties, the early sixties. We all had a much more . . . how to put it? Not *formal*, but, polite. Public. Way of speaking then. The women in our group—black and white alike—had a sense of a public . . . vocabulary, really."

"All I'm saying is, that wasn't a black vocabulary."

"It wasn't black vernacular, if that's what you mean. Nor was it white vernacular, necessarily."

Marcea made a slight noise.

"My father, for instance," Lily said. Her voice was louder, and strained. She's furious, Linnett thought. "He was brought up on a farm, in Maine. His mother spoke in a way he was perfectly comfortable with, and he dropped into that way—that vernacular—with her. And at home, occasionally, with me and my mother. To express certain things. As the black women in our group dropped into their vernacular, a countrified vernacular really, on occasion. To emphasize certain things. Perhaps only slightly less often than they did at home, I'd argue." She looked at Marcea, expecting a response.

There was none. Her pen had stilled as Lily got more wound up. When Lily began to speak again, her trembling hands rose slowly from the arms of her chair. "It was not a rhetoric yet, you see? It had no political meaning for them to speak one way or another, just as it didn't for my father. It simply allowed them to refer easily to experiences outside our group, to signal those, in a way, to us." She leaned forward a little. Her mouth worked. "And you must remember that they were, after all, integrationists too. They imagined a world, as I did, in which we would *all* be changed. Yes. Not exactly in the twinkling of an eye, but yes, changed. That had implications for all of us."

"More implications for them than you, I'd guess."

"It had implications for all of us," Lily said again. Her voice broke. *She's torturing her*, Linnett thought.

Marcea pressed her lips together. Linnett saw the wings of her nostrils arch slightly.

Lily began again, her voice weaker, more whispery. She was speaking faster too, and more breathlessly. "Let me explain. These were middle-class women. Teachers. Social workers. The black English you refer to became important a few years later, and it was a lower-class English. The insistence on its importance was, in effect, already a repudiation of the experience of the women—the kind of women—in my group. Was part of an argument that said my friends were Toms, were not true blacks, because they spoke as they did." Lily seemed to be pleading with Marcea. "You see the result now when black school children feel that to learn anything, to be good at school itself, is capitulation, is trying to be white."

"But don't you feel your friends *were* trying to be white?"

Marcea's head tilted slightly. Her eyes, amused, briefly met Linnett's. She had no idea what this was costing Lily.

Linnett felt a strong pull of allegiance to the old woman, drawn by her effort, her pain. She watched Lily pull herself together for one more try.

"I would agree they were trying to leave a certain world behind, yes—as we all do when we try to move along, move up. And perhaps they were leaving the language of home behind, as we do when we grow up, when we're socialized. But there was an unfortunate conflation of class and race that happened right then, in the early sixties. *To be black* meant you had to act and sound like a lower-class black, a rural black. But the problem is there aren't completely parallel black and white universes. If you want to be, say, a teacher, you handicap yourself by talking like a Mississippi sharecropper. As my father would have handicapped himself by insisting that he should be able to speak as his mother did at board meetings."

Marcea nodded. "But what I'm saying is, the language he learned to speak at board meetings was white too. He didn't have to leave his whiteness behind to speak that language."

"But my friends didn't feel any less black—I know they didn't—because they were educated and could speak an educated language. Look here, if you go around and talk to ... Well, there are a whole lot of black ladies my age and older, women who fought to be educated, to become doctors or teachers or whatever. And they *can* sound remarkably white, I suppose, if by white you mean grammatical, educated. But I would be very interested to hear you or any other young person tell them they were less black because of what they achieved. How they talk."

The rain was steady now, with an occasional wind-whipped slap across the glass. Linnett had poured herself a third glass of wine. As she looked up now, she saw Alan's car pull out from under the cover of the driveway and park, next to hers, under the beech tree. She watched as he got out, his head hanging between hunched shoulders, and ran to the stairs. His loud footsteps mounting them caught Lily's attention. She looked outside.

"Ah," she said. *"Here* he is!" And in her voice was such a sense of joyous recognition, such relief, that Linnett was startled. Did she imagine Alan as a white knight, come to rescue her? And then, at that image in this context, she smiled to herself.

Now Alan burst into the room, the screen door banging shut behind him. His shoulders were darkened with rain, his curly hair was slightly flattened. "Jesus," he said. "I thought this was supposed to head out to sea." And then he took them in. "Hi," he said. "Just a second."

He crossed the room to the kitchen island, opened a drawer, and took out a towel. Wiping at his face, his hands, he came over to them. He said hello to Linnett, and introduced himself to Marcea.

Lily whispered to him sharply now. He bent over his mother, listened, looked quickly back at Marcea and Linnett. Linnett heard him say, "I'll ask Gaby, Lily. I need to get her up."

Lily pulled at his sleeve, and he bent close again. He stood up, answering her patiently: "I think that's fine, Mother, but I want to check with Gaby first."

He turned to Marcea. "Lily imagines I can shed light on the Blackstone Church scandals."

Marcea nodded, politely. "Anything you'd care to tell me."

"Well, who knows? But I need to wake my wife up first, and make sure she doesn't need me. I usually help her at work about this time. She's got a shop in town to close up."

Marcea nodded pleasantly, and Alan excused himself and went down the hall.

Linnett looked at Lily. Exhausted, collapsed back, hands trembling.

Perhaps hearing Alan, Noreen had come out again now from whatever she'd been doing at the back of the house. She began to ask Lily about her nap in a loud, cheerful voice. Lily's lips pressed together, she shook her head.

Linnett got up, clumped down the long hallway past Gaby and Alan's bedroom to the bathroom. She felt the muffled, pleasant sensation of too much booze. She'd have to slow down a bit, she thought. All she'd had to eat today was the sandwich. She could hear the murmur of Alan's and Gaby's voices as she passed their room.

In the bathroom, she splashed water on her face. She looked at herself in the mirror, seeing herself with the cruel clarity sometimes afforded the slightly drunk. She was getting old, the little vessels that had pinked her nostrils and cheeks were blooming elsewhere too. Linnett fumbled in her purse and got her makeup pouch out. Carefully she applied foundation and rubbed it in. She put on lipstick. She leaned close to the mirror and looked at herself. Then, slowly, she lifted her hand. She slapped her own face, hard. Momentarily, tears stung her eyes. She smiled fiercely at her reflection, and opened the door.

When she came back into the living room, Noreen seemed to have gone. Yes, when Linnett looked out, her tanklike station wagon was no longer there. Alan had taken charge of things. He was moving around the kitchen area, opening and closing the refrigerator, setting things out. Marcea was standing by the island, talking to him, explaining her presence, her research. Alan's amiable, loud voice punctuated her softer one from time to time. Linnett sat down by Lily, in her chair. The teapot and wine bottle had been removed. She picked up her tape recorder. It had finished and turned itself off. She looked at Lily. The old woman's return glance seemed not to recognize Linnett.

Alan brought over a plate of cheese and thin white crackers and set it down. He went back to the kitchen and returned with a newly opened bottle of wine and some glasses. Marcea came and sat down too, and Alan poured for everyone but Lily, who shook her head when he held up a glass to her.

Gaby came out from the hallway now, wearing an old crew-neck sweater over baggy jeans. She looked like a strong young boy. Alan looked over her. "So you think it'll be okay, you can manage," he said.

"Of course," she said.

He turned to Marcea. "Have you met . . . ?" He gestured toward Gaby.

Gaby stepped over to the little group. "No, we didn't." She extended her hand across the table to Marcea, who stood again. The younger woman towered over Gaby. "I was asleep already when you arrived."

"Marcea," Alan said. "I'm sorry, I didn't get the last name."

"McKendrick," Marcea said.

"I am pleased," Gaby said. "I am Gaby, Alan's wife." She made a little formal shaking motion with her hand, and then stepped back. "Linnett," she said cordially, and bobbed her head by way of greeting.

Linnett raised her glass.

"It *is* awful, isn't it?" Gaby said. Linnett was startled for a moment, and then realized Gaby was looking outside, that she meant the weather. Linnett looked out too, to where the trees slowly moved under their burden of wind and wet.

"You'd better take a parka," Alan said. He sat down on the long built-in couch under the window, his strong-featured face shadowed harshly by the lamp next to him.

As Gaby clumped back and forth in her clogs, Alan and Marcea began to talk again.

How long had it been, Linnett wondered, since he'd entertained a black person in his home? And then she thought that was unfair. She had no idea. Maybe he had black colleagues where he taught. Or clients. They wouldn't be neighbors, though. She couldn't recall seeing a black person in town. She reached over and carefully spread some cheese on one of the fragile crackers.

Now Gaby stopped outside their circle again on her way out, snapped up in a bright green parka. "Anyone who is still here on my return must stay for supper."

"That's not a punishment," Alan said. "That's an invitation."

"It's a *reward*," Linnett said.

"I'll have to get going by then," Marcea said. "But thanks."

"Oh, I am sorry," Gaby said. "But maybe you'll change your mind. You could wait the storm out with us. And you, Linnett." Gaby turned her brown eyes to Linnett. "It's too terrible outside to go home and eat alone. We count on you."

"Thanks," Linnett said. "I will."

Gaby flipped the hood of the parka up and left then, shutting the inner door, too, on her way out. And it was suddenly quieter in the room.

There were a few seconds of silence. Then Alan said, "Well, what has Lily called upon me to bear witness to?"

chapter 15

Later it would be hard for Alan to remember many of the things he said—so much else went on that night and for the next few days. The young woman, Marcea McKendrick (when she called him months later he instantly remembered her name, how she'd looked, the firm grip of her hand), had described the basic argument between them. Lily had exhausted herself already, he could see, but she had insisted on having Noreen sent away without going in for her nap, and she sat through Marcea's explanation, stony-faced, drained-looking. Marcea was clear and concise, and, he thought, fair-sounding in her summation.

"So, if your perspective could offer us anything new . . . " she said. He thought there was something faintly amused in the way she suggested this possibility.

He remembered later that he talked about his high-school friend, Clayton Davis, his one good black friend. He remembered telling Marcea about the time he'd said to Clayton that he'd felt overwhelmed by the rapid influx of black kids straight up from the delta into his grammar school. That Clayton had said to him, "*You* were overwhelmed. Imagine how *we* felt." That it had not occurred to him until then that the great migration happened also to a stable, middle-class and working-class black community with much to lose. He knew, even as he told this story, that part of the point of it was to let her know that he'd had a black friend. *You see, I am not prejudiced.* He felt again the odd sense of falseness and shame about Clayton—who had disappeared, whose name was included on the list of the lost at class reunions. "We'd appreciate having any information about the following class members, who have dropped off the face of the earth." If Clayton was his friend, why didn't he have any idea what had happened to him? Why had he moved so completely beyond Alan's ken shortly after they both graduated from college?

As he thought about it later, it seemed he must have been talking about Clayton by way of agreeing with Marcea that yes, there was a black language that middle-class blacks were cut off from, that connected more directly to the black experience.

But what of Clayton's black experience then? Had Alan said he thought it was inauthentic? He couldn't have said that, could he? And not to Marcea, surely, with her smooth delivery, her barely accented voice?

Maybe he mentioned Clayton as a way of agreeing with Lily that the notion of integration could work as long as the black community aspired to the middle class, maybe he said that his comfort with Clayton had to do with that.

He couldn't remember, he couldn't remember. What he remembered most clearly was Lily earlier when she asked him to speak for her, whispering with dislocated urgency over the sound of the rain and wind outside. She had dropped her charm. She seemed merely insistent, and physically wasted. Gone. "Tell her," she whispered when he bent over her. "I want you to tell her how it was."

But insistent on what? What had she wanted from him? What could he have given her that would have helped?

At any rate, he hadn't. He talked of Clayton, yes. And he knew he'd spoken of his relief when the black power movement essentially threw whites out of the civil rights business, that he'd said, in fact, that the clarity then was like a good hard kick in the head. In the ribs? He couldn't recall. He'd met

Linnett's eyes, though, and saw that she recognized his reference. And this is what set things in motion. Something lighted
in her face, and after a few minutes of his talking of other
things, she leaned forward, set her glass down, and spoke to
Marcea.

Her voice was pleasant, conversational. "You know, maybe
the difference, the difference in the way Alan and Lily feel, has
to do with his having been beaten up, did you know that?"
Alan could tell that she was excited, she saw dramatic possibilities here. Instantly he regretted having brought it up, even as
obliquely as he had. Especially as obliquely as he had. "By
black kids," she said. "As a kid. When he was a kid."

Marcea's expression tightened, closed. "Oh?" she said.

Alan felt his pulse thicken. He was angry at Linnett, furious
at himself.

Lily whispered fiercely, "You're not going to flog that old
horse again, are you?"

And instantly, freshly, Alan's rage was redirected and he
felt it once more as his anger at Lily's silencing him then, as the
true rage he'd felt at the time and not been allowed to shape in
words. "I'd like a chance to flog it *once*, Lily," he said, with
forced geniality. And then his voice grew harder. "I'd like to be
able to say, just once, in front of you, that yes, I was beat up,
and yes, that it was wrong, it was wrong."

Her trembling hand waved vaguely in front of her. She
croaked, "It's hardly even relevant in the sense of larger
wrongs, larger . . . "

"But it's relevant to me. To what goes on between me and
you."

"But you mustn't seize on that. That isn't . . . "

"Mother, I don't think I did. I didn't. But don't you see . . . "
She started to shape a word and he held his hand up. "No, here
it is. You felt there was this one black community to respond to,
which you insisted I respond to. You heard one message from
the black community. One." He raised a finger. "But I grew up
hearing, I don't know. Four or five? Sure, at first, 'Be my

friend.' But then 'Stay away from me.' Sometimes 'Help me.' Then 'Hands off.' Then 'Fuck off.' That's what the beating said, Lily. It said 'Fuck off. Fuck off, and die.'"

It was as though some final peg that held her together had been pulled. Her mouth slackened, her hands hung, wildly dancing. They all sat in silence. The rain pelted the window. Finally Lily whispered hollowly, "I wish you'd felt more as I did."

Alan looked away sharply. He understood that Lily had spoken from her heart, and he was instantly ashamed. And he felt—her tone, her collapse made him feel, viscerally—how alone she'd been too, deeply alone, in much of what she'd lived through. He felt, in spite of his anger, a sense of understanding her. He was silent for a long moment. Then he reached forward and touched her dangling, trembling hand. He said, "How much easier life would have been for all of us if I had."

She didn't respond. After another few seconds' silence, he stood up. "I'm going to take you in for your rest now, Lily. No arguments. Let's go." He reached down and pulled his mother up next to him. They didn't speak as he guided her to the bathroom. He waited for her outside the door as he always did in the mornings, and then he led her to bed. She seemed barely able to move, to recognize him. He took off her shoes, he lifted her legs onto the bed, he eased her back against the mounded pillows. Her eyes didn't meet his, but this didn't seemed deliberate. She was long gone in exhaustion, beyond anger or mischief.

He could hear the voices from the living room as he spread the afghan over Lily, and he wondered what they might be talking about, Linnett and Marcea. What they might be saying about him, about Lily.

When he came out, Marcea stood up immediately. "I really need to go," she said. "I'd like to get home before it gets too dark." She gestured. At this time of evening the sky was usually still lemony blue. Today the rain had brought an early night. There seemed to be no sky at all above the black, tossing trees.

"We can't persuade you to stay for dinner?"

"I'd like to," she said. "But really, I can't." She was already putting her notes away.

Alan watched her. "I hope what I said . . . Well, that I haven't offended you."

"Not *me*," she said, and laughed. As though, what? she was beyond taking offense. Perhaps as though it was only Lily he'd offended. Or none of the above. She was a child after all. Thomas's age. Most likely just that careless too, about the tone of what she said, about the ways people might understand it.

She and Linnett were saying goodbyes, chatting briefly. She'd look for the article. Linnett wished her luck with the thesis. Alan went to get an umbrella from the coat closet in order to walk her out to her car. They went through a ritual of insistence and refusal, but in the end, of course, he walked with her across the dark yard and held the umbrella open above the car door while she slid in. After she'd shut it, she rolled the window down partway. "Thank you," she said primly, politely.

He looked at her. He felt she had stumbled into something that might have been painful for her because of his anger at Lily, because of his shabby effort to flirt with Linnett. He didn't want her to leave. "I'm sorry," he said.

"What?" She squinted up into the wet air at him.

"I'm sorry." He spoke loudly over the noise of the driving rain. "I'm sorry to have talked about that. About being beaten up. It wasn't important. It wasn't . . . to the point. It was stupid."

She looked up at him steadily, measuring him, he felt.

"It was a stupid thing to say. To talk about. It was aimed at Lily, to hurt her."

"I think I knew that," she said.

Alan put his hand on the door handle and smiled at her. "It's just I was raised to feel being white was itself a kind of sin, and I've never figured out how to expiate it."

"Well," she said. She didn't smile back. She looked away, toward the lights of the house through her windshield. She

shrugged. "I hope one day you do." And then she bent forward
and turned on the engine.

As she drove away, Alan stood alone in the dusky down-
pour, watching the red lights disappear into the shrubbery of
the driveway. Then he turned under the umbrella and looked
back at his house, the warm yellow lights inside, Linnett sitting
on one of Lily's chairs looking blindly back out at him. He had
never felt less drawn to it, to its comfort and warmth. He
started back across the wet, dark yard.

He avoided talking to Linnett when he went in. He put a
CD on, one Thomas had recommended to him, and excused
himself to work. In the kitchen, he got out a thick, yellow-
pepper soup Gaby had left in the refrigerator, and turned the
heat on low under it. With deliberated care, he chose bright red
paisley placemats for the table, matching napkins. Slowly he
laid out the thick white plates and bowls, the old silver from
Gaby's family. He washed the mâche, the frisée, as Gaby had
asked him to do, picking carefully through the pale green
leaves.

By the time Gaby came back, breathless from her run across
the yard, he'd settled himself a little. She fixed him coffee,
which they usually had together when they came back from the
shop, and Alan offered Linnett more wine. She accepted.

Gaby had asked about Marcea, and Linnett explained her
departure. Now she was trying to explain, too, the basic issue
between Lily and Marcea, the point about black English.

Gaby seized on it. She was sitting with Linnett. As Alan
came over to join them, she began to speak of her sense of losing a part of herself in English.

Linnett argued that this was different, that black English
wasn't a different language, but a different dialect.

Still, still Gaby said. Alan watched her. She was gesturing
broadly, she was excited. One cast oneself as differently in a different dialect surely, she said, as in a different language. The
French of Paris caused her to pitch her voice higher, to be less
determined in her enunciation, more rhythmic. "There is a par-

ticularly feminine way of speaking French. It's a much more sexually divided language than English, which men and women speak just the same way. I have always felt . . . less female, less attractive, when I speak English. Listen." And she translated those words into French. Alan could hear the rise in pitch in her voice, the slightly singsong quality. He wondered that he hadn't thought about this before, about what she had lost when she decided to become his wife. To become American. And hearing her speak in French now reminded him that it was also his loss. He was shocked that he hadn't realized this, and for the first time was aware of how much he too missed her, the Gaby who spoke French.

"But doesn't Alan speak French too?" Linnett asked. "Can't you be sexy, anyway, with him?"

"Oh no," Gaby said. She looked at him. "Alan had a little French, and we used to try to talk together, remember dear?"

"I remember the struggle," he said.

She smiled broadly, and turned back to Linnett. "But you see, after all, we had made our choice. We were in America. And I think you have to choose, one language or the other. So he lost it, his French."

"Still," Linnett said, "your accent in English is mighty sexy."

Gaby waved her hand dismissively. "Ah, but I don't control that, you see. It's purely accidental that I sound one way or another. I felt . . . I don't know how to say it—*in charge of* my own sexiness, in French."

Linnett nodded drunkenly, a diminishing series of bobs of the head. "Yeah, I see your point."

After a moment, Alan said, "There must be an up side to this, Gabs."

"Oh, I am not complaining," Gaby said. "Only observing."

"It gives you a lot of freedom though, if you think about it."

"What do you mean?"

"Well, the accent marks you as foreigner, of course, and therefore . . . I don't know. Not part of the American dialogue."

"Well, thank you very much," Gaby said, in mock affront.

"No, you know what I mean, I think. There are, for instance, rules for Americans, we're sort of silenced about this and that. Particularly, like this afternoon, the racial stuff. And you don't have to honor that silence."

"I was not even aware of it."

"That's what Alan's saying, I think, Gaby," Linnett said.

He laughed, sharply, and after a moment, said, "But also, more than your being unaware, I don't think a person like Marcea would hold you so accountable for what you might say."

"Pffft," Gaby said. "There's nothing I could possibly say that could offend Marcea anyway."

"Well, I'd argue that with you, but not effectively, I think."

Gaby had just opened her mouth to answer when Lily's bell rang, a faint tinkling under the sound of the storm. "Ah, excuse me," she said. She got up and crossed the room.

Instantly Alan got up too, and pretended to be busy again in the kitchen. He didn't want to have to talk to Linnett.

It turned out that Lily felt too tired to come to the table. Alan helped Gaby fix a tray, and she took it back into the guest room. When she came back, Alan poured the soup into the warm tureen and brought it to the table, and they sat down and started their dinner at last. Outside the storm was steady. They spoke of it, of Marcea driving back to Providence.

Gaby got up and began to sauté the scallops for the warmed salad. Above the hiss and sizzle, she spoke loudly. "This will just be a moment. I hope you're not starving to death."

"No, no," Linnett said. "The soup was so good." Then, after a moment she began to speak about her impending departure, at the end of the week she thought. She had to report for jury duty.

In the way she pronounced *du-ty*, Alan heard that she'd crossed the line into true drunkenness. Either he or Gaby would have to drive her home.

"Well, you can always hope they'll reject you," he said. "If you're at all educated, they usually do."

"Oh, but no, I love jury duty," she said. "Just the circumstances of it. You know, getting up in the morning and going to a place where there are other people, and grousing about the weather or someone or other's incompetence. It's like the real world again. Like having a job. I hope they *do* pick me."

"Last time Alan was called, he was turned away," Gaby said. She'd brought the salad bowl to the table. A citrusy aroma rose from it as she began to dish it out onto their plates.

"No," Alan was saying. "Last time I *did* serve. And it was the stupidest thing I ever heard. Remember? It all centered on a curb cut. This guy was suing the town because his neighbor got a curb cut. I'd never truly understood what boredom was before that trial."

"I'd forgotten that one," Gaby said. "I was thinking of the one when we were still in Boston." She passed their plates.

"Ah, that one." He turned to Linnett. "That one was a homicide. Murder. I was glad not to have to decide it."

"God, no. Someone's whole *life* in your hands."

Gaby sat down and they began to eat.

Linnett began to tell a jury-duty story, one of her own, but Alan was barely listening. He was remembering the kid, the black kid charged with murder. He was powerful-looking, short and thick-necked. It was the early seventies, an era when he might have been expected to have an Afro, but his hair was clipped short. He wore glasses, horn-rimmed glasses, and a suit. He and his lawyer, a white woman in *her* glasses, *her* suit, conferred briefly about each potential juror, and Alan remembered their eyes on him as the judge, a polite, seemingly off-hand man, asked him a few questions about what he did, about his training as an architect. Though he was relieved when the judge said he was dismissed, he was oddly disappointed too, as though his ability to be impartial, to be fair to this young man—to be his defender, if that's the way it played out—had been questioned. He wanted to explain himself. "I believe in innocence," he wanted to say.

Later Alan had looked in the paper for news of the kid, but he never found a mention of the trial. Apparently it was an ordinary murder, a routine case. Whether the kid was guilty or not, it wasn't worth writing up.

When Linnett got up to go to the bathroom, she started walking before she was fully settled on her crutches, and one of them flipped out from under her arm. She nearly fell, and Alan and Gaby half-rose simultaneously, and then slowly sat down again as she adjusted herself and moved away down the hall.

"I'll drive her home if you like," Alan said in a lowered tone. "She shouldn't go alone."

Gaby smiled. "I don't like."

"Oh, come on, Gaby."

"No, it isn't that, really. It's just so awful out. I mean, just look." They sat for a moment looking mostly at their own reflections in the glass, but suddenly conscious too of the noise of the storm around them. "We could just put her in Thomas and Etienne's room," Gaby suggested. "The beds are made up."

"If she'll agree."

"I'll insist. I'm very good at that. With my adorable little French accent."

"All right," he said. He stood and began to clear the table.

Gaby lowered her own voice. "She likes to drink, I think."

"It's probably easy, when you live alone, to get in the habit of having too much."

"Yes, but we held dinner off for too long. I feel responsible."

"Well, but who knew about Lily?"

After a moment's silence, Gaby said, "She seems completely exhausted. Poor old thing."

"She has for a couple of days, don't you think?"

"Still. Was she terribly upset this afternoon?"

"I don't know." They heard the bathroom door opening and Linnett starting down the hall toward them. "She was so tired it was hard to tell. But she wanted me to defend her, I think. The way she sees things. And I couldn't."

Gaby nodded and touched his hand as Linnett sat down again.

They were still sitting at the table at about nine-thirty when the telephone rang. Alan answered it. It was Marcea McKendrick, apologizing if she was interrupting or bothering them.

"Not at all," Alan said. He felt an odd excitement at hearing her voice—perhaps that her goodbye hadn't been the final one, that he might have another chance. To what? He didn't know.

"It's just, I had the radio on," she said, "fixing a snack, and I heard that this storm that's coming in? That it's like a hurricane. Hurricane force, anyhow. And it didn't seem like you knew that. It's supposed to hit the whole coastline tomorrow. That's what they said." Her voice thrilled as the bearer's of bad tidings often does.

"When?" Alan asked. "Tomorrow?"

"Yeah, they think like late morning or early afternoon? Anyway, I wanted you to know."

"Well, yes, thanks. We sure *didn't* know. We're still just sitting around the table."

"Well, I'm glad I called then." There was a pause. "Good luck," she said after a few seconds.

"Yes," he said. "And thanks again."

He had barely finished telling Gaby and Linnett when the telephone rang again. Thomas. He'd been watching TV with a friend when they interrupted the program with an alert. "They showed it on the map, Dad, the possible trajectories. And you're sitting right in the middle of one of them." His voice was nearly breaking in his excitement. Behind him, Alan could hear Gaby doing her insisting to Linnett.

"Do you want me to come down?" Thomas asked.

"Definitely not," Alan said. "It's got to be very bad driving, and there's not that much to do anyway. I want you to stay right there."

"We could get hit too," Thomas said enthusiastically.

"Well, you can always hope," Alan said.

"It *is* kinda cool," Thomas said.

"I'm glad you think so."

"Hey, you kinda think so too, don't you?"

"I do and I don't. But I know what you mean, son."

By the time Ettie called at a little past eleven, Lily and Linnett were sleeping. Alan and Gaby had been busy for an hour or more. They'd brought all the deck and yard furniture into the house. The living room was crowded with the odd collection, there was barely room to move around. They had started to tape the windows.

Gaby answered the phone, and Alan could tell by the way her voice widened with pleasure who it was. While she spoke to Ettie, she moved around the kitchen area, loading the main dishwasher, wiping the countertops. They didn't talk very long, though Alan heard her ask about the internship, and about when he would come home. She laughed then, and said, "Yes, if we're still here."

When she came back to help Alan, she said, "He saw it on the eleven o'clock news."

"How is he?" Alan asked.

"He sounds very good," she said. "But then, he always does."

Alan was struck by the truth of this.

Before they went to sleep, Alan and Gaby lay in bed for a while listening for news of the storm on the radio. (The television was in Thomas and Etienne's room because Gaby disapproved of it. One of Alan's occasional and intense pleasures was lying in sheets that smelled of his sons, and watching whatever it was Gaby wasn't interested in, usually sports.)

A few seconds after Alan turned off the light, Gaby said, "Well, we have done what we can."

"Not quite," Alan answered. "I've got the Admundsens' house to think of too, and it's a lot more exposed than we are."

"Oh, Alan, of course! And the windows are just in! What will you do?"

"I'm going to head over in the morning, if it seems like there's going to be time."

"I will come and help you," she said instantly.

After a moment, he said, "What about Lily?"

"Oh, Lily!"

They lay side by side. The rain drummed steadily on the roof and the deck.

Gaby spoke. "I'll see if I can bring her to Noreen's." She had turned to him, he could hear the change in her voice. "That would be better anyway, Alan. It's that much farther inland." Noreen lived in North Bowman, seven or eight miles up the road, in one of several developed areas of neat, nearly identical small houses.

"Yeah. You're right. If Noreen will take her."

"I'm sure she will. And then I'll come over and help you."

"Well, we'll see. There may not be time for any of this."

After a few minutes, she said, "It was sweet that the boys called, wasn't it?" Her voice was slow. And then her breathing thickened, elongated, and he was alone. The rain drummed and pocked the roof, slowed, then sometimes struck it fiercely, a watery bludgeon. Alan thought of the day ahead of him, of the confusion of the day past.

It *was* sweet that the boys had called. He saw their faces in his mind's eye, the curious way they looked like brothers without resembling each other in the least.

He thought of Marcea then, of her call, her voice relaxed and open on the phone. He remembered the way her face had closed when Linnett told her he'd been beaten up. But she'd called, called to warn them. He'd felt, he realized a kind of blessing when he heard her voice again, the sense of something having been forgiven. He had spoken, and she'd forgiven him.

He thought of his own father suddenly, that last time he'd seen him, the gray-yellow death color of his skin, the tears that rose in his eyes when he coughed. How he stopped Alan from speaking then, from saying what he felt.

Which would have been what?

After all, he really didn't know, he realized. Maybe, in his youth, he had just wanted to hurt Paul, as he felt then that Paul had hurt him.

Rebecca had had a fight with Paul once, at the dinner table. Paul had casually asserted that all whites were guilty of racism, and Rebecca had turned on him, had said something about how in her childhood, Paul would have defended her passionately against such a charge. When, she asked him, had everything changed? How was it that she had somehow, magically, become a racist? Was it conferred on her with adulthood? Or maybe when she got her period?

Alan had been thrilled by this. Lying in bed now, he remembered Rebecca, as he hadn't in years. He saw her face, handsome, dark. The long Maynard nose. Thomas looked a bit like her, he thought.

She was personalizing things, Paul had said. He was talking about something else, something larger.

"Oh, Daddy, it's always something larger, something larger. I'm tired of there never being any small truths. That's what I believe in."

Alan had never come close to such speech. Or the closest he'd come had been tonight, uselessly, with Lily. He saw her again, her utter collapse when he spoke the truth at last. His small, small truth. In the dark, he winced.

Was this his revenge, he wondered, to speak it, this overdue truth? Or had he just been showing off—for Marcea? for Linnett?

And what truth anyway? Surely he wasn't interested in *that* small truth, that wasn't the issue, that he'd been beaten up.

What hope was there anyway in his life, at this point, and with that audience, for anything like a larger truth that connected to his story?

He turned in bed. He was suddenly seeing in his mind's

eye himself as a young man, encircled on the dark street, the shocking, naked hatred on the faces as they began to hit him. He remembered his own sense of innocence then, confused at first—how could this be happening, *to me?*—and then, as the blows fell and the plume of pain unfurled, blinding and raging and clear. After they left, after the last stabbing kick against his head, the piercing pain in his jaw, he'd lain there, curled up at first, and then on his back, looking up at the night sky, black behind the angry screen of orangy city light, and he felt the relief, the pure joy, of having survived. But much more. The hard bright clarity of his own pain, of knowing that this, this could not be altered or confused or taken away from him. *Mine*, he had thought, tasting his own blood, swiveling his tongue against his yielding teeth. Mine.

chapter 16

Lily woke to the wind, its song calm in her limbs. She lay still and watched its long, sustained swing in the branches outside her window. In answer to it, it seemed, she was changed, her body felt transformed, magically—heavy and powerful. She had a sense of responsive muscle and sinew that she would have said she didn't remember, but now that it had been returned to her, was as deeply familiar as her sense of her own weight. The rain had stopped in the night, but the sky was a pearly gray-yellow, a beautiful, dangerous color. The wind was slow and deep, and Lily understood that she was held in it, as through it were a boat on a slowly rocking ocean, that its dragging rhythm was what had brought her body peace.

She held her hands up, veiny and knobbed and steady, the only ornamentation a ring of her grandmother's. There was nothing in their splayed, still strength that even hinted of her disease. This miracle had happened to her a few times before, sometimes in response to music, more often to weather. Once sailing on a boat in Lake Michigan. The child of an old friend had taken her and his parents out, and the singing rhythm of the water coursing through her body had steadied her. They had laughed about it, about her *cure*, but of course, as soon as she was walking on land again, the Parkinson's had reasserted itself, and her gait back up the wooden dock was trembling and festinate.

With the next long exhalation of wind, she swung her arms suddenly out and then together again and up, a conductor signaling the music to start. She laughed out loud.

She could hear noises in the kitchen. Alan, she assumed. She pushed the blanket off her legs and lowered them slowly to the floor. She put her weight down and felt her legs muscularly receiving it.

She'd surprise him, she thought, he who considered her so helpless. And as she moved around the guest room and bathroom, getting ready for what the day would bring, she imagined Alan, his startled face when he found her dressed—how he would look, how she would look, what she would say. Then she thought of how he had looked yesterday, talking to Linnett and that Marcella person.

So much like Paul!

She had mistaken him for Paul actually, she realized now, and she stopped, dumbfounded, a hairpin in her hand, her jaw gone slack.

She had actually thought—it was unbelievable!—that it was Paul coming in from the rain, and she'd thought—here's what it was, she remembered in amazement—she'd thought for a moment he would take her part, explain it to them, how it had been, the excitement of that world. The moment Alan spoke to her, she had known him, of course, and she'd come quickly back into the world where Paul was dead and their time together was years in her past. And she'd utterly forgotten her mistake, she'd somehow pushed any awareness of it from her mind.

Until now. She looked at her old, old face in the mirror. Was this the kind of thing she would descend into more and more?

She saw her father suddenly, wearing a soiled tablecloth like a cloak around him, turning in fear from her approach, his gaze milky and unknowing. It wasn't bearable. She stuck a pin savagely into her hair, then another, and another. She stared at herself coldly, the tears rising in her eyes from the streaks of pain on her scalp.

She filled the basin and viciously washed her face, then patted it dry. Carefully she applied powder and her lipstick.

There was a sharp knocking on the bedroom door, and Lily padded to it, opened it.

Gaby stood there, holding a tray. Lily saw coffee and her oatmeal. Gaby's face opened in astonishment at the sight of Lily, dressed and tidied up. "Lily!" she cried.

Lily made a slight curtsying motion. "Yes, if you'd waited a few minutes more, you could have had the full effect. Shoes were next."

"But I'm amazed. How did you do this?" She crossed the room and set the tray down on Lily's table. She turned and looked Lily up and down as the old woman moved smoothly too, after her.

"Every now and then the Lord gives me such a day." Lily gestured to the windows. "I think today it has to do with the weather. The wind."

"Well, I'm delighted for you. Though I'm sorry the Lord had to give the rest of us a hurricane for you to have a good day."

Lily looked dubiously outside to where the trees' tossing had picked up. "This is a hurricane?"

"This will be one a bit later on." Gaby shrugged. "This is what the weatherman tells us, so it must be true. And I have a great deal to do, as you may have guessed, so it is good luck, in a way, that you can do more for yourself today." She gestured to Lily's chair, and Lily moved to it and sat down. Gaby slid the table in toward her.

Lily had just begun to eat when the thought occurred to her: "But where's Alan?"

Gaby was reaching over Lily's bed, flipping the sheet and blanket back. "Alan has gone to the house he's building, to see what can be done to protect it." Vigorously she smoothed the bottom sheet out. She looked over at Lily for a moment, watched her lift a spoonful of the oatmeal to her mouth and tilt her head slightly back to begin the process of swallowing. Gaby's lips tightened, and she turned and finished making the bed, her strong arms pulling everything smooth. She plumped the pillows and set them in place.

"Now," she said. "I'll be back in a bit. I'm going to take some coffee to Linnett."

"Linnett is here?" Lily stopped, her spoon halfway to her mouth. Everything was topsy-turvy.

"Yes. She spent the night last night."

"Was this on account of the hurricane too?" Lily asked.

"No, no, no. She simply had too much to drink." Gaby smiled grimly, remembering. Then she frowned. "Well, perhaps it was actually a little on account of the hurricane, because the rain was so heavy then that we didn't wish to drive her home through it. Anyway. She spent the night here, in Thomas and Etienne's room." She watched Lily take another slow spoonful. "I'll be right back," she said.

Lily could hear her in the kitchen, though she worked more quietly than Noreen. She strained her throat to close, then sipped gratefully at the coffee, which went down so much more smoothly. She stopped to rest. The pine branches on the tree outside bowed slowly, ceremoniously, and then slowly lifted.

Lily cried out faintly at their beauty, and closed her eyes momentarily in prayer, in her own slow sweep of gratitude for her cleared sense of her body, of herself. *Help me, God. Help me make use of your gift to me today*, she prayed.

And suddenly she understood what she had to do, what she felt now she'd been struggling not to understand for days, what she'd known was waiting for her, but doubted she'd have the strength to accomplish. How could she have doubted? How could she not have guessed she would be given the means, the power, when she most needed it? Her heart welled in sorrowful gratitude. When she opened her eyes, tears stood in them, and Gaby was in front of her.

She was frowning. "Lily, I am afraid I shall have to ask you to, really, to hurry a bit. I'm going to take you to Noreen's for the day—you'll be safest there—and I need to get over to help Alan. So you see, I am waiting for you."

Lily didn't have to think, the words were there. "Surely you don't need to wait. Why can't Linnett take me? You can see perfectly well I don't need much help today."

The idea startled Gaby, Lily could see this, but now the younger woman began to think it through. Lily took another mouthful of the cereal and lifted her chin so Gaby could see her slow effort, would take it into account—how long she would be if she had to wait for Lily to finish.

"Do you really think you could get to her car by yourself?" Gaby asked after a moment.

Lily swallowed once, then again. Dramatically she lifted her hand to her throat for a moment. Then she said, "Look at what I've already accomplished. A person who dresses herself. Who puts on her own lipstick. What is there that I can't do?" she asked. "Except eat quickly, apparently. But everything else is possible with the Lord."

Gaby sat down on the foot of Lily's bed and stared out the window, weighing the idea.

"I feel very bad keeping you from Alan," Lily said.

"It isn't your fault, Lily."

Lily took another spoonful, again exaggerating her own slowness. When she'd swallowed, she said, "You could draw Linnett a map."

"I will ask her," Gaby said, rising abruptly.

She came back beaming and brusque. "She said she will. I told her you'd be a little while, but that is fine with her. She'll shower and the like. And I have a few things I'm doing—I've started to draw a tub of water, in case the electricity goes off and the pump won't work. And I want to pack some lunch for Alan, and then I'll be going."

"I'm glad, dear," Lily said.

Gaby paused. "You are sure you can manage."

"If you'd like, I'll get up and do the cha-cha-cha for you."

Gaby smiled, and then looked around the room. "Are there things you'd like with you at Noreen's for the day?"

"I think not. Watching the hurricane will surely be amusement enough for the likes of me."

"Well, then." Gaby stepped forward and quickly bent to kiss Lily's cheek. "I'll see you this evening."

"Yes," Lily said. "Be careful."

As she made her way through several more spoonfuls of oatmeal, she could hear Gaby going in and out, the bang of the screen door three or four times. And then her car started. Lily could see it moving across the yard and disappearing into the driveway under the bending, swaying branches.

After a while she realized that she was hearing the water singing in the pipes behind her bathroom wall: Linnett, showering. She waited until it stopped, and then about five minutes more, and then she pushed her table away, got up, and—as she felt it—floated smoothly out of her room and down the hall to her grandsons' room. She knocked.

"Just a sec," Linnett's voice called back.

And in a minute or so the door opened. Linnett stood with her crutches tucked under her arms, her hair hanging in long damp ringlets, her blouse dotted with water, her face clean-scrubbed. She looked older and tired without the makeup. "Lily!" she said.

"No canes, even," Lily said, raising her empty hands.

"Are you ready to go now? I'll be a few more minutes." She waved her hand vaguely behind her, back into the room.

"No, no. That's the point. That was Noreen on the phone."

"Oh! I didn't hear it."

"Well, maybe because you were in the shower. Anyway, she's coming for me."

"But Gaby wanted me to take you."

"Well, it turns out Noreen has to go out and get some things, candles and batteries and the like," said Lily, thinking quickly. "And she said she'd just as soon swing by at the end of all that, since she's not sure how long it will take, you know, they may be out of them at various stores and she may have to drive around a bit . . . " A part of Lily was admiring her own improvisational skills. "So she'll just get me whenever. And in all honesty, though I didn't want to say so to Gaby since she was in such a hurry to get going"—she made her voice sound slightly irritated—"I think I could make use of the able-bodied Noreen. No insult intended, of course."

Linnett was frowning. "Maybe I should just call Noreen back and confirm all this."

"I told you, dear, she was going out," Lily said impatiently. "And I should think you'd be grateful. You probably have things you should get too. And you should hurry home and draw some water."

"Water?"

"Yes. If the electricity goes, you'll have no pump, and you'll need water to flush and wash up with. That kind of thing."

"Ah," Linnett said. She still looked dubious.

Either it would work or it wouldn't, Lily thought. She turned. "I've got to get back to my oatmeal," she said. "I need to try to finish up by the time Noreen gets here."

She was aware of Linnett's watching her as she made her way back down the hallway. After she'd sat down again, she was even more intensely aware of listening for Linnett, for her noises in the house and what they might indicate, but the wind had picked up now and was audible as a steady low sound through which Lily could hear nothing else. She was startled then, when Linnett appeared in her doorway. She'd put on makeup, and—Lily's heart leaped!—she had her backpack on.

"I'm off, Lily," she said. "Off to fight the storm at my house."

"Well, good," Lily said. "And if we all survive, I shall see you tomorrow."

"Maybe," Linnett said. "Actually, I was thinking I might just stay home and start writing. Unless you need me, of course. I mean, I don't really have any more questions for you."

"Oh no," Lily said. "I'll have no need. And I'm glad you feel ready to move ahead. That's very good, very nice." She paused, and then smiled slyly. "You imagine you have plumbed all my mysteries then."

"I'd never claim that," Linnett said. "Never." She was grinning back. "But I do think I'm in good enough shape for an article for *The New Yorker* anyhow."

"Well, good. Good for you."

"You sure you don't want me to stay until Noreen gets here?"

"My dear, the truth is, I'd relish the time alone. I literally can't remember when I was last alone, you've all been such conscientious baby-sitters. So run along."

"Hump along, anyway."

"I'd never say it."

"See you soon, Lily."

"Yes," Lily said. She listened carefully again as Linnett left. But she could hear nothing, and couldn't tell whether she was truly alone until she saw Linnett in the yard tilted into the wind on her crutches, making her way laboriously to her car. She was aware of her heart, suddenly, pounding heavily in slow excitement.

It took Lily another half an hour to finish the oatmeal, and in that time the wind's clamor picked up and the telephone rang twice. *Noreen*, she thought, and hoped it wouldn't occur to the girl to get in her car and come see why Lily hadn't been delivered to her.

A few branches lay in the yard now, Lily noted as she stood up, and the trees' bending was more extreme, more violent. Surely they would all break, forced this far? There was rain blowing now too, spattering the windows. The noise of the storm agitated her curiously, she noticed she was a little breathless. But as she lifted the bed jacket from its hook in her closet, she had the comforting sense of another self, a consoling self accompanying her, and she spoke out loud, as though to a frightened child. "It's perfectly all right now. It will be fine."

With a sharp scissors Gaby had loaned her for her desk work, with sure fingers at her command—at the wind's command, they were as steady as you could wish—she slit open the worn silk lining of the bed jacket (the slice of the blade through the ancient cloth as easy as the sigh of the wind) and spilled the bright-colored capsules onto the bed. Children's colors. *Mexican jumping beans*, Lily murmured, remembering the children's fascination with those mysterious, bright-colored things and their ceaseless dance. Her eyes unexpectedly filled with tears, and she spoke to herself reassuringly again.

She had far too many. In her wish to be thorough, to avoid the bad luck of being pumped alive again, she had seen several different doctors for prescriptions. She knew she risked being ill if she took too many, but she wanted a few more than the book recommended anyway, just to be safe. Carefully she counted what she thought was the correct dose into a pile, then fetched her water glass from the bathroom and scooped them into that. The rest she threw away.

While the wind shuddered against the house, she floated on its force into the kitchen. She found a knife to cut the capsules, heavier and sharper than any she'd used in her life. She barely needed to grip it to push it through the bright little shells. How useful, she thought, to have such a knife! And her own hands, how useful they were today too! She made herself admire their sure grip on the tiny, pretty pill-cups of powder, the way they turned each one so neatly out, pouring its contents into her glass.

When she'd emptied them all, she went in search of vodka to the cupboard where Gaby kept liqueurs. Yes, clear and cold-looking. And then to the freezer for some ice cream. It had been there awhile—it glittered with crystals when Lily opened it. But she dug down below the twinkling surface and scooped out enough to fill a small bowl with the stuff.

Her problem, she knew, would be eating fast enough to get all the pills down before she passed out. She had thought it all through, that she'd let the ice cream get good and soupy before

she started, that she'd wait to drink the vodka until the very
end.

She set everything down on her bedside table and went into
the bathroom, whispering encouragement to herself. Carefully
she repinned her hair, and put on lipstick. She sat on the toilet,
then, and waited to move her bowels. She had read of the loos-
ening of the sphincter at the moment of death, and wished, if
she could, to avoid that indignity.

When she was through, she came out and arranged her pillows. She shut the door to her room; she came back to the bed
and opened the edge Gaby had smoothed down. She sat down
and slowly lifted her legs up and stretched them out. *"There
you go,"* she murmured. She pulled the covers neatly across
her midriff. Then she reached for the ice cream and stirred it
until she could no longer see the granules of the drug. She
began to eat.

Of course, Lily had planned too what she would think of
during these moments. She had assumed that she wouldn't
have arrived at this point unless there were losses, sorrows,
that brought her here, but she had been determined not to
dwell on those—they were inevitable, after all—and to remember instead all the places she'd loved being in. And this is
where she traveled now, as she drank the ice cream spoonful by
spoonful (in spite of its odd, bitter taste, it went down more
easily than she could have hoped) and then sipped slowly at
the full glass of vodka.

She remembered sitting in the tent formed by the skirt of
her mother's dressing table while Violet got ready to go out. A
wonderful fleshy light came through the sheer pink fabric of
the table, making Lily's hiding place seem like the inside of a
shell. And the dizzying floral smell of Violet's perfume! Or perhaps it was her powder. Everything, at any rate, that was safe
and encircling and female.

And then the nearly empty bedroom in the parsonage in
Belvaine—they had so little furniture then. The astonishment of
physical love in the long afternoons they stole together that

first summer of their marriage. The girl who did the laundry couldn't be persuaded to use less than far too much bleach, and the trousseau sheets, dampened with their sweat, transferred that odor to Lily and Paul. Later in the day Lily would often catch a whiff of herself smelling bleachy and innocent, a well-scrubbed woman, and she'd blush in the midst of whatever else she was doing.

The nave at Blackstone Church, soaring and dark. The creak of the wooden pews, the little four-holed trays for the tiny communion glasses—the children loved to poke their fingers through them—the deep red-velvet cushions, worn to white on the welting and around the buttons. The woolly, wet smells in winter of people's coats and scarves and gloves, the welcome chill of the dark, damp space in summer.

Lily's eyes were closed now, and she'd stopped reaching for the vodka. The storm around her raged fully. Her room had darkened, and the windows were smeared with a paste of seawater and rain and the leaves the storm had stripped from the trees and chewed alive. As she slipped deeper into her drugged slumber, her will was affected too, her grip on her visions loosened. Her father was there, silent and angry at something she'd done. She couldn't get him to speak to her, he kept his face averted.

And then she was a bride, young and also old somehow, faltering on her canes as she made her way down the long dark aisle at Blackstone. The faces, black and white, were turned to her in judgment, in dislike. She whimpered. Someone was waiting for her—the bridegroom—at the end of the rows of pews, but she couldn't see who it was, every step forward drew her somehow farther back, she was losing control of her limbs.

Perhaps it was the noise of the branch falling thunderously on the front stairs, splintering them, that called her back. Perhaps not. But suddenly she resisted the pull of her own ending. There were things she had left undone, and her mind struggled now to make sense of them. It was Paul, calling her, telling her that she'd left one of the children—the boy she thought—left him alone in his room somewhere. She stirred, her hands fluttered on the coverlet. She struggled back up to near consciousness.

And then the center of the storm passed over her, and there was a great, hollow stillness. Lily had recovered just enough of herself to know what this was: the eye.

The *I*, she thought. *Lily*.

And was amused at this joke. Her joke. God's joke. A nearly invisible smile twitched on her face.

Though after a few minutes the storm moved on, for her, miraculously, usefully, the world stayed as still as it had been in that moment, as still and deep as a lost meadow. She heard a voice she took to be her mother's calling *"Lily? Lily?"* And she rose from the sunstruck field she sat in. "Coming," she thought she said. "Coming."

But she didn't.

As she'd pulled out onto the main road from Alan's driveway, Linnett watched a car with a boat on a trailer behind it pass, going in the other direction, away from the sea, the boat swaying wildly, ominously, in the wind. Already limbs were strewn here and there on the road, and Linnett's own car moved sideways frequently with the slam of the storm. She was hung over, she was frightened, and she decided not to stop anywhere for batteries or bottled water. Several other cars driving inland passed her as she drove along, one other of them also pulling a rocking boat. Of course, she thought, you'd want to get them out of the water.

The village was deserted except for two teenage boys on rollerblades, holding up what looked like towels as sails to catch the wind. Their yelping, breaking voices were swallowed by the din of the storm, they sounded like distant barking dogs.

The Thayers' house looked abandoned. All the lawn furniture, antique-looking, white-painted wooden chairs and tables and curving benches—all of it had been removed. A lone shutter on an upstairs window banged repeatedly against the house, its sound diminished by the storm's roar, a faraway tocking hammer.

At Linnett's cottage, the deck table and chair had been removed too. Or perhaps had blown away, she thought. She parked as close to the deck as she could, directly on a little garden of some kind of ground cover. She braced herself carefully against the wind on her crutches before she moved beyond the shelter of her car. Even so she was nearly blown over as she took the three or four steps to her door.

Inside she went to the bathroom to run water into the tub and get some aspirin. When she turned on the faucet in the sink though, there was a little burst of water, then only a suck and gurgle and the slow weakening dribble of what had been in the pipe.

"Shit," she said.

She took the aspirin to the kitchen area, and opened the little half-refrigerator. The light, of course, did not come on, although what was left of the seltzer water was still cold in the bottle. Linnett took three aspirin with a glass of the water, and returned the bottle to the refrigerator.

Something fell hard on the roof of the house and she started wildly and cried out. When she'd calmed a bit, she said aloud, "Jesus!" and moved directly to her bed. She leaned her crutches against the wall next to it and got in. Her head throbbed with her pulse and her mouth felt dry even though she'd just had the water.

How tired she was of this! Of herself, of this endless cycle of vague remorse, quasi-resolution, and then within a week or two, another night like the last one. "Quasi-resolution," she murmured, and swung her head slowly on the pillow. The storm's roar was steady now, an astonishing constant racket. She opened her eyes for a moment, and saw that the tree outside her window had been completely stripped of its leaves. Its branches were sharply articulated, an old woman's limbs. It looked barren and wintry. She shut her eyes against the sight, and for a short time crooned softly to herself.

Then she slept, through the thud of branches above her, through the peeling away of part of the roof.

It wasn't until the eye passed over, that sudden, shocking peace, that she was jolted awake. "What?" she cried aloud, jerking herself up. And then lay back. Something grievous and painful pulled at her, she didn't know what. Her leg, trapped in its heavy carapace. Her drinking. Her emptiness. Tears formed in her eyes, and her throat ached. Something she hadn't done, all the things she had. She wept.

There were no large trees around the Admundsens' house—it stood in what had been a field dotted then with cows lazily making their way down to the river—so the only real risk from the storm was that the wind itself would take apart some of the pieces Bill and his crew had so painstakingly nailed and bolted together, would break glass, or throw the remaining piles of lumber and materials around, at worst, of course, through the new windows.

By the time Gaby got there, Alan was taping the window wall. He'd already climbed the scaffolding and thrown the boards down from it. Then he'd brought them into the house, along with the other loose lumber lying around. They worked together on the windows as long as they could, and when the wind got too strong, they came inside to watch what would happen. They were wet and cold, but Gaby had brought towels and blankets. She'd brought a portable radio too, and food— thick sandwiches of cheese and basil leaves and green olive paste, and cookies and berries. She'd brought three thermoses too, one of water, one of coffee, one of the yellow-pepper soup. They stripped and wrapped up in blankets, and sat huddled against the back wall of the house, eating their picnic and listening to reports of the hurricane's progress on the radio—the litany of power outages, roads washed out, dunes breached, phone lines down, harbors ruined.

Alan imagined he could hear a certain logic in this

announced chaos—the logic of the hurricane's chosen path. But he knew there was an element of luck, even within that path. There were those places which would feel the first brunt of the wind's force, and others which would escape. By luck—or the exact angle of the wind, or the rise of the land, or the distance to the open sea. It was this he hoped for.

And the Admundsens were lucky. Alan and Gaby could watch their luck hold as the wind hit the top half of the other bank of the river and a swath of trees—a wide stripe mounting the crest—was felled in a kind of thrilling and violent slow motion. The house vibrated with the wind's force, and the new windows buzzed in place, but that was all. A little later there was the astonishing quiet of the eye, and then slowly, slowly everything grew calmer and the sky began to lighten. They had been sitting for perhaps an hour.

Alan got up, cramped, and walked around, holding his blanket like a cape over his shoulders. "I think that was it," he said. He stood in front of the wall of windows and watched the river below. "That *was* it," he said finally. He turned and grinned at Gaby. He began to dance, Isadora-Duncan-like in his blanket-robe. "That was it, that was it Gabs, Gabs, Gabs." He swept the blanket this way and that. Around him, and then away, swirling sawdust and wood shavings along with it, dramatically revealing, then concealing himself. He cast the blanket on the floor and leaped back and forth across it, his long skinny body in sharp articulation, his penis flopping and dancing wildly on its own. He ended with a dramatic flourish, on one knee, his body thrust forward, his arms and head arched back.

Gaby had been laughing, crying out for him to stop. He stood and shook his blanket out, rewrapped himself in it, and came to sit down beside her again. She was wiping tears from her eyes. The radio jumped to another reporter, on Point Judith, his rapid-fire account of damage.

"That was terrible, Alan," Gaby said. "How can I take you seriously?"

"Why should you take me seriously? It's nothing I've ever been interested in."

"But why not? Everyone wishes to be taken seriously."

"Not I. I had entirely too much of that growing up. So serious. So lofty. So elevated. I say the hell with it."

"Lily doesn't."

"The hell with her then."

"Alan!"

"I mean it."

"Hush," she said. She put her arm around him. "Oh, you're shivering."

"My cold upbringing. Just thinking of it."

"Ah, Alan," she said.

Her body was hot, and she welcomed him into it, opening the blanket-tent around her. He slid forward, wrapped his legs around her hips, pushed his cold hands under her arms. "God, what would I be without you, Gaby?"

"Shhh," she said.

"My little heat pump. My hearth."

"Heart?" she asked.

"Yes," he said.

After a few moments, Gaby tipped back on her buttocks, lifted her solid legs up, swinging them above Alan's, and pulled herself onto his lap. He saw her thick brown fur, the injured-looking purple of her genital flesh.

He clung to her, rested his head between her small round breasts. He felt his penis stiffen against her. "You looked like one of those Rodin nudes doing that," he said. "So proud of her cleft."

"Good," she said. "I am." She adjusted herself onto him, holding her blanket around his head.

Inside the tent she made, he watched their bodies fit together, he arched forward slightly and she helped him come into her. "Can we do this?" he whispered.

"Not without some pain perhaps," she said.

"Ah, the best way," he said. "Mine with pain, please." It

was another joke. They'd seen a sign once in Boston: *Body Piercing: With or Without Pain.*

They rocked together slowly for a long time, Gaby sometimes pulling herself forward and back against him, sometimes letting Alan shift them. His big hands moved freely over her body, holding her, turning her. Near the end he slid them under her solid buttocks, and his fingers found their way into her. She moaned and arched her back to open herself wider to him. He could feel his own fingers through the wall inside her, he moved them in and out against her, against himself, and she whimpered over and over and he pushed into her.

When they were done, they collapsed against each other, letting their blankets fall. Their flesh was sticky with sweat. Alan released Gaby, stroked her slick back, kissed her. After a few minutes, she slid backward, off his lap, to the floor again. She hugged her knees and sighed, gustily. Their breathing slowly settled.

"Look," Alan said. "The sun."

She turned and looked out the wall of windows. The clouds were shredded open, moving fast across the blueing sky, and the sun shone above them. The wet field and the water of the river sparkled in its light.

"Mmm!" Gaby said. "How lovely!"

They sat side by side for a while, watching the scudding clouds.

"This will be a wonderful house, Alan," she said quietly.

"Do you really like it?" he asked.

"This will be a wonderful house," she said, more slowly this time.

After a moment, he said, "I wonder how ours survived."

"This gives me hope," Gaby said, gesturing around her.

Alan didn't say what he was thinking, which was that there wasn't necessarily any connection.

"I suppose we should pull on our wet clothes," he said after a while.

"Yes."

He got up and went to where they'd both been standing when they stripped down. He bent over his own pile. "Wet, and cold," he said.

"I should have brought extras," she said. She was packing the food back into the basket she'd brought it in. Alan tossed her clothes to her and they hit the floor with an ominously loud *whack*. He was pulling his own pants on, whooping with cold, jumping up and down.

By the time they'd shaken and folded the blankets and packed the leftover lunch and thermoses back in the car, they'd warmed up a little, though the cool breeze gave Alan goose bumps every time it struck him. Gaby drove him to the top of the Admundsens' driveway where he'd left his car, and they started home, Gaby following him.

Before they'd gone half a mile, though, they came to a tree lying across the road, tangled in wires. A utility truck was parked beyond it, and several men in hard hats were moving around. Alan could hear a chain saw.

He leaned out his window. The man walking toward him was shaking his head, *no*, and gesturing Alan back with his hand.

"I've got to get to Bowman," Alan called. "Can I get around by Cobbtown?"

"As far as I know there's no wires down there, but the bridge over the pond washed out."

"So you're saying I can't *get* to Bowman."

"Not till we're done, I'd say."

"How long do you guess you'll be?"

The man turned and looked behind him. "Hard to say. At least an hour. Could be longer."

Alan and the man grinned at each other. "Okay," Alan said. He got out and went to Gaby's car, pulled up behind his. "We're stuck, it looks like. Till they get this cleaned up."

After a moment, taking this in, Gaby said, "What do you propose we do?"

"Finish our picnic, I'd say."

She shrugged and made a moue.

And so it was that they turned around and drove back to the Admundsens'. More formally, more ceremonially, this time they made a bed for themselves out of the blankets. Alan had a sense almost of shyness as they undressed on either side of this pallet, as though they were teenagers, doing something exciting and illicit. Much more tenderly, they made love again, and slept for a while afterward on the hard floor. When they woke the sun was gone, and the sky was a dramatic deep pink. They lay side by side, slowly eating the one remaining cookie, the last of the berries, and when they dressed, their clothes were almost dry. Alan helped Gaby carry the things back to her car once more. The air felt rinsed and cold. They stood for a moment leaned against the car, not talking, reluctant to let go of this time. Then Gaby reached up and touched Alan's cheek. "I have missed you, Alan. Lily . . . she divides my loyalty, I'm afraid."

He nodded. "Well, today was a reprieve."

"Yes. And I'm glad. I don't like to feel that way, but I do. She is not easy, poor old woman." She sighed and opened the car door, and Alan moved off to his car.

They passed the spot where the men had been working. The tree had been cut just enough to open the road, and the pale round ends winked white in the twilight on either side of it. As he drove, Alan squinted into the shadows around him. At some places along the road everything looked normal, and then there'd be an open cut in the woods carved by the wind, trees would be uprooted or felled for the length of its long swipe. When he passed houses he looked even more carefully. He saw some damage, and every yard was littered with branches, but it didn't seem as bad as he'd imagined it. Candles or oil lamps made a weak yellow light in some windows, and here and there people were working outside in the near-dark.

Their own driveway was open and clear except for a carpet of leaves and sticks his tires crunched over. When he pulled out

into the opening at the bottom of the drive, there was just
enough light to see by, a light unfiltered by leaves, which were
utterly gone. The yard was a mess, a deep tangle of branches.
He pulled over to make room for Gaby and turned off the
engine. Then he saw the huge limb fallen across the porch and
steps. He groaned and got out of the car. Carefully he picked
his way across the dark yard. He dragged the limb back off the
steps. They had splintered beneath it, as though someone had
taken a huge, dull axe and chopped them down the middle.

He grabbed the iron rail and climbed the stairs, putting his
weight along their outer edge. The decking on the porch was
intact, and he walked around to the front of the house, looking
for damage. The glass in one of the French doors to the living
room was broken, but that seemed the extent of what he could
see tonight. Tomorrow he'd get up on a ladder and check the
roof. He came back to the steps and helped Gaby up them.
"This looks like the worst of it," he said.

Inside, the house was dark and still, free of all the unnoticed electrical noises that usually hummed and ticked along
with their lives.

"I'll get candles," Gaby said.

"We've got a flashlight somewhere too," Alan said.

While Gaby set the lighted candles around on the counter,
on the table and the collection of yard furniture, Alan felt his
way through various drawers in the kitchen, searching for the
flashlight.

"What do you think, Alan?" Gaby was saying. He looked
over at her. "I'm going to call Noreen, but I think we should
wait until tomorrow to get Lily, if Noreen can keep her. We'll
never get her across the yard or up the stairs, particularly in the
dark."

"Absolutely," Alan said.

"If the phone is even working," Gaby said.

While Gaby made the call, Alan swept up the glass in the
corner of the living room. He could hear her voice rise sharply
in alarm, and he stood and waited for her to finish.

She put the phone down. "Lily isn't there," he said.

"But you took her there," he said.

"No," she said. "I asked Linnett to. Lily was having a very good day, and she thought Linnett could manage. But according to Noreen they never made it."

"Well, then, where the fuck are they?" he asked.

"Noreen thinks maybe Linnett took Lily to her house, that maybe the roads were already impassable then."

"Christ. Okay. So Linnett. Do you have her number?"

"No." Gaby rubbed her forehead. "And it won't be listed either, since it's a rental."

"Maybe Lily has it in her room somewhere." He picked up the flashlight.

"Or, no. Wait a minute. Who was she renting from?"

"The Thayers," he said.

"I'll call them. They'll know."

"All right. That's the easiest."

And while Gaby went back to the phone, Alan took the flashlight down to the storage closet at the end of the hall to find some cardboard and cut it for the broken pane of glass. He had just gotten out the Exacto knife when Gaby called sharply to him.

"Lily isn't there either," she said as he stepped out of the closet. She stood by the phone in the candlelight at the other end of the hall. She looked frightened.

"What do you mean?"

She lifted her hands. "She isn't there. Linnett didn't take her. She says Lily told her Noreen was supposed to pick her up."

"But that wasn't ever the deal, was it? Was it?"

"No. No. And Noreen. Well, she knew nothing of such a . . . "

"Jesus, this is crazy. Where is she?" They stood frowning at each other in the strange yellow light. "She can't just have disappeared."

Then Gaby's face shifted. "Alan! She's here!" she cried. "She must have misunderstood somehow . . . "

But Alan had already turned back into the utility closet for the flashlight, and now he was striding toward her and then past her, across the room, the skittering oval of the flashlight dancing on the floor in front of him. Gaby was still explaining it to him, to herself, as he stepped to the door and pushed it open to find Lily.

chapter 17
—

Every builder and workman in town is booked for at least a month with hurricane repairs, so Alan decides to fix the front steps himself. Since Ettie and Thomas are both home for the ten days or so until school starts, Alan and Gaby decide that it may be better to wait until they are gone to begin—this is one of those projects that Ettie could do well but Thomas would have trouble participating in, for fear of hurting his hands. Three or four times in the days he is home, Ettie asks about the steps. "I mean, it'd take us, what? a day? a couple of days?" But Alan leaves the small stepladder tilted into place against the deck next to the ruined stairs, and that is how they all go in and out. It isn't until after the boys have left, and Gaby, who closes the shop for two weeks right after Labor Day each year, has flown to France on what has become an annual visit, that Alan begins the work.

Carefully he unbolts the painted iron rails and lays them on the deck. Then he begins to take apart the stairs. All the risers and treads are gone, he knew that the moment he saw them—crushed in the center by the branch's fall. But he discovers when he gets down underneath that only one stringer will need to be replaced. He draws up a careful list for the lumberyard.

Even so he spends a long time there in its shadowy, cavernous interior, looking over grades of wood, buying the materials. He looks too at specialty woods, at hinges and locks, at tools he has never used, and now, he supposes, never will. Alan worked for a contractor during the summers in architecture school, and occasionally after that until he had a stable income, and he loves everything about the working end of the business. He has been looking forward to this project. Perhaps some of the reason he didn't want to begin while Ettie was home has to do too with this: he has wanted to be alone, he realizes now, with wood, with tools. He wants to work slowly and carefully and in silence. He wants to lose himself in this, not have it be part of any human connection. He wants the consoling reasonableness of measurement, the logic of fit and exactitude, the pleasure of the smell and smoothness of wood, its shapeliness under saw and plane, under his hands.

On Tuesday he brings his tools out from the storage room— his circular saw, plane, clamps, level, hammer, drill. In the odd, December-like sunlight under the stripped trees of the summer yard he works, fastidiously measuring and remeasuring angles, cutting the jagged jawline of the stringer, slicing and stroking the decking, the risers, smoothing every edge before setting wood in place.

The air is warm and windy, the curls of wood dance away across the yard. The glimpses of the water in the river below sparkle. Alan takes his shirt off after a while and the bare sunlight heats his flesh. The naked wood and its shavings smell of beginning, of hope. The magic of building things, he thinks.

His mind wanders freely, unattached, unfocused, over his life. Gaby, his children, Lily, death—even his own death: how it will come to him, whether he will ever be tempted to make Lily's choice.

His hands perform their repetitive tasks, and he thinks of his work, of his comfort in it. Of Gaby, with her family in France. Clary, Lily's ashes. And then Lily's face, as it was that night. He sees the flashlight's trembling dance once more on its slack, gray surface—the eyes slitted open and milky, the jaw slung agape. He stops working, he stands straight for a moment, looking around the empty yard.

Of course, the logical time to scatter the ashes would have been the day of the memorial reception (no service, as Lily's will had dictated), but Clary had the idea that Rebecca might somehow show up, or make her presence known, and so they waited. During the three days they were gathered in Chicago, Alan often watched her, his sister—big-boned like him, blond too, her hair carefully frosted and shaped—watched her eyes nervously surveying a room, watched her jump eagerly whenever the telephone rang. Even at the memorial reception as she greeted the straggling arrivals, her glance swung several times around the room, as though Rebecca might be hidden among the elderly people gathered to remember Lily. Now, standing in his yard, he suddenly remembers Rebecca clearly, how she looked: the one of them with dark hair, like Lily's. Perhaps, like Lily too, he thinks, she went white early. Perhaps then Clary wasn't so foolish to look; Rebecca could have been moving among the other white-haired guests.

He stops again now, to think of Rebecca, as he hasn't in years. He remembers the way, periodically, she and Clary would descend to rescue him from all they saw as *wrong* in his life, how for a while he would be swept into their world, never understanding it or their impulses. He remembers a game of Monopoly played with them one night when he was about eleven or twelve. He was in his pajamas, they in their underwear. And it was such innocent underwear, really, as he thinks of it now. Nothing lacy or gauzy, the underpants waist-high, the bras big as halters, everything a nurselike white cotton. Nonetheless he had been in a state of anxious struggle with his arousal, aware of the few curling strands of pubic hair he could glimpse at their crotches from time to time, conscious of the shifting shapes of their breasts as they reached forward to roll the dice or move their pieces around the board.

Clary explained their theory later to him: their behavior

was to be an antidote to Lily's coldness. Their relaxation would help to make him more comfortable, easier, about women and sexuality. He laughs out loud now in his sunstruck yard, thinking how very wrong they were, how comical the scene was.

They scattered the ashes on the last day in Chicago, he and Clary, while Gaby and the boys were packing up for the return trip. It was windy, too windy a day for such a chore, but they had no choice, and so they made their way out to the rocky edge of the point, a thumb of green projecting into the lake at 55th Street. The water slapped at the rocks, the wind pushed against them. Clary insisted on a prayer to mark the moment. While her lips moved, Alan looked at her hands, aged, veined, holding the plastic bag of ashes. He looked at the powder within, dotted with the stonelike bits of bone. He could faintly hear the drift of Clary's voice murmuring the Lord's Prayer with its familiar rhythms, and he was grateful to her. He felt a sense of some necessary ceremony being enacted.

When she was done, they stood for a moment, buffeted and rocking slightly. Then Alan threw the first handful out. And felt it blow back onto him, into his eyes, his hair, his opened mouth. He blinked. He swallowed. He ran his tongue over his lips.

He turned to her. "This won't work," he said.

In the end, they had to come around to the 57th Street side of the point to get out of the wind, and Alan crouched on a rock and more or less turned the plastic bag out. Lily's ashes poured forth, some sinking, some floating away, white on the lake's dark surface. Within a few seconds, though, they all disappeared in the lively water.

Clary was tearful at that moment, but she recovered herself quickly. On their way back across the grass, she sighed and said, "God, I hate to say it, but Mother died in the absolute nick of time for me."

"What do you mean?" Alan asked.

"Money, dear boy." She held her hands up, rubbing her fingers against her thumbs. "Filthy lucre."

Alan, in spite of his own confusion about Lily, was startled by Clary's finality, her coldness: Lily seemed *done* for her.

An hour or so later, settled in the plane on his way home, he saw Clary's odd gesture again in his mind's eye and recognized abruptly what it had reminded him of—the repetitive motion of Lily's hands when she was at her most tired. He looked at his own hands then. There was a dark crescent curving under each fingernail of the right hand. He started to trace under one with his left forefinger, scraping it clean, and then he realized what he was scraping at—Lily's ashes. He turned his hands quickly then, palms up in his lap, as if supplicant.

The telephone rings four or five times while Alan is working, but he doesn't stop to answer it. He eats his lunch outside, sitting on the deck, and works until late in the afternoon. It's cool by then, he's put his shirt back on. The fall shadows across the yard are long, even in the bright light. It isn't until early evening, after he's showered and poured himself a glass of wine, that he pushes the message button on his machine and stands waiting, pen in hand, to record whatever comes.

The first voice is Peter Admundsen's, with brusque condolences about Lily. Then he says, "Now that you're back, I wondered if we could meet at the house to go over a few details." Alan groans aloud.

There's a dinner invitation for him and Gaby for the end of the month from the Mercers. It will be the first time that they've seen them since before Lily came.

Then a call from Linnett Baird.

Her voice startles Alan, and he sets his wine glass down. "Hello, Gaby. Hello, Alan. I hope everything was . . . went . . . smoothly, at the memorial service. Alan, I wondered if I could talk to you. I thought I might come down maybe Thursday or Friday if that would work for you. There's a little bit of final fact-checking kind of stuff I'd like to do. Could you call me back?" And she recites a number with a western Massachusetts area code.

Ettie has called too, with a list of items he left at home by mistake. Can they be mailed to him? Like, soon?

Alan goes through the calls in order, answering them. When he calls Linnett back, he gets her machine and tells her either day is fine, he'll be working at home. He sets the phone down and takes a sip of the wine. It's almost dark outside. He has turned on several lights by now, and he's suddenly conscious of his reflection in the windows, raising the glass, setting it down. Why is he nervous? Why is he a little excited at the thought of seeing Linnett?

It's nothing, he tells himself. The mild flirtation they had earlier, the fact of his solitude now. The connection with Lily. He was drawn to Linnett, certainly. Attracted by her. But not finally interested in anything, he's sure of that. And he reminds himself too of how angry he was at her the night before Lily died. Very angry.

Alan finishes the stairs the next day, and with reluctance cleans his tools and puts them carefully away again. It takes him several hours to apply stain to the new wood, and then the job is done. He has a sense, as he rinses the brush and then his hands with paint thinner, of a return from a distant place—of his life, his complicated but pleasant, ordinary life, calling him back. That night, before he goes to bed, he finds a carton and searches Ettie's and Thomas's room for the things Ettie asked for: a stack of photographs Alan flips through, most taken in New York, young people Alan doesn't know. A textbook Ettie was reading, underlined heavily for the first twenty pages or so and then pristine. His soccer shoes, a box of CDs, a green sweater hanging on a hook in his closet. Alan looks around the room just before he turns the light off. Every year it seems less his sons', more just an extra space. When they took down the last batch of posters—sports figures, rock groups, a beautiful young pianist named Hélène Grimaud—they didn't put any more up to replace them. There are framed family photographs hanging on the walls now, and a sketch of the harbor done by a friend, but these are Gaby's choices. Their lives, their choices, are being made elsewhere. They are gone, he thinks, and there is so much he failed to say to them, failed to give them.

But doesn't every parent feel this way? He thinks of Lily again, of how hard it must have been for her, being a parent, incapacitated as she was by her rigidity, her coldness.

And then is startled by this idea. Lily, *incapacitated*. Startled by the sympathy, by the forgiveness, the word implies. As he carries Ettie's carton to the kitchen and begins to tape it up, he thinks of how often his own feelings have startled him since Lily's death.

Linnett comes on Friday, mid-afternoon. Alan is rearranging trays of slides for his fall lectures. He's in his study, at the back of the house, and the projector makes a whirring sound, so he doesn't hear her car pull in. The doorbell surprises him.

When he comes into the hall, he can see her standing in silhouette in front of the screen door. For a moment, he doesn't recognize her. And then he realizes, walking toward the door, that she isn't carrying her crutches. Or they aren't carrying her.

He is struck by how tall she is, how, somehow, larger than he remembered her. She's wearing jeans and an undershirt top, with a big, unbuttoned red linen shirt like a jacket over that. Her hair is in a ponytail at the nape of her neck, but silvery strands have pulled loose and they dance in the light breeze.

When the door opens, she snatches off her sunglasses and extends her hand. "Alan!" she says. And after a pause: "I was just so sorry, about Lily."

Should he kiss her? Alan no longer knows the rules. Their hands grip firmly, but she doesn't bend forward in any way, so he just tightens his grip slightly for a moment. "Thanks," he says. "It was . . . difficult."

"And so unexpected," she says.

They still stand on either side of the threshold. Now Alan steps back. "Well, come in," he says.

She walks past him, a sure, long stride. She's only a few

inches shorter than he is, he sees this for the first time, and she carries herself with a masculine vigor that surprises him. He's thought of her injury, he realizes, as part of her.

"I'm really grateful you could see me," she says.

"With the usual stipulations, of course," he answers, trailing her.

She turns back and grins at him. "But of course."

She's standing in the living room. Alan has crossed to the kitchen. "Sit down," he says. "Would you like something?"

"I'd take a beer if you've got one."

"Coming up," he says. He gets a beer out for her and pours himself a glass of seltzer. When he brings them over, she's seated on the built-in couch in front of the windows, turned sideways to look out at the yard.

"The hurricane really did a number here," she says.

"Yes. Well, actually, there's no real damage. And the trees will all come back. This is our winter light." He gestures. "An early guest this year."

"Mmm," she says. "Thanks." She takes the beer and sips it.

Alan sits down opposite her, in one of Lily's chairs. "You've recovered completely," he says.

"Oh!" She looks down at her leg. "Almost," she says. "I've got a bunch of exercises I have to do. But I can't jog yet, and I miss it. I've gained about five pounds since the *ordeal* began."

"It's odd to see you, castless."

"It was the only way you knew me, I guess."

"Exactly."

She looks over at him, framed in the ornate curve of carved wood around the back of the chair. "It's odd to see you here without Lily."

"Yes. Well. The only way you knew *me*, I guess."

She smiles. "True."

A little silence falls.

Then Linnett stirs herself. "The service was in Chicago?"

"Such as it was. I mean, there was no service. Per Lily's orders. We had a kind of . . . " His hand circles. "Reception."

"Oh!" She nods. "Like a wake or something."

"No, exactly *not* like a wake." Alan laughs at the memory of the party, that gathering of the lame and halt in the rented space, the watery sound of the roomful of elderly voices. "Like a ladies' tea or something. And then Clary—my sister—and I scattered her ashes over the lake. In the lake." He's still smiling, remembering that the hotel called the rental space a "function room," that the boys delighted in that name.

Linnett, looking carefully at him, thinks his response is odd. Distant. "So that's that," she says, trying to move into what seems his mood.

"Well, there's still a lot to do with the estate and so forth, but yes, that's that."

"What did she die of, exactly?" She planned earlier to lead to this question much more slowly, but that doesn't seem necessary given what she reads as Alan's present frame of mind.

Alan is startled, but he shrugs, as though casually. "Old age. Parkinson's disease."

"No, but I mean, there has to be a cause. What was on her death certificate?"

"Heart, I think. I didn't read it." Surely this isn't the sort of thing she wants to know.

"Heart? I didn't know she had heart problems."

"I didn't read it. I think that's what the doctor thought it might have been. In the short run." He sets his glass down. "Look, you're not writing about her death, are you?"

"Well, yes. Obviously I need to include it. I mean, I can't exactly ignore it, can I? I mean, in a way, it becomes, almost, the *point* of the story."

"Maybe you shouldn't do it at all, then." He's frowning. "The story. The article."

"Oh, I have to do it, even to get the kill fee."

"The kill fee?"

"Nice term, huh? Yeah, I mean, I have to turn something in to get paid for my time. And I put in a lot of time. If they take it, obviously, I get full price. If they don't, I get less, but something. That's the kill fee. Naturally I'd like more. I live, just a little *bit,* hand to mouth. I could use it. And they want the death, obviously. It's the hottest part, now."

"This . . . language is ludicrous."

"It is the language, nonetheless. I didn't invent it." Linnett has realized by now that she made a mistake being as casual as she was about Lily. Whatever he feels, it isn't as simple as she assumed. But there's something prissy too, old-maidy, she thinks, about his tone, that she resists sympathizing with. She decides to plunge ahead. "Did you find her?" she asks.

"I don't want to talk about it." He shifts forward in the chair, abruptly, rests his elbows on his knees and grips his hands together for a moment. "Look," he says, "I think this is a mistake, my seeing you."

"Well, what did you think I was coming for, anyway?"

"I don't know. Facts, you said. I guess I thought date of birth, date of marriage, places, names. That kind of thing."

"Well, it is that kind of thing, really. I mean, date of death, cause of death, circumstances. That's the same kind of thing."

He sits back and looks at her. He makes his voice businesslike. "Okay, date of death, August 26th. Natural causes, died in bed."

"She was in *bed.* What was she doing in bed?"

"Jesus, I don't know. Resting? She lay down and she died. Can't you leave it at that?" He sounds genuinely angry, Linnett thinks.

"Well, I suppose I could. It's just that she lied to me, you know?"

"What do you mean? She lied to everyone, a little."

"No, I mean, that day. She told me Noreen was coming for her, and that was simply not the case. I've spoken to Noreen."

"Oh, fuck it, Linnett. There was a hurricane. All of that, all of those . . . arrangements, got confused that day. *I* was confused. I thought Gaby had taken her to Noreen's. It's not surprising Lily got confused."

"This wasn't confusion. It was a lie. She told me Noreen

spoke to her. Called her, spoke to her. Told her things. And it just never happened. Period. That's different, that's *way* different, from not being sure of what Gaby told her. And it implicates me." After all, she can be angry too. She can take the high moral ground here as well as he can. "Do you think I'd have left her by herself if I wasn't sure Noreen was coming? It made a difference to me that Noreen had supposedly called her. And as it turned out, she hadn't."

"Lily was ill. She was sometimes confused, even about what happened. As opposed to what didn't. She . . . You didn't see her over the weekend. The weekend before she died. She was very confused. She was having . . . She was *in*, a bad time. A bad time." And suddenly the memory of Lily entering the room on her canes, spiderlike, grotesque, her features drawn on with palsied strokes, comes clearly back to Alan. He turns away from Linnett.

Linnett can see that he is affected, somehow. She gentles her voice. "You know, Alan, I knew her a little too. And I think I could tell you something about the nature of Lily's bad times. And I can also tell you that the day of the hurricane was not one of those times. It was, if anything, a good time."

After a moment, he says quietly, "Even if you're right, even if she lied, what difference does it make?"

"If I'm right, she was not confused. That's what difference it makes."

"And so? So what?"

"Did she kill herself?" Linnett asks.

"What are you talking about?"

"Because that's my theory. *My* theory. That Lily arranged to be alone, by lying to me, and somehow killed herself when she was alone."

"If you write, or publish, anything like that, I will sue you." He has picked up his glass again, and now he sets it down, too hard.

"Hey, come *on*, Alan. I'm just *talking* to you. To *you*. This is *me*."

"You're talking about my mother. I wish you would remember that. Not just some fascinating . . . subject."

"I do. I do remember that. And this piece will be nothing, I can promise you, if not sympathetic to Lily." She thinks of a new tack. "Did you know she couldn't write anymore?"

He looks over sharply at her. "What do you mean?"

"Well, you know how she'd kind of taken me on as a secretary, in exchange for the interviews?"

He nods.

"And I was supposed to help her write a story. That was the deal. She had this story all mapped out, in her head or whatnot. And maybe others too, for all I know. Anyway, we tried about six different ways and we couldn't do it. *She* couldn't do it. She couldn't . . . I don't know. It felt like she couldn't hold on to a train of thought. That wasn't, you know, concrete. Real. She couldn't . . . access her imagination, somehow. It felt neurological. And she actually said she thought it was, that it felt that way to her, as though the disease, the Parkinson's, had destroyed whatever the connections were that let that happen."

After a moment, he says, "I see."

"This all happened that week before the hurricane. We tried that whole week, one way or another. I tried taking dic*ta*tion, I tried leaving her alone to talk it into the *tape* recorder. Nothing."

Alan's gaze has turned out the window.

"So you see, that's why it seemed to me that she might feel . . . at the end of something. She might have thought her life, or a substantial part of her life, was over."

"Lily didn't kill herself, Linnett." He's looking back at her. He seems, suddenly, old, fatigued.

"Okay." She waits. "I just wanted to explore my theory."

He nods stiffly. Linnett believes he is still angry at her. He isn't. He isn't really even thinking of Linnett, just of what she's said about Lily, the increase of emptiness it's brought to him. That, and then a sweeping, bitter pity, the purest emotion he's felt for his dead mother.

"Did she leave, like papers and letters?"

He looks at her. "Some."

"And what will happen with those?"

"The letters I destroyed." He hears her intake of breath, but her face doesn't change. "She'd been going through them, you knew that. There were only a last few she hadn't destroyed herself. Recent ones. Not very interesting."

"And the papers? What were they?" A quick thought. "You didn't chuck them too!"

"No. She has a literary executor. Trix, I guess you say. Her agent. I sent them on to her. So some of them may find their way into print, I suppose. I don't know, though. It seemed like old stuff to me. Very early things. Story starts. Things like that. Juvenalia, really. As if she'd ever been young."

He tries smiling at her, but she's all business now. "I'll probably call her then. The agent."

"Sure, that's fine."

"And the rest of her estate is, like . . . ?"

"Furniture, books, jewelry. A trust. All to be divided three ways."

"*Three* ways."

"Yes, Rebecca has her share. In case she ever comes back. So she won't feel deprived."

She shakes her head. "Jesus. After, what? Thirty-five years?"

"Well, you know the line. 'There is more joy in heaven over one sinner that repents than ninety-nine righteous people who don't need to.'" He is surprised, and then not surprised, that he can call this up, something he would have said he didn't remember, something lost to him forever.

After Linnett leaves, Alan tries to work again, but can't. The bright buildings, their forms, their interiors rising up against the blank wall of his study, mean nothing to him. He turns the projector off, he roams the house.

He goes into the guest room, Lily's room, and stands staring out the window. He thinks of what Linnett said, that Lily couldn't write. He wonders why he didn't want to tell Linnett that Lily took her own life. Killed herself. Why does it matter whether Linnett knows?

It does. Not from shame. But it does.

In part, Alan supposes, because he wants to impose some limit for himself on how much of Lily's life can be made public. She might not have minded, but he is in charge of this part of the story—her silence about it has given him that right, he feels—and he has decided, he realizes, that it will remain private, something only his family will know. He smiles, understanding that there may be an angry aspect to this kindness too, that this may be the very opposite of what Lily would have wanted.

Also (he's trying to be honest with himself, thinking of Linnett now, of how newly and differently attracted he was to her without the cast, without the crutches), perhaps it was useful to him, in an immediate and tawdry sense, to have the wedge of indignation to drive between himself and her. If so, he isn't sorry.

He doesn't know. He feels he doesn't know anything.

When the doctor finally arrived that night—their family doctor, an old friend—they went together into the guest room. Gaby had taken away the dishes Lily had used by then, had closed Lily's eyes, and then her jaw too, by tying a kerchief around Lily's head. She'd set several candles around in the room so that the doctor—whose name was Greg Halliday— could see. It looked like a nineteenth-century deathbed, and Lily looked completely at peace, her features thrown into deep shadows by the flickering light, her hands resting on the sheet at her bosom.

Alan was still in a kind of hysteria of disbelief, unable to stop talking, to stop telling his story, full of the most irrelevant details—the way the raw tree ends on the road had looked in the twilight, the way the hurricane had moved, the series of phone calls they'd made trying to find Lily.

Greg was used to this kind of thing, though, and he listened politely to Alan as he moved around. He did a cursory examination, asked a few questions, and called an ambulance. He gave Alan instructions about contacting the funeral home in the morning. He said he was terribly, terribly sorry. He had a quick bourbon with them, sitting in the crowd of extra chairs in the candlelit living room, and then he left. He said his house was a real mess.

After the ambulance took Lily's body away, Gaby and Alan sat up in the candlelight until almost four, talking. Alan felt, as he told Gaby three or four times, that at any moment Lily could just walk into the living room and begin to speak to him.

In bed, Alan fell into a strangely light sleep, full of waking dreams of all that had happened. And then, sometime after dawn, a deep, bottomless slumber.

Gaby woke him at about ten. She'd been to the shop and found that, as she'd expected, their electricity was off too. She'd made a sign and posted it. Then she came home, and when she opened the trash can to dump out the grounds from her earlier cup of coffee, she saw the brightly colored plastic casings of the capsules lying over the top of yesterday's garbage. She reached down and picked up one of the little halves. Then she went to the sink and picked up the dishes Lily had used—she'd left them there, unwashed, the night before, since there was no running water. She smelled them, noted the peculiar odor in the bowl. She sat awhile by herself, thinking it through, before she woke Alan.

They talked about it together for several hours. About whether they were honor-bound somehow to call Greg and start Lily's death again.

No, they decided. Gaby was especially firm. It was done. It was obviously something Lily had planned to do for a long time. There was no point in complicating it now. It was a kind of achievement, really—*ahsheevmante*, she said, and for a few seconds Alan didn't know the word—that Lily had managed it as well as she had. Alan called the funeral director and arranged for a cremation. Then he and Gaby went for a long walk.

When they got back, Alan went into Lily's room. Gaby had stripped the bed, he saw, and he was grateful. Lily's bed jacket was tossed casually over the back of her chair, and he hung it up. A file folder lay on her worktable, the papers sliding out. The wastebasket was full.

Alan began to go through the papers on her desk, looking for a note to him, a farewell, an explanation.

There was nothing. The last letters, the ones she hadn't read, were from fans, people who were moved to tell her something of their stories too. Alan read two or three with interest, but then began to sense the repetitive quality in them. There were a few other letters too, he saw as he flipped through this last folder, from newer friends, from her agent. Nothing important. He dropped them all into the wastebasket on top of the letters she had herself dropped there.

He moved around the room, picking up any scrap of paper. There were reminders: *Tell Linnett no talks. Letters:* and a list of names he didn't know. *Call Dr. Freilich.* A list: *Toothpaste, Gaviscon, calcium.* And then one with his name alone, at the top of the little sheet. It said "Alan:"

He could hear Gaby's voice on the telephone in the next room. He looked out over his ruined yard, the bare branches of the trees, the smeared windows. "Alan:" He imagined Lily's voice, saying it, saying his name. Her old voice, before the Parkinson's, strong and deep and urgent. "Alan!" What might have followed? He stared again at his name.

And then he crumpled the paper and dropped it too, into Lily's wastebasket, and went to get a trash bag to throw it all away.

By now Alan would have said that he'd thought about Lily's death, explored it from every angle. Confronted it. But the pity, the sympathy he felt when Linnett told him that Lily couldn't write, when she offered him this new reason for Lily's choosing death, has made him realize he hasn't. That he's not done. That he can still, even now, have new feelings about Lily, feelings he doesn't fully understand.

When Gaby comes back from France, she has four days before she needs to return to work. She has come back early, in fact—rearranging her ticket at some expense—because she wants to take this time to be with Alan. But she finds herself glad to leave earlier than planned on other grounds too. Her father, while he wasn't quite sick, wasn't quite well either, and the days in France were long ones of the entire household's servitude to his comfort, his endless round of petty complaints. The house needed work, and everything in it looked shabby and grimy to Gaby. The kitchen hadn't been thoroughly cleaned in years. And Paris itself seemed noisy, crowded with cars. The air stung her eyes, she imagined it coating her lungs.

When the plane landed at Logan and she looked across the yellowing marsh grass to the white frame houses and the clear, piercing blue of the sky behind them, she felt at home, eager for her life here.

Alan has missed her and is glad for her return, but he finds he can't respond to the sympathy she offers about Lily, he can't make use of it. His feelings about his mother have gotten too complicated, too difficult, for Gaby to reach. They talk about her death a little, and each time he finds himself trying to change the subject, to move on to something else. He doesn't think she notices this. He hopes not, at any rate. Though sometimes after one of these exchanges he feels her eyes lingering on him.

He continues to work a little through these days of her vacation, but mostly in his study at home—on his lectures, primarily, but also on the plans for the addition to the big house in the village, the project he has gotten. (The church in Vermont is mired in politics and has put off trying to raise the funds for a while. Three different people have written Alan of this decision, "so I guess maybe they really, really mean it," he tells Gaby.)

He usually stops work in time for lunch. They go swimming twice. They make love each afternoon, and then they lie in bed and talk together—about the children, about what they might do with the money from Lily's estate, about a cookbook Gaby thinks she might try to write.

They have friends over one night, and on their last free evening, they take a walk together after dinner, all the way into the village. It's nearly dark when they turn from the dock and start back. Two black dogs who rose from the sidewalk in front of one of the old houses in town and trailed them companionably lag a little behind them now, sniffing at the various delights of the docks; but then catch up. The windows are lighted in only about half the houses—the summer people have gone, though the air off the water now is still humid and warm. In the houses that are occupied, they can hear the music and the portentous intonation of television dialogue, sometimes with human conversation rising above and around it. Far out over the water a bell clangs. In the distance a dog starts barking, and the two black dogs begin barking too, in response, circling Gaby and Alan as though protecting them.

A few other dogs here and there in the village pick it up, and the black dogs run excitedly ahead into the dark, into the calls sounding back and forth. Gaby and Alan pass a house where someone is practicing the piano, a beginner's piece. The air smells heavily of the sea.

They haven't talked much on their walk, just pointed here to a stand of fall flowers, there to the birds lined up on the telephone wires in silhouette against the fading light like so many quarter-notes. Now Gaby pulls her sweater tighter around her and sighs. "Ah, Alan, this is such an *American* night."

What part of his history, of his surprising grief, of his abiding connection to Lily, is at work in him then to make him want to say that this is not America, this dream?

But he doesn't. Because he loves her, he doesn't. "Is it?" he answers.

chapter 18

The months go by for Alan, months of forgetting and remembering, forgetting and remembering. In mid-November, Lily's chairs come back recovered. Gaby has chosen a very rich, brocadelike fabric for one, and a silk stripe for the other. Alan didn't notice when they left, actually, but on the day of their return, he stops as he's crossing the living room, and stares at them, as though, literally, seeing a ghost. Lily is there, it suddenly seems.

And then the feeling is gone, and what he is aware of is the mystery of the difference between the living and the dead, the absolute closing of the door between them, the finality—why should it be so amazing from time to time?—of her being gone.

When he goes in to wake Gaby and the light from the hallway falls in across the bed and onto the old quilt, across her strong hands lying on it, he remembers the flashlight's beam on Lily's face when he found her, that terrible final relaxation that left her looking shocked and yet waxy, her eyes slightly open in the deepest sleep. He bends over Gaby and smells her familiar yeasty smell, feels the heat of her life, her responsive stir and whimper as he touches her. He feels nearly as though he has willed this awakening, and he is so grateful for it that when her eyes open to meet his, she sees tears in them.

*   *   *

In December, Gaby and Alan drive up to Boston on a Sunday afternoon to hear the *Messiah* performed. Ettie is still in school, not due home for ten days, and though they have invited Thomas, he's not going to join them—he has tickets to something else that day, a performer they have never heard of, in a tiny hall whose name they don't recognize. They have agreed to meet him afterward for dinner.

It's a bright cold day, with a frosty, light, early snow lying like glittery powder on the ground. White gulls circle high above the city buildings, calling, something Alan always loved about Boston. On Newbury Street they sometimes landed outside the mansard windows, startlingly huge and ugly, a primordial, nightmare version of *bird*. And then flew off into grace again.

Under the marquee at Symphony Hall, the crowd shuffles and stamps. It's pleasant to move into their hubbub, to feel encircled by their body warmth, their groomed smells, their bursts of laughter. They slowly press with the group into the warm building, then beyond, into the sanctuary of the large performance hall with its huge, twinkling chandeliers high overhead, the brightly lighted stage with the rows of chairs across the back for the singers. Alan and Gaby find their seats, arrange their coats, scan their programs. Their conversation is only intermittent, as it has been in the car on the way up too. Alan is preoccupied with end-of-semester problems at school, with the last interior details at the Admundsens' house, which they want to be in for Christmas.

Gaby is just tired, having catered a big party in town the night before. She is thinking, too, though she hasn't told Alan this, of selling her share in the business. This fall the routine has suddenly seemed too demanding to her—overwhelming, really. She might continue to work, just part-time, she thinks, and perhaps at last start to write her cookbook. She has no idea yet whether all this is practical, but she's begun to make inquiries.

And so they sit side by side in the hall full of the dull roar of thousands of conversations, the underlying sibilance as others too flip through their programs.

The performers enter and settle themselves, and then the soloists and the conductor. The music starts.

Alan finds himself not as moved as he thought he'd be by the first section, or then the second. Perhaps this is because the music is being played on early instruments, which give the impression of great restraint. The voices too must apparently be controlled, to mix with the more subdued instrumentation. Alan is used to the no-doubt musically incorrect *Messiah,* the overblown, overdramatic version—it was what he heard and thrilled to several times in his youth at Rockefeller Chapel. This version feels curiously bloodless to him.

He lets his mind float while the beautiful, distant music traces Christ's birth and betrayal, his death, his resurrection. He is seeing the work left to be done at the Admundsens'; he is imagining the face of the student he particularly dislikes, who will, he is sure, protest the grade Alan is going to give him, probably taking it to higher levels.

After the Hallelujah Chorus and the second intermission, about a quarter of the audience doesn't return. Alan and Gaby, actually, are alone in their row, and she makes a joke about the possibility of lying down and having her usual nap before dinner.

The music in this section is less familiar to Alan, he hasn't heard it piped in seasonally at grocery stores and bookstores as he has the choruses from the first two sections. He opens the text to follow the words, and is struck, when he gets to the phrase about our being changed, "in a moment, in the twinkling of an eye," by the homeliness of the expression. And then realizes that the expression is as homely and familiar as it is precisely because it comes from Scripture. The bass is singing his beautiful duet with the trumpet now. "We shall be changed," he sings, over and over, in hopeful insistence, the trumpet eloquently punctuating his claim; and Alan is hearing with Lily's ears, hearing this promise she believed in—praying for her, in some sense, with his intense listening, but also feeling his own sorrowful distance from this certainty, and from her.

And now the contralto and tenor move into their duet, "O death, where is thy sting? O grave, where is thy victory?" Their voices twine, calling again and again, "O death!" "O grave!" He is undone by the beautiful rending harmonies, the plaintive but joyous dance the voices do, the belief. The belief. And for him, the end—of Lily, of Paul, and of all they kept alive for him. *In* him, he sees. His throat swells. He bends his head, closes his eyes, and keeps his head bent through the chorus's sprightly thanks to God, through the joyful pronouncement of Christ's great worth, through the amazing, soaring last amen. Through the beginning of the applause, which doesn't end it for him.

It's dark when they come out, and lightly snowing again. They walk south on Mass Ave, past the subway station, past the bowfront brick houses, most thick with apartment life, the fluorescent lights inside many, where once there were chandeliers. They have agreed that the music was wonderful, they have both claimed their favorite performers. And now Gaby, as though she had some sense of what was happening to him, speaks of the passage that stirred his feelings. "It's odd, truly, to speak of death's 'sting,' isn't it? 'O death, where is thy *sting*.' "

Don't, he wishes to say. But he keeps his voice conversational. "What's odd about it?"

She wrinkles her nose. She looks, for those few seconds, like a girl. "It's an odd word. It's little, and puny. I know! It's like *stink*, that's it!" He doesn't answer. "At any rate, it doesn't sound . . . correct, to me."

"What is it in French?" he asks after a moment. "Sting?"

"It's . . . I think in the Bible, in that passage, it's *aiguillon*. And that's better, isn't it? It has more . . . depth than *sting*. More meaning of power, really." Their feet make regular crunching bites in the snow. "I almost felt like giggling a bit when they were singing."

"I didn't," he says. "It moved me."

She looks at him quickly then, and quickly turns away. She feels chastised and angry, shut out, again, from his sorrow, if sorrow is what it is.

The wind cuts through Alan's wool coat, and he hunches his shoulders against it. They pass a bar, a pizza place. The black faces. Except for the architecture, he could be in Chicago.

They turn down Columbus Avenue into the South End. They're meeting Thomas at a restaurant here, one Gaby has read about and wants to try. This neighborhood was marginal at best when Gaby and Alan lived in Boston. It has come back a good deal by now, but still varies from block to block, house to house. It feels familiar to Alan, he likes it.

The restaurant is in a storefront on the ground floor of one of the brick town houses. It's warm and crowded, bright with noise. When they come in, Thomas stands up at a table in the front window and waves to them. After they hang up their coats, they weave their way through the tables to him. He is buoyant and energetic, thrilled by the music he's heard, even excited a little by the snow. As though he were still a child, Alan thinks.

Alan feels remote, locked away in his own earlier experience. Gaby and Thomas appear not to notice. They are talking of the music, then of the upcoming holidays, then of the menu—what looks good. Alan is facing the street, Gaby and Thomas are turned in to him. As they talk, Alan stares out behind them at the snow, carried sometimes nearly horizontally on the wind. Under the streetlights the air is thick with the mothy flakes, but in the black valley beyond their light, the snow seems to disappear, or to become just a light fog through which he can see this world—the tall red buildings, the lighted apartment windows, the bundled pedestrians. The thought of home, of the house he has made, seems, from here, isolated and chilling—the long, lonely ride back, the wooded dark drive, the house set by itself on the cold, black river. He wishes he could stay here, in these lights, this city.

After dinner, they take a cab back to the parking garage,

and Alan gives Thomas money for the rest of his ride. Silently they retrieve their car, drive to the expressway and head south on it, toward home.

Gaby speaks, finally, even though she knows this is dangerous. "What are you thinking, Alan? About the music, still?"

Alan looks over at her. The heater has finally gotten the car warm and she has relaxed, unbuttoned her coat, and taken off her gloves.

"Some, the music. Boston, I guess."

"Mmm."

"Would you ever think of moving back?"

Ah, here it is. She shifts in her seat, looks out her window. "No. I wouldn't. I like my life precisely as it is."

"Just a question."

She turns to him quickly. "No, it's not, Alan. It's more than that and you know this."

He is startled. "What is it, do you think?"

"I don't know." She shakes her head. "I wish I did, so I could help you. But I don't. It's part of Lily's death, I think. But since we cannot talk of that . . . "

He doesn't answer her. She is watching him, but he keeps his eyes steady on the dark road ahead.

She shrugs, finally. "At any rate, no, I have no wish to change my life."

And he realizes, suddenly, what he has been asking her. Realizes that the version of life he has offered Gaby—their life together—is a gift he has given her and has no right to take away. He reaches over and touches her hand. "Of course you don't."

The boys will come home for Christmas, Thomas for five days, Ettie for two weeks. They will sleep late every morning, and then wander the house until at least noon in pajamas and slippers, carrying sections of the paper into odd corners. Gaby will leave bags of scones out for them, of muffins, of what she calls "breakfast cookies," and they will carry these around, along with orange juice or coffee, scattering crumbs, leaving sticky circles. The house will ring with Thomas's music from noon until evening, and sometimes Alan will thrill to it, and sometimes he will think of it simply as noise to be endured.

Ettie will switch to the guest suite the second night of Thomas's stay, "because he talks in his sleep. God. All night." And reaching deep into the drawer of the nightstand there one evening—he never says for what—he will find at the back of it an ancient, flowered-silk pouch of Lily's. Inside will be a pair of reading glasses, two buttons, around twenty dollars in fives and ones, an old family ring she wore occasionally, and a locket with pictures of her parents within, one on each side of it.

He will look embarrassed, almost ashamed when he brings this out to Alan, who is sitting in the living room. Wordlessly he will hand it to his father.

"A reticule for Christmas, Ettie?" Alan will ask, smiling.

"Open it, Dad."

Alan will pull wide the strings at the mouth of the bag. "Oh!" he will say. He will lift out the items one by one, setting them on the arm of his chair. He will shake his head slowly at what is odd, what is touching in this collection.

Ettie will understand this as grief, and quickly reach out to grip his father's shoulder. But what Alan will be feeling is that Lily has somehow just forgotten this, that he needs to find a way to get it to her—as though she were a traveler who had left something necessary behind. He will have a strange sense of puzzlement and obligation, of incompleteness.

On a bitter-cold winter day, Alan will decide, for reasons he isn't clear on, that it is time to read Lily's book—her fiction, her collection of stories. He will take it with him to his office, where, he feels, he can somehow be more alone with it. He plans to read it story by story, when he has the odd moment free.

But of course this isn't what will happen. The steeple clock will say almost three when he begins the first day, and he will still be reading when he looks up and sees that it is time to go and wake Gaby. The next day, Alan will simply sit down and begin to read as soon as he arrives, acknowledging to himself his eagerness to take in Lily's words.

He has read most of these stories before, as they have appeared separately in magazines, and he was affected by them then mostly as they reflected some aspect he could recognize of Lily's life, or Paul's, or the whole family's.

In the aggregate, though, they will affect him differently. He will feel, after these few days, immersed in a sensibility that he might not have recognized as Lily's. He will feel that he is drawing closer to a sense of her, of how she understood the world. He will feel incapable of describing this, even to himself, except by contrasting it to the way he understood her before: that she seems, as the writer of these stories, somehow softer, more forgiving, than he knew her in life, or in her memoir. There is a kind of mysterious generosity in the despair of these pieces.

In the last story—the one published the previous spring in *The Atlantic*, she wrote of her character, an old woman:

Imagine her as she imagines them. [Her children, whom she left long since.] She sits in her studio apartment—what they call a studio, it's really a rented room with a refrigerator and hotplate installed. From next door through the thin walls she hears the sordid, night-long battle between her neighbors begin, as it must each evening, whatever the trigger this time. Money, food, drink, sex, cleanliness, the use of language. She feels a kind of gratitude, for this is her trigger too, the beginning of her true night. She has the telephone book open to the map of the United States divided into area codes. 202—Washington, D.C.: the white buildings, the wide groomed paths and flower beds. 802—Vermont: the rolling hilly green of old farms. 312—Chicago: the famous buildings, the gray lake. And in each place, she sees the face of one of her children, costumed now one way—as a doctor or a lawyer—now another—artist, teacher. But always youthful, the way they were when she left them.

It's no wonder that when she calls the numbers listed by their names, the voices are always wrong. Too old, too defeated, too brusque. She has given them perfection, in memory. She has imagined them unembittered, unsaddened, undiminished, unchanged. What else, poor woman, could she do? Because of course, the first change she would have to imagine would be the one wreaked by her departure, and at that time and whenever she thought of it later, she had argued to herself that it wouldn't change anything. They were launched, they were accomplished and safe and happy. They would have the memory of her, but none of them needed her person anymore. They were done with her, she felt, and her departure might even be construed as a kind of gift to them. If she could have spoken to them, she might have said, "All I did, truly, was to move earlier than I should have into memory."

How could she have so misunderstood things? It is the right of the children to leave the parents, it is what they need to do, in order to be adult.

And the transformation into memory of a parent is a gift we give gladly only to the dead, receive gratefully only from them.

Alan will be sitting by the window in his office as he reads this. The day will be bright and windy outside. The grass on the town green across from his windows will be stiff-looking, rimed in frost, the limbs of the winter trees as black as India ink drawn with a broad nib against the blue of the clear, cold sky.

*   *   *

Linnett's article will come out in mid-February. One of Gaby's employees will bring the magazine into the shop to show her, and Gaby herself will stop on the way home at the drugstore to buy a copy for Alan.

It will be shorter than Alan would have thought, given the time Linnett spent with Lily, and on the whole, more adulatory than anything else. It will begin with the death.

> Lily Maynard, the noted memoirist and short-story writer, died last August in a Massachusetts coastal town while a hurricane raged around her. This somehow seems entirely appropriate, that the elements themselves should protest her death. For even though she was old, and on some days nearly incapacitated by Parkinson's disease—a fact which she had by and large kept a secret from her admiring reading audience—Lily Maynard was an intriguing and vital and complex presence—beautiful, astonishingly alert, deliberately mysterious, quick, funny, and occasionally even downright mean.

After that, in part because of his relief, Alan will find the rest unremarkable, a fairly predictable summary of Lily's career and achievements. These will often be set cleverly, Linnett describing Lily very well—a gesture for instance, or a turn of phrase with which Lily dismissed whole decades of her life. She says of Lily's Parkinson's voice:

> The effect of this rushed, smooth, nearly inexpressive quality is that she seems to be trying to slip her often outrageous opinions past you. You hear a remark as the modestly presented, idle thought of an elderly woman, and only somewhat later do you realize she's said something profoundly insulting, or wildly politically incorrect, or shockingly intimate.

On the whole though, the fresh slant that Linnett wanted

will seem absent to Alan. Maybe the death *will* make it hot enough to be well-received, he thinks. He doesn't wish her ill.

In the late spring, he will finally get around to rearranging the guest suite back to the way it was before Lily came, something Gaby will have asked him several times to do. First he will move out the table Lily worked at, and then he will start to shift the bureau next to it back to its original position. And he will see under it a letter that escaped Lily's destruction.

This is special, this is a gift, Alan will think, and sitting alone on the bed in the guest room, he will let himself read it. It is from Lily's mother, mailed, clearly, early in Lily's marriage.

My dearest girl [Violet wrote],

This is written in haste, as I will try to get it to the mailman when he comes by—too soon! I hear the ticking of the hall clock as I write.

By now you will be completely settled in. I am grateful for all the detailed floor plans, the swatches of fabric, and the account of furniture arrangements, so that I can imagine you in your life there. How exciting it must all be, especially after the quiet life here at home with just me and your father! The amount of entertaining you have done in just the first few weeks is almost literally staggering to me.

I do think it's a good idea to keep a record of menus, not just so that you don't serve the same group the same thing twice—how clever you are to have thought of that!—but also so that you can remember what dishes were especially successful. I am wondering if you have quite enough china? I have that set of twelve dinner plates I never use anymore, from Cousin Laurie. Would they be of more use to you? This is an offer, dearest, so think about it.

We have had Auntie for another week. She just wasn't well enough in my opinion to make the trip back home.

So I sent a telegram to Uncle Patch and we kept her. She just left today, your father took her to the train. And I will pack her things and send them on after her in a day or two. It was hard on Henry to have her here so long—he likes his privacy, as you know, but I felt we couldn't in good conscience let her go any earlier.

And now I must close, my darling, for the clock is striking the quarter hour and Mr. Bement is nothing if not punctual. I would need the window measurements by next Friday to get Mrs. Stickley to do the curtains you would like, and I would very much like to do that for you.

I miss you terribly and look forward with great eagerness to my first visit to you in your new life. Please give my love to dearest Paul, and know that it is always flowing toward you, my darling daughter.

Your loving, Mother

There is no news here, nothing even interesting, really, but Alan will be moved to tears by the presence and the absence of this new Lily, waiting so patiently to make herself known.

But what is so new?

He isn't sure. That her mother thought of her as a child, when she was twenty-six or twenty-seven? That she was so deeply loved, adored even, in a way she was somehow so incapable of passing on? That her life with Paul had begun with such ordinary and familiar steps—arranging furniture, making curtains, having over the first guests?

The letter is on frail onionskin paper, tissue almost, which rustles and whispers as he handles it. The ink is black, faded to yellow-brown. The writing is strong, vertical and shapely, the hand of a person who wrote, no doubt, four or five letters a day. His own hands will tremble as he tears it in half, then into quarters, before throwing it too away.

This must be the last, he thinks. The last surprise, the last gift.

*   *   *

Early the next fall he will get a telephone call from Marcea McKendrick. He will recognize her voice before she says her name, as though it were only a day or two since he saw her.

She will say, almost shyly, that she was sorry to hear of Mrs. Maynard's death.

He will thank her for that.

"I guess it was just shortly after I talked to her."

"Yes," he will say. (He will not say, "It was the next day.")

Well, she will say, she is coming the next weekend to the state beach nearby, and she wonders if he might like the copy of her thesis she had intended to give his mother. "I promised everyone who talked to me I'd send them each a copy. It was kind of, like, part of the deal? It's just a Xerox that I did myself, I couldn't afford bound copies, but it does belong to her, if . . . " Her voice will trail off.

And Alan, who will be glad simply to hear from Marcea McKendrick, who will be touched that she so honors her bargain with Lily, and who will think that she may, somehow, bring him something from Lily too, will say, "Oh, please do stop by. I'd be delighted to have the thesis. I'd be interested to read it."

"Okay, great," she will say. "I'll be with some friends, though, they've got the car, so it really will be just to drop it off."

They will arrange a time, late on Saturday afternoon.

Alan will be home a good hour before she is due. He will check to be sure there is wine, seltzer, beer, iced tea, in case they should all want to stop.

But as Marcea promised, she will get out of the car alone and cross the yard (it will be green again, in full leafy shade). She will wear a loose pink cotton smock, a beach dress, and her unpinned hair will fall free over her shoulders in amazing tight coils, dark brown touched with gold at every twist.

He will open the door before she rings, and they will stand for some moments, talking. She will refuse his invitation to come in, gesturing back at her waiting friends (black and white together, Alan will note). Just before she leaves she will say again how sorry she is and she will give him the thesis, in a black binder.

Then she will say, "Oh, and I had a kind of funny message, I might as well give to you. I found a couple of the women, you know, from the church group? And one of them, Iva Lewis, did you know her?"

Alan will nod, remembering Iva, who had a fat son his age, Charley, and who ran the youth choir with an iron hand and a limitless supply of chocolate chip cookies.

"Before I realized she didn't know your mom was dead, she was remembering her and all? And she said to tell her, 'Girl, how you been.'"

She will say this woodenly and for a moment Alan will be confused, trying to make meaning from it.

Marcea will laugh, then, a little uncomfortable, a little shy. "Well, what she actually said was"—and here she will change her voice deliberately, make it Southern, black, pitch it, perhaps even a little higher—"*Gi*-rl! How you *bin?!*"

And Alan will laugh too, hearing in these words, said this way, tenderness, endearment, the warmth that Lily had drawn from her life at Blackstone Church, the affection Iva felt for his mother, the woman she thought of as "girl."

And Lily will be born for him again, as though she had been waiting for this moment too. And he will understand that all these loving moments, these births, are things he holds within himself and always has, though he couldn't have felt them until they were released by death. By the gift of memory. Hers to him.

His to her.